Bailey's
Research for
the Health
Professional

THIRD EDITION

Bailey's Research for the Health Professional

THIRD EDITION

Angela N. Hissong, DEd, OTR/L, CMCP, CMMT
Program Director
Occupational Therapy
The Pennsylvania State University
Mont Alto, Pennsylvania

Jennifer E. Lape, OTD, OTR/L
Assistant Professor
Occupational Therapy
Chatham University
Pittsburgh, Pennsylvania

Diana M. Bailey, EdD, OTR, FAOTA
Professor Emerita, Tufts University
Medford, Massachusetts

 F.A. Davis Company • Philadelphia

F. A. Davis Company
1915 Arch Street
Philadelphia, PA 19103
www.fadavis.com

Printed in the United States of America

Last digit indicates print number: 10 9 8 7 6 5 4 3

Senior Acquisitions Editor: Christa Fratantoro
Manager of Content Development: George W. Lang
Developmental Editor: Karen Carter
Art and Design Manager: Carolyn O'Brien

As new scientific information becomes available through basic and clinical research, recommended treatments and drug therapies undergo changes. The author(s) and publisher have done everything possible to make this book accurate, up to date, and in accord with accepted standards at the time of publication. The author(s), editors, and publisher are not responsible for errors or omissions or for consequences from application of the book, and make no warranty, expressed or implied, in regard to the contents of the book. Any practice described in this book should be applied by the reader in accordance with professional standards of care used in regard to the unique circumstances that may apply in each situation. The reader is advised always to check product information (package inserts) for changes and new information regarding dose and contraindications before administering any drug. Caution is especially urged when using new or infrequently ordered drugs.

Library of Congress Cataloging-in-Publication Data

Bailey, Diana M., 1942- , author.
  Research for the health professional / Angela N. Hissong, Jennifer E. Lape, Diana M. Bailey. — Third edition.
    p. ; cm.
  Preceded by: Research for the health professional / Diana M. Bailey. 2nd ed. c1997.
  Includes bibliographical references and index.
  ISBN 978-0-8036-3916-4 — ISBN 0-8036-3916-3
  I. Hissong, Angela N., author. II. Lape, Jennifer E., author. III. Title.
  [DNLM: 1. Research Design. 2. Data Collection—methods. 3. Data Interpretation, Statistical. 4. Publishing. 5. Writing. W 20.5]

R850
610.72—dc23

2014025756

For students, practitioners, and educators
embarking on the research journey . . .
It is easy to think of an idea.
It is challenging to make your idea a reality.
It is inspiring to see the idea change lives.

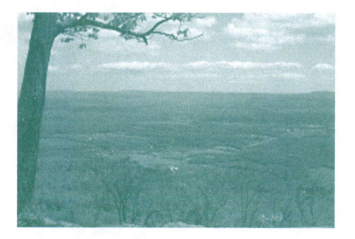

There are blue skies and
endless territory to explore.

Preface

Research for the Health Professional was designed to be a practical and informative guide for research and evidence-based practice for a variety of healthcare students and professionals. The text will guide you to:

1. Differentiate research from evidence-based practice
2. Discriminate between quantitative, qualitative, and mixed methods research methodologies
3. Access and critically evaluate literature related to your practice area
4. Ignite your passion for your profession or chosen practice area to inspire participation in research and evidence-based practice activities
5. Apply principles of research and evidence-based practice to design, implement, and evaluate meaningful research studies or innovative evidence-based practice projects
6. Share research and evidence-based practice findings through a variety of methods
7. Engage in collaborative and self-directed learning activities to become researchers, evidence-based practitioners, and professional leaders

We have taken a straightforward, positive, and engaging approach to research and evidence-based practice that draws upon our combined 25 years of teaching experience, from the associate to doctoral levels. Understanding and engaging in research and evidence-based practice can be challenging, but with use of a structured process and a passion for the chosen topic, both can be extremely rewarding and enlightening. The philosophy of the text is to learn by "doing," meaning that mastery of the content is facilitated via hands-on activities, engaging assignments and discussions, and collaboration with others.

Our intention was not to write a comprehensive research text, but rather to lead you through each phase of the research process in a simplified and systematic way. This text is appropriate for those just beginning in the research or evidence-based practice journey, but can also be an effective tool for more advanced students and practitioners or those needing a refresher course. With these goals in mind, each chapter contains several features.

First, **Learning Outcomes** define the chapter goals and let you know what you can expect to learn in each chapter. Second, **Skill-Building Tips** are included at the end of each chapter in bulleted format to summarize practical suggestions for understanding and applying chapter content. These tips have been accumulated through our experiences in conducting research and evidence-based practice and in teaching others to do the same. These tips should allow you to avoid some of the common pitfalls and to move through the research process with greater ease. Third, **Learning Activities** conclude each chapter and provide opportunities for critical thinking about the chapter content. These questions can serve as a foundation for each phase of the research process, by allowing you to consider chapter content from the perspective of your clinic, practice, or research situation. Finally, **additional resources and templates** are available within the chapters and in the online resources through DavisPlus to guide you through the research process. In addition, a variety of examples from multiple disciplines have been included throughout the chapters to demystify more complex concepts.

Reviewing the chapters in chronological order reflects the approach we have found to be most effective for research in traditional, online, and blended academic settings. For those more interested in evidence-based practice, we recommend reviewing sections in the following order: Section I, Section III, Section II, Section IV. In either case, we hope this text will guide you to design and conduct a successful study or project, and to pursue grant writing or to present and publish to share your work with others.

One final feature that we chose to include is the **inspirational quotes and photos** that open each chapter to set the tone for a positive and engaging learning experience. Research and evidence-based practice can be challenging and time-consuming, but we believe that it can also be inspiring and fun with proper life balance. Balancing competing activities and finding time to enjoy the simple leisures is fundamental to a healthy and fulfilling life, and we remind our students of this frequently. The chapter photos were taken throughout our writing journey for this book, as we tried to stay true to our own philosophy. We hope you enjoy the journey and embrace the joys of research and conducting evidence-based practice! The process will surely change you if you let it!

Angela N. Hissong
Jennifer E. Lape

Reviewers

Diana M. Bailey, OTR, EdD, FAOTA
Professor Emerita
Tufts University
Medford, Massachusetts

Joseph A. Beckett, EdD, ATC
Chair, Department of Sports Medicine &
CAAHEP-accredited Athletic Training Education
    Program Director
University of Charleston
Charleston, West Virginia

Nicceta Davis, PT, PhD, MSPT, MPH
Associate Professor
Doctor of Physical Therapy Program
Loma Linda University
Loma Linda, California

Deanna C. Dye, PT, PhD
Physical Therapist
Wound Care Department
Eastern Idaho Regional Medical Center
Idaho Falls, Idaho

Vickie S. Freeman, PhD
Department Chair and Professor
Department of Clinical Laboratory Sciences
University of Texas Medical Branch
Galveston, Texas

Rita M. Heuertz, PhD, MT(ASCP)
Professor, Director of Departmental Research
Clinical Laboratory Science, Doisy College of Health
    Sciences
Saint Louis University
St. Louis, Missouri

Shirley J. Jackson, MS, OTR/L, FAOTA
Associate Professor and Former Chairperson
Department of Occupational Therapy
Howard University
Washington, District of Columbia

Frances E. Kistner, PT, PhD, CEAS
Assistant Professor
School of Physical Therapy
Massachusetts College of Pharmacy and Health
    Sciences
Worcester, Massachusetts

Rosemary M. Lysaght, PhD, OTR/L
Assistant Professor
Department of Occupational Therapy
University of Utah
Salt Lake City, Utah

**Cheryl A. Manthei, NCTMB, MT, MS-IDT,
    BBA, AAS MSG, AAS CHEM**
Program Director, Therapeutic Massage and
    Bachelor of Health Services Administration
Department of Health Sciences
Baker College of Allen Park
Allen Park, Michigan

Kevin C. Miller, PhD, AT, ATC
Associate Professor
Department of Athletic Training
Central Michigan University
Mount Pleasant, Michigan

Maralynne D. Mitcham, PhD, OTR/L, FAOTA
Professor and Director
Occupational Therapy Educational Department
Department of Rehabilitation Sciences
College of Health Professions
Medical University of South Carolina
Charleston, South Carolina

Annie Morien, PhD, PA-C, LMT
Lead Instructor
Florida School of Massage Therapy
Gainesville, Florida

Stanley Paul, MD, PhD, OTR/L
Associate Professor
Department of Occupational Science and Therapy
Keuka College, New York
Keuka Park, New York

Kimberly S. Peer, EdD, ATC, FNATA
Athletic Training Education Program Coordinator
  and Associate Professor
School of Health Sciences
Kent State University
Kent, Ohio

James R. Roush, PT, PhD, ATC
Associate Professor
Department of Physical Therapy
Arizona School of Health Sciences
Mesa, Arizona

Victoria Schindler, PhD, OTR, BCMH, FAOTA
Associate Professor
Department of Occupational Therapy
Richard Stockton College of NJ
Galloway, New Jersey

Holly Schmies, PhD, ATC
Assistant Professor
Department of Athletic Training
School of Physical Education and Athletic Training
University of Wisconsin—Stevens Point
Stevens Point, Wisconsin

Karen Sladyk, PhD, OTR, FAOTA
Professor and Chair
Department of Occupational Therapy
Bay Path College
Vernon, Connecticut

Frank B. Underwood, PT, PhD, ECS
Professor
Department of Physical Therapy
University of Evansville
Evansville, Indiana

Janet H. Watts, PhD, OTR, CRC
Associate Professor and Director of
  Post-Professional Graduate Studies
Department of Occupational Therapy
Virginia Commonwealth University
Richmond, Virginia

Michael B. Worrell, PhD
Assistant Professor
Department of Occupational Therapy
Indiana University and University of Indianapolis
Indianapolis, Indiana

Acknowledgments

Our deepest gratitude goes to:

Joe and Jere, for understanding our need to flee to the woods, the ocean, or the spa in order to make this book a reality. We couldn't have done it without you.

Our family and friends, for your concern and support along the way.

Our faithful and loving canines, Chloe and Sophia, who slept on our laps as we wrote and gently reminded us to take time to enjoy the simple things in life.

Christa, Karen, and Liz, for believing in us and guiding us throughout the journey.

Finally, to our students—past and present—who inspired us through their journeys of research and evidence-based practice, to write a sensible and lighthearted book to ease the process.

A special thank you from Angela to Dr. Julie Beck for contributing to the Adult & Transformative Learning Influences on the Inquiry Process dialogue in Chapter 2.

Photographs

The chapter opener photos taken during our writing journey are:

EPIGRAPH:	The Cabin, Breezewood, Pennsylvania
CHAPTER 1:	Harbor of Christiansen, St. Croix, U.S. Virgin Islands
CHAPTER 2:	Breathe & Balance Lecture, Philadelphia, PA
CHAPTER 3:	Seaside Mahoe Tree, Carambola Beach Resort, St. Croix, U.S. Virgin Islands
CHAPTER 4:	Osprey Nest, Westport, Ontario, Canada
CHAPTER 5:	Grandfather Mountain, Linville, North Carolina
CHAPTER 6:	Woody Pines—Whitetail Mountain Forest, Beech Creek, Pennsylvania
CHAPTER 7:	North Atlantic Ocean, Island of Bermuda
CHAPTER 8:	Enchantment Resort, Sedona, Arizona
CHAPTER 9:	Moais Stone Head, Valparaíso, Chile
CHAPTER 10:	Cape Hatteras Lighthouse, Buxton, North Carolina
CHAPTER 11:	Snowy Stream, Springwood Farm, Pennsylvania
CHAPTER 12:	Butterfly, Dupont State Forest, North Carolina
CHAPTER 13:	Bald Cypress Tree in the Bayou, New Orleans, Louisiana
CHAPTER 14:	Wright Brothers National Memorial, Kill Devil Hills, North Carolina
CHAPTER 15:	Bee & Lily, Garrison Institute, New York

(Photos taken by Angela Hissong, Jennifer Lape, and Joe Lape.)

Brief Contents

Contents

Section 1

Beginning the Journey

Chapter 1

Concepts of Research: Embarking on the Journey

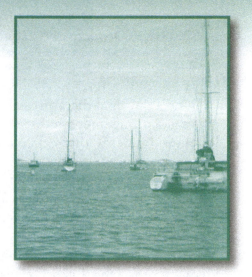

The universe is full of magical things, patiently waiting for our wits to grow sharper.
—*Eden Phillpotts*

LEARNING OUTCOMES

The information provided in this chapter will assist the reader to:

- Understand the components of engaging in the research process.
- Define the steps required to complete a research process.
- Identify potential challenges in the research process.

Introduction to Research

Research can be an enjoyable, stimulating, and fascinating activity to engage in along one's professional journey. Often anyone who is required to write a research thesis starts out overwhelmed by the idea, yet comes to enjoy the challenge and ends up feeling proud of the results. Great satisfaction can be derived from completing this exacting, often complex, and always stimulating process.

Unfortunately, some people avoid research because of their preconceived notions. Research is the systematic investigation of a problem, issue, or question undertaken to increase our knowledge. This includes reviewing numerous sources of literature on a given topic and drawing new conclusions about that topic, manipulating certain variables to see what happens to other variables, or searching for the meaningfulness of a variable to an individual or group.

Systematic investigation involves the process of logic, often called *deductive* and *inductive* reasoning. Deductive reasoning starts with a general theory and ends with a specific conclusion; this is sometimes called a "top-down" approach. For example, the researcher starts with a general theory, forms a hypothesis based on the theory, tests the hypothesis, assesses the results, and forms a conclusion (Box 1-1).

Inductive reasoning starts with a specific observation that eventually forms a general theory; this is sometimes called a "bottom-up" approach. In this type of reasoning, the researcher starts with an interesting observation, then looks for a pattern of similar observations. From this pattern, the researcher develops a hypothesis, which forms the basis of a general theory (Box 1-2).

When using inductive reasoning, one accepts or believes a finding about a situation and then applies that belief to all similar individuals, assuming that the finding will be true for all. For example, if a healthcare practitioner finds that having clients complete a

BOX 1-1 ■ Deductive Reasoning

Theory → Hypothesis → Observations → Conclusion

An occupational therapist believes that positive encouragement improves patient outcomes (**general theory**) and **hypothesizes** that positive reinforcement will decrease stroke recovery time. The therapist tests the hypothesis on 100 patients and finds that stroke recovery time decreased by 50% (**observations**). The therapist concludes that positive reinforcement decreases stroke recovery time (**conclusion**). This confirms the original theory.

BOX 1-2 ■ Inductive Reasoning

Observation → Pattern → Hypothesis → Theory

An occupational therapist **observes** that a patient's ability to climb stairs improves when preceded by a balance task (e.g., standing on one leg with eyes closed). Over the next several months, the therapist **looks for a pattern** whether the balance task causes improvements in other areas (cognition, motor skills, etc.). After observing improvements in other areas, the therapist believes that the balance task should be performed at the beginning of every occupational session (**hypothesis**) and implements this as standard protocol for all therapists (**theory**).

specific questionnaire about their health history is beneficial during an initial evaluation, the practitioner may choose to give all subsequent clients the questionnaire to fill out.

The point of consideration with deductive reasoning is that, although the principle is usually true, there may be exceptions. The point of consideration with inductive reasoning is that the individual upon whom you have based the principle may be the exception, so that the principle will probably not apply to all other cases that follow.

Journey of Exploration in Research

Research in the health sciences is a challenging task; however, it can be accomplished with the proper tools and guidance. Human behavior is extremely complex and, therefore, difficult to isolate and measure. Because we are working in the health field, added dimensions must be considered when working with and conducting research with clients. These may include time constraints of the client and the healthcare practitioner, complicated medical diagnoses, working within the many layers of the healthcare system, and the numerous ethical issues involved when doing research with people. With that said, we are nonetheless seeing more support for healthcare practitioners as they conduct research in the community setting with a focus on preventative or wellness programs.

When considering your research agenda, keep the following six points in mind:

- First and foremost, explore and understand the types of research and determine which type best fits the question you are pondering (Table 1-1);
- Be aware that finding collaborators who are interested in your research is time-consuming;
- Give considerable thought to the type of research project you want to engage in;
- Learn as much as you can about the embedded systems or structural rules that will affect, and at times overrule, how you conduct your research;
- Be willing to compromise and accept that perseverance is a key asset during the research process;
- Finalize your research question, then sit down and write up a time line (Figure 1-1).

Estimate Time to Complete a Research Project

Practitioners often ask, "How long will it take to complete a research study?" or "How long should I devote to conducting research each day or week?" In my experience in advising graduate occupational therapy students in their thesis preparation and writing, the time frame is an average of 6 to 12 months. This includes

Table 1-1 ■ Description of Categories of Research

A	Basic	Applied
	Abstract, general, and concerned with generating new theory and gaining new knowledge for knowledge's sake.	Designed to answer a practical question to help people do their jobs better.
B	Experimental	Descriptive
	Manipulate a variable to see its effect on another variable, control for as many other variables as possible, and randomly assign subjects to groups.	Describe a group, a situation, or an individual to gain knowledge that may be applied to other groups or situations, as in case studies or trend analyses.
C	Clinical	Laboratory
	Performed in the "real world" where control over variables is quite difficult.	Performed in laboratory surroundings that are controlled.

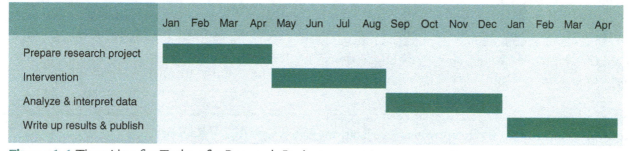

Figure 1-1 Time Line for Tasks of a Research Project

conceptualizing the issue to be studied, carrying out the project, and writing the study. Students are usually not carrying a caseload of clients or tied to a 40-hour work week; however, they do have classes to attend and often are working full-time on an affiliation.

Research conducted by practitioners tends to take longer—about 1 year to 18 months—with some time spent on the project each week. Of course, different phases of the research demand more or less input. For example, if a new treatment approach is being investigated, the practitioner must adhere to the number and length of treatment sessions stipulated in the research protocol and put time into preparation and record-keeping. Activities such as reading the literature and writing the results are done on one's own time and on a less precise schedule. A therapist who works from 9 to 5 should plan on reading and writing in the evening and on weekends because few clinical situations afford

therapists enough free time during the day to do the extra work required to complete a research study.

Steps in the Research Process

It is helpful to remember that research is a circular process. The researcher starts with a question in mind, goes through the investigative stages, and ends up with an answer to the question. More often than not, further questions arise during the analysis and interpretation of the data, leading to yet more research ideas.

There are different points of entry into the research process. Some people enjoy starting afresh at the question identification stage; others may discover some study results that they question and feel they would like to investigate for themselves. Still others enter at various phases along the way. Whatever the entry point, the steps required to complete a research project follow a logical sequence:

1. Identify a problem that needs to be solved or a question that needs to be answered.
2. Review the existing literature related to the problem or question.
3. Formulate a question or hypothesis about the problem based on the literature.
4. Design a procedure that will address the question or hypothesis.
5. Carry out the procedure.
6. Collect and interpret the findings.
7. Present findings to one or more committees.
8. Publish your research so that others may benefit from the identified knowledge. It is very helpful to talk to your committee and peers about where to publish your research.

This process will be addressed step by step later in this text. As each step is explored, practical hints are offered that explain each step, along with suggestions on how to get over the hurdles that frequently present themselves.

Remember that, if you persevere, you can carry out a research project from its inception to publication by using this book as your step-by-step guide. This book is designed to guide you through each stage of negotiation and navigate through your own and other people's questions about the research process.

Research Process Challenges

When one begins with a research project there is a time of balancing out new tasks with everyday activities. We have compiled a list of common challenges that may be encountered prior to starting and/or in the initial stages of the research process:

- Balance commitments to allow for time to complete all stages of a research inquiry.
- Underestimate how much assistance or cooperation you may need from all the people involved in the research inquiry.
- Sort out how much time you need to complete each phase of the project.
- Say no to "tempting" opportunities that come up while you are engaged in the research inquiry that you really want to do.

- Understand the reality that your social life will be limited secondary to engaging in a research inquiry.
- Construct support systems to help you complete the research agenda in a timely and cost-effective manner.

Synopsis of This Book

The following is a *picture in preview* of the forthcoming chapters of this book. You have just read Chapter 1, which gives you an overview of how you should approach your research journey. The four chapters in Section I will assist you in beginning the research process. Section II of the book addresses research methodologies and designs, whereas Section III addresses evidence-based practice. Section IV gives you detailed information regarding common tasks along the journey related to preparing to implement your project, analyzing your findings, presenting the research to committees, and finally publishing and presenting the knowledge to the larger community.

SKILL-BUILDING TIPS

- As you begin to navigate and negotiate through various research processes, do not fault yourself or others.
- Remember that others around you may not be as passionate about your topic as you are and that they may not understand the research process or your research project. It isn't their fault. Be kind to them and yourself.
- Don't worry too much about the rules when you begin the research. You will not do everything correctly the first time and will have to go back and redo a few things. This is part of the learning process.
- Be humble and honest during the process from start to finish. If you need help, ask for it.
- Keep excellent notes.
- Find these four key people to assist you with the following tasks:
  - A person who understands the technical aspects of your research

- A person who is familiar with various writing styles such as APA (American Psychological Association) or MLA (Modern Language Association)

- A person who will read your manuscript and correct grammar and spelling (that's right, the computer still does not pick up everything!)

- A kind person who will take you out for dinner, bring you a chocolate cupcake, or sign you up for a massage when you most need a break from your research project

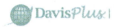

⌀ LEARNING ACTIVITIES

1. What is your mission statement (i.e., why do you want to complete your research project at this point in time)?

2. Are you ready to give up social time for research time? If the answer is yes, how will you accomplish this? For example: Rather than going out for dinner with friends three nights a week, you might go out only on Friday night.

3. List five reasons why you are passionate about completing your research study at this point in time.

Chapter 2

Identifying a Topic: Purpose Balanced With Passion

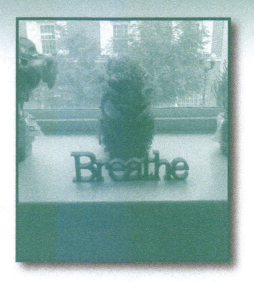

The shape of one's knowing becomes the shape of one's being, doing, and becoming.
—*Unknown*

LEARNING OUTCOMES

The information provided in this chapter will assist the reader to:

- Explore the process of identifying topics that elicit a professional passion for inquiry.
- Appreciate the influence adult and transformative learning provide when aligned with the processes of engaging in an inquiry.
- Acknowledge the need for a balance of personal and professional obligations while engaged in an inquiry.

Identifying a Topic: Passion Within One's Profession

An idea for an inquiry project typically begins from a grounding experience you have had in your field of study, although it may start anywhere. One key starting point to remember, and one that will consistently guide you through the inquiry process, is to begin with, maintain, and end with a passion for what you are studying. Think about a professional grounding experience that has been a guiding force in your life

as a student or practitioner. Ironically, this grounding experience will not only guide your inquiry, but will also fuel your passion to plan and execute your inquest. It will truly assist you in coming to know, understand, and engage in evidence-based practice and inquiry.

Post the process of looking within to discern what you want to study, and take time to consider the many philosophies and pedagogies of practice that you have been exposed to over the years. First, philosophical perspectives of evaluation, intervention, and care have helped shape and guide your practice more than you may think about on a daily basis, secondary to them becoming engrained in your work and second nature. Next, consider the experience you have in practice with your clients in terms of the teaching–learning process. Each time we engage in practice with clients there is a teaching–learning component to the session. A few pedagogical methods for any given session may include collaboration, critical reflection, transformation, and replication of a therapeutic modality or exercise. Again, it is very important to take time to ponder the philosophical and pedagogical perspectives and notions that have influenced and enlightened you on areas of practice that you want to explore further. Note that coming to know and understand why and how these notions fit into your agenda may take some time, but giving them deep thought and the courtesy to form a base for your inquiry is time well spent. Once you have established the role these two points will play in your inquiry, the next step is to consider how your learning is situated in the process.

Adult and Transformative Learning Influences on the Inquiry Process

Adult education theorists—extrapolating from and building upon cognitive, social, behavioral, and humanist learning, as well as developmental theories—highlight the diversity and complexity of adult learning needs as well as environmental influences upon these needs (Kasworm, Rose, & Ross-Gordon, 2010). Historically, Knowles (1984) emphasized the impact of self-concept, orientation to learning, experience, time perspectives, and motivation on adult learning processes, whereas Mezirow (2000) expounded upon the importance of critical reflection, as influenced by cultural beliefs and attitudes, on the transformation of perspectives and the development of new understanding. He believes adults resolve contradictions and move to more progressive conceptual constructs by:

- Becoming disoriented with existing beliefs
- Self-examining and critically assessing assumptions and knowledge
- Searching for new roles
- Acquiring new knowledge and skills
- Building competence and confidence in these new roles
- Reintegrating the components of life in response to these transformed perspectives

Developmental theories explore the diversity of ego and moral development, learning preferences, life events, and neurophysiological changes on the readiness, willingness, and selectivity of adults to engage in learning activities. A firm and steady level of commitment to embark upon the inquiry, aligned with the establishment of a time line, may seem like a small feat, but it is essential to your success. Even during the brainstorming stage of the process, it is wise to look at your calendar and determine what social events, family gatherings, and vacations you are going to forgo to conduct and complete the inquiry. The ole' saying, "Something's got to give," applies to anyone who decides to engage in a small or large scale inquiry. It is next to impossible to balance both, so some things need to wait or be significantly reduced in order to accomplish your goal. Looking forward a bit, Table 2-1 is a typical time line for the final four months of a small scale inquiry.

As noted by Mezirow (2000) and Taylor (2007), adults who engage in a significant transformative learning experience will exhibit the following characteristics: (1) display a sense of selves; (2) be intricately influenced by their professional identities and levels of social, emotional, and cognitive development; (3) bring a wealth of personal and clinical experience; (4) seek refinement of knowledge and attitudes; (5) search for immediate applicability of newly acquired skills; (6) juggle multiple personal and professional responsibilities; (7) undergo stages of perspective transformation; and (8) desire active participation in directing their own learning experiences. Adults' particular learning styles and stages of development should mold to the styles of their active participation and direction of learning. Again, in order to accommodate this diverse and complex learning, the inquiry process should be designed to invoke enthusiasm and passion alongside its method for achieving the stated objectives outlined by the investigator. For your first inquiry, you should select a topic and formulate an agenda that not only fulfills a need in your practice area, but touches your heart.

Furthermore, when you begin to consider engaging in inquiry, it will take time away from your other daily tasks. This can't be overstated or pointed out more intently, because this is a common downfall to completing the inquiry. Therefore, give yourself permission to stop and pause in order to explore the space between your professional and personal life. You must be honest with yourself and discern how important it is for you to engage in an inquiry. It is important to look inward and consider the pace of your current day and determine how you are going to balance an inquiry with all of your other responsibilities. In addition, you must be prepared to be changed by the experience and

Table 2-1 ■ **Example of Daily Tasks During Implementation and Evaluation Inquiry Stages**

Date	Specific Task	Date	Specific Task
Sept 1	Final Review of Outline of Implementation	Oct 4/5	
Sept 2	Week 1 Implementation	Oct 6	Week 6 Implementation
Sept 3	Conduct and Write	Oct 7	Conduct and Write
Sept 4		Oct 8	
Sept 5		Oct 9	
Sept 6/7		Oct 10	
Sept 8	Week 2 Implementation	Oct 11/12	
Sept 9	Conduct and Write	Oct 13	
Sept 10		Oct 14	Write Final Implementation Section
Sept 11		Oct 15	
Sept 12		Oct 16	
Sept 13/14		Oct 17	
Sept 15	Week 3 Implementation	Oct 18/19	
Sept 16	Conduct and Write	Oct 20	Oct 20 Submit the following: Implementation Section Implementation PowerPoint Slides (3–4)
Sept 17			
Sept 18		Oct 21	Week 1 Evaluation of Inquiry
Sept 19		Oct 22	
Sept 20/21		Oct 23	
Sept 22	Week 4 Implementation	Oct 24	
Sept 23	Conduct and Write	Oct 25	
Sept 24	Conduct and Write	Oct 26/27	
Sept 25		Oct 28	Week 2 Evaluation of Inquiry
Sept 26		Oct 29	
Sept 27/28		Oct 30	
Sept 29	Week 5 Implementation	Oct 31	
Sept 30	Conduct and Write	Nov 1	
Oct 1		Nov 2/3	
Oct 2		Nov 4	Week 3 Evaluation of Inquiry
Oct 3			

Continued

Table 2-1 ■ Example of Daily Tasks During Implementation and Evaluation Inquiry Stages—cont'd

Date	Specific Task	Date	Specific Task
Nov 5		Nov 27	
Nov 6		Nov 28	Happy Thanksgiving—Day Off!
Nov 7		Nov 29	
Nov 8		Nov 30/Dec 1	
Nov 9/10		Dec 2	■ Last Day to Get Paper and Poster to Printers ■ Start Gathering Things Needed for Formal Presentation of Inquiry
Nov 11	Week 4 Evaluation of Inquiry		
Nov 12			
Nov 13		Dec 3	
Nov 14		Dec 4	
Nov 15		Dec 5	
Nov 16/17		Dec 6	
Nov 18	Week 5 Evaluation of Inquiry	Dec 7/8	Last Day to Submit PowerPoint via Moodle Dropbox
Nov 19			
Nov 20		Dec 9	
Nov 21		Dec 10	Last Day to Submit Article or Grant via Moodle Dropbox
Nov 22			
Nov 23/24	Final Week of Evaluation of Inquiry	Dec 11	Travel to All-State University Celebration Begins
Nov 25	■ Finish PowerPoint ■ Evaluation (2–3 slides) Summary (1–2 slides) ■ Design and Finish Poster ■ Finish Article or Grant Proposal (3–20 pages; depends on what you are doing—can copy and paste a lot of information)	Dec 12	■ Poster Set-up Starting @ 10 a.m. ■ 4:00–5:30 p.m. Poster Round Robin to Healthcare Practitioner Community
		Dec 13	■ 10 a.m. Present PowerPoints ■ 5 p.m. All-State University Celebration ■ Dinner or Celebrate Downtown at Elbow Room!
Nov 26		Dec 14	Ah—Feel the Glow!

notice how you are changing alongside the inquiry processes. As noted in the previous paragraph, the process will more than likely be a transformative learning experience for you; therefore, you should not only pay attention to the work you are doing, but also how

the work is changing you as a practitioner. Because this is very important, let's take a bit more time to appreciate transformative learning.

Mezirow, Taylor, and associates (2009) note that transformative learning can be broken down into two fundamentally different views. One viewpoint stresses the personal transformation that focuses on the individual. This view looks at the person's growth through reflection and self-critique but it does not look at the impact that the social context has on the learner at all. The other viewpoint sees transformative learning essentially linked to social change and awareness of power within the purview of the learner. It is further noted by Mezirow, Taylor, and associates (2009) that "transformative learning may be defined as *learning that transforms problematic frames of reference to make them more inclusive, discriminating, reflective, open, and emotionally able to change*" (p. 22). It is very important for the practitioner to embrace and acknowledge how his or her previous knowledge is dovetailing with new knowledge. Southern (2007) further explains the transformational learning environment as follows:

> Once we accept the invitation to participate in new ways, we create the possibility to become fully engaged in the process. When this engagement leads us to question assumptions and see the limitations of old thinking and the opportunities in new possibilities, creative energy is set free; students and teachers alike begin to share the learning space, taking responsibility for creating the necessary conditions to become a true learning community. Those conditions include meaningful relationships, purposeful work, shared leadership, and communicative and cultural competence. (p. 332)

The shared experiences with peers, mentors, and clients during the inquiry process will be the changing agent or significant learning process that will transform the way you view and conduct practice from that juncture forward. Once you have gathered the literature, facilitated a therapeutic experience for individuals or a group, compared it to your personal knowledge, and illuminated perspectives, your professional and personal journey will be transformed.

Educational Aims During the Inquiry Process

You are more than likely reading this book because you are involved in a formal education process or taking on an inquiry process for your own educational benefit. From an educational perspective, practitioners

come to understand and engage in an inquiry in order to (1) critically assess inquiry literature influencing practice; (2) develop strategies for conducting inquiries; (3) determine the effectiveness of their own theoretical constructs and practices; and (4) critique interprofessional collaborative practice techniques. Additionally, through the inquiry process, practitioners develop clearer and more concise writing skills consistent with accepted healthcare practices. Professional engagement in an inquiry also helps when communicating to other professionals and consumers about the analyses of the research and evidence-based outcomes related to their evaluation or intervention protocols.

Developing a Topic of Interest

To develop a topic and align its purpose with a professional passion, you should formulate a question that you are excited about. What do you really want to investigate? Start by thinking about your everyday work. What issue or problem keeps coming up during your daily practice? Is there an area of practice that you are not involved in that you would like to explore? Maybe there is a group in your community you would like to explore practice options with, or an area of inquiry that you explored earlier with someone and now you would like to revisit the topic to dive deeper into the literature and engage in an inquiry agenda. Begin by pondering an inquiry agenda by writing down words that are part of the question you are seeking and then begin to formulate draft questions (Box 2-1).

Once you have brainstormed key words and possible inquiry questions, you should then go to a literature database. Type these words and your draft questions into the query to seek out available information. As Creswell (2014) notes, "A common shortcoming of beginning inquirers is that they frame their study in complex and erudite language . . . good, sound inquiry projects begin with straightforward, uncomplicated thoughts, easily read and understood" (p. 2). He further suggests the following questions:

- Is the topic inquiry able, given time, resources, and availability of data?
- Is there a personal interest in the topic in order to sustain attention?

> ## BOX 2-1 ■ Example of How to Ponder an Inquiry Using Key Words to Formulate Questions
>
> ### Key Words
>
> - Adolescents With Disability or Involved Disease Process
> - Social Justice
> - Self-Advocacy
> - School-Based Practice
> - Occupational Therapy
> - Counseling
>
> ### Draft of Inquiry Questions
>
> - How do adolescents with a disability or disease process learn to self-advocate for accommodations or adaptations during the transition planning process of their academic career?
> - How does occupational therapy assist adolescents with a disability or disease process in understanding social justice in the educational environment, in order for them to learn how to self-advocate for accommodations or adaptations?

- Will the results from the study be of interest to others (e.g., in the local region, state, region, nation, global)?
- Is the topic likely to be publishable in a scholarly journal? (or attractive to a thesis committee)?
- Does the study (1) fill a void, (2) replicate, (3) extend, or (4) develop new ideas in the scholarly literature?
- Will the project contribute to career goals?

You have almost arrived at discerning what you want to do for your inquiry. To finish, consider the processes and needs of engagement in a research or evidence-based inquiry by answering the following questions:

- Is there something from your past experience, current interest, or an area of practice you want to move into that is influencing the route you are following?

- Who do you want or need to engage in the process with you?
- What is the true question you are trying to answer? Is it more about the clients, the practice area, the environment, or a particular intervention?
- What resources do you have available to you to carry out the inquiry?
- Who do you want to influence, assist, or affect by engaging in the inquiry?
- How much time do you have to invest in the process? What is the time line and are there financial implications if you take longer than the allotted time?

Once you have answered all of these questions, you can situate the purpose of the inquiry.

Embracing and Situating the Purpose of the Inquiry

The purpose of the inquiry is different for every inquiry; however, the journey of the process is a way of learning and coming to know more about a topic of interest. To some extent, all of us conduct informal inquiries every day, so we are familiar with the processes of investigations and conclusions. It is extremely important to *stay in the moments* of the process and to document them so you can learn even more from the process when you review the notes. Also, remember to seek wisdom along the way when you need it from friends, colleagues, and resources. Try not to just walk through the experience, but embrace it, get excited about it, and consistently move forward with your agenda. You will be in the *inquiry-space* for months and sometimes years, so it is important to find enjoyment during the time. It is common, while gathering data and then writing the evaluation of the inquiry, for people to get bored, complacent, and lonely. Therefore, it is essential for you to reach out to people who will support you during the experience. Further, during the engagement phase, people tend to be stressed by managing all the components and time lines and tending to the participants' needs; however, this time tends to be the most uplifting and collaborative time of the inquiry. Now that you know to *stay in the moments* as you move through the inquiry process, let's take a look at how to situate your inquiry. There are endless options, but here are a few that make the most sense in healthcare practice.

Therapeutic Intervention

Through an action inquiry, you will expand your knowledge of:

- Assessing client and facility programming needs.
- The process of implementing a therapeutic program or project.
- The compatibility of the recommended program with the overall objectives of the client(s) program.
- The strengths and limitations of the recommended program or project.

Management of Healthcare Program

Through a narrative inquiry, you will glean a better understanding of:

- The mission and goals of the facility.
- Staffing issues relevant to the project.
- Knowledge of the legal issues involved in the provision of services at this facility.
- Assessment of the impact of recent changes in delivery systems of this facility. (These might include health care, education, welfare, penal systems, etc.)

Environmental and Technological Adaptations for Clients

Through a participatory action inquiry, you can gain a better understanding of the:

- Expansion of knowledge of appropriate environmental and technological adaptations for the client population.
- Expansion of knowledge in identifying environmental and technological adaptations appropriate to the client population's lifestyle and values.
- Ability to determine the strengths and limitations of the environmental and technological adaptations used or proposed.
- Ability to identify funding issues relevant to the populations served and at the site.
- Ability to provide clients and staff with new knowledge on environmental and technological adaptations.

Evaluation of Healthcare Evaluation Procedures

Through a quantitative methods inquiry, you can determine the expansion of:

- Knowledge of appropriate evaluation procedures for the site's client population.
- Knowledge about the level of expertise required to administer the selected evaluation procedures.
- Ability to determine the strengths and limitations of the selected evaluation procedures.
- Competency skills in administering the selected assessment tools included in the evaluation process.

These are just a few of the thousands of options available to situate the purpose and plan for your research or evidence-based practice inquiry. As previously noted, you must start from a place of passion when engaging in an inquiry. If you are not vested in the topic from the start, it will be difficult to stay motivated to engage in and complete the task. Good luck, and most of all—enjoy the moments along the journey of inquiry.

Chapter Summary

This chapter gives the reader insight into the needs of preparing for a research inquiry. The transformative nature of adult learning, which typically takes place during the research process, is explained to assist the reader in understanding the feelings, emotions, and learning they may encounter along the journey. It explains the learning path that led to and contributes to the process, as well as ideas of how to balance one's time and energy alongside of an inquiry.

SKILL-BUILDING TIPS

- Explore everything that fills you with passion in practice before you begin the inquiry. Don't settle on something just because you are able to easily find a literature base to support your efforts. Explore-pause-ponder-pause-then make the final decision on your topic.

- Your project will not flourish if you do not take risks and move forward every day.

- You can't enjoy what you don't work for.

■ Don't delay pieces you feel are going to be difficult. Make sure to put a pen to paper or fingers to keyboard every day for at least an hour while engaged in an inquiry.

■ The average person wastes 2 hours per day procrastinating. If you get stuck, figure out some way to create a shift in your mindset so that you can move forward quickly and swiftly.

💬 LEARNING ACTIVITIES

1. Write your professional mission statement on engaging in an inquiry. Why is it important to you personally and professionally?

2. List at least 10 ideas you have for an inquiry. Now write a defense for each one—why do you want to explore more about this topic? Select two of your ideas and write a question of inquiry for each. Write down why you are passionate about these two topics. Lastly, sit back and ponder—which one fits you best at the moment?

3. Write down 10 reasons why you are committed to engaging in an inquiry.

REFERENCES

Creswell, J. W. (2014). *Research design: Qualitative, quantitative, and mixed methods approaches*. Thousand Oaks, CA: Sage.

Kasworm, C., Rose, A., & Ross-Gordon, J. M. (Eds.). (2010). *Handbook of adult and continuing education* (2010 ed.). Thousand Oaks, CA: Sage.

Knowles, M. (1984). *Andragogy in action*. San Francisco: Jossey-Bass.

Mezirow, J. (2000). Learning to think like an adult: Core concepts of transformation theory. In J. Mezirow (Ed.), *Learning as transformation: Critical perspectives on a theory in progress* (pp. 3–33). San Francisco: Jossey-Bass.

Mezirow, J., Taylor, E., & Associates. (2009). *Transformative learning in practice: Insights from community, workplace, and higher education*. Jossey-Bass: San Francisco.

Southern, N. L. (2007). Mentoring for transformative learning: The importance of relationship in creating learning communities of care. *Journal of Transformative Education, 5*, 329.

Taylor, E. W. (2007). An update of transformative learning theory: A critical review of the empirical research. *International Journal of Lifelong Education, 26*(2), 173–191.

DavisPlus | For additional materials, please visit **http://davisplus.fadavis.com, key word: Hissong.**

Chapter 3

Reviewing the Literature for Research and Practice

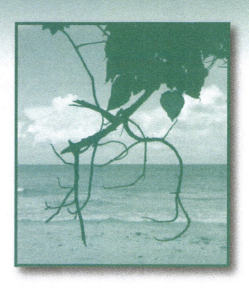

When nothing is sure, everything is possible.
—*Margaret Drabble*

LEARNING OUTCOMES

The information provided in this chapter will assist the reader to:

- Understand the process of approaching and undertaking a literature review.
- Identify potential resources to facilitate the research or evidence-based practice literature review process.
- Conduct a literature search.
- Organize self and material in order to write a literature review.

Reviewing the Literature

Now that you have explored some research questions and settled on one that you would like to answer, the next step is to conduct an overview of your topic to determine if the question has already been adequately addressed. If so, then you need to modify your question. If not, then your process moves into a review of the literature. Many novice researchers ask, "Why is this necessary? Why can't I just start in on my project?" There are several reasons:

- Perhaps someone has already researched your question, or one just like it, and the answer is already published. You certainly would not want to waste your time and that of your subjects by repeating what has already been reasonably well researched.
- Perhaps someone has tried to investigate your question or one very similar and met with insurmountable problems (e.g., not finding a test instrument sensitive enough to measure one of the crucial variables or not being able to prompt adequate narratives to show the depth and breadth of your question). This information would be useful before embarking on a similar project.
- Perhaps someone has investigated your question or a very similar one, but not in the same way that you intend to investigate it. You may plan to use slightly different methods or subject characteristics. You would, however, want to benefit from the information that could be gleaned from the previous study.
- Someone may have already studied one component of the topic, and you can build on that research, thus saving yourself time and energy.
- You might wish to place your study in context with similar studies so that the reader will know how to perceive your work.
- You must place the study within the theoretical base that informs the question(s) from the perspective that you feel gives the optimal insight to the problem (e.g., biomechanical, occupational

science, or social constructivist theory). An increased understanding of the topic and the literature will assist you in the process.

- It will be reassuring if you find reasons in the literature to suggest why the study you propose will address the problem and how your study is capable of solving the problem or answering the question.

- While searching the literature, you will likely find evidence that will prompt you to revise or change your question. It may need a different emphasis; for example, you may decide to look for a correlational effect rather than a cause-and-effect or you may refine your prompting questions.

In any profession, there are strongly held impressions about various areas of practice, things with which most practitioners would agree. However, impressions are not enough. A basis for research and documentation of these beliefs through the literature is constantly needed. Furthermore, a thorough review of written material on the proposed topic of study is essential if the researcher is to design a relevant, original, and timely research study. In addition to articles and books that pertain strictly to your chosen subject, it is important for you to read related material and to be well-versed in the topic being studied. Some examples of such reading are given in Boxes 3-1, 3-2, and 3-3. From these examples you can see that breadth of reading is as important as depth of reading in preparing an effective research proposal. We typically tell our students they will actually spend 70% of their time researching and reading, then spend 30% of their time writing, while doing the entire study–literature review. We get some raised eyebrows when we make this statement, but it's knowledgably based on supervising hundreds of successful research and evidence-based projects.

How to Do a Literature Search

You are likely to find material relevant to your topic in journals, books, global websites, and government documents. Because much of the material relevant to healthcare professions is found in the medical, social,

> ### BOX 3-1 ■ Statement of Research
>
> In studying the temporal adaptation of individuals who have chronic psychiatric conditions, therapists reviewed literature in the areas of use of time in the "normal" population and in the chronic psychiatric population. Areas addressed were the human drive to explore and to master the environment, purposeful activity, the environment, demographics of people similar to those in the sample, and methods of measuring temporal adaptation.

> ### BOX 3-2 ■ Research Abstract on Improving Healthcare Quality and Safety
>
> In a study by McCrory (2012) on improving healthcare quality and safety, you can see the depth and breadth addressed and gleaned from an excerpt from the abstract: The experimental results of four studies used to develop and assess laparoscopic surgery instrumentation, practices, and procedures were addressed. In the first experiment, a novel hand-controlled electrosurgical laparoscopic grasper was developed and evaluated to eliminate the use of foot pedals, reduce surgery-related discomfort, and minimize the risk of actuation errors. The final three studies compared the emerging technique of single-incision surgery to conventional laparoscopic surgery to determine whether there were any technical, physical, or subjective performance differences across the two surgical techniques. In all, these studies contribute toward the improvement of the quality and safety of minimally invasive surgery.

educational, anthropological, psychological, and engineering sciences, the best place to locate material is in institutional libraries, such as those found in universities, postgraduate medical centers, training

---

BOX 3-3 ■ Research Abstract Related to Physical Therapy and Prosthetic Use

In a study related to physical therapy and prosthetic use by older adults, the literature survey may include statistics on the whole population, followed by those in the elderly population who are undergoing amputations; conditions commonly leading to amputations; and review of the literature concerning whether or not to fit elderly amputee patients with prostheses. Topics may include costs versus benefits, physical limitations, motivation, training time, and the likelihood of patients using the prostheses upon discharge; and finally, an overview of studies describing functional outcomes of prosthetic use by elderly people. Additionally, the authors stated that they had limited their literature search to the past 15 years because of recent changes in surgical procedures and rehabilitation care and improvements in prostheses.

---

institutions for healthcare professionals, and other institutions of higher learning. Although this may cause a minor problem for the practitioner who is isolated geographically, frequently material can be found through the public library by using the services of interlibrary loan. Most of the information found can be accessed online and in full-text via e-mail or electronic warehouses. You may be able to gain access to information by becoming a member of your university alumni association. Many universities offer use of the library as a guest when you join the alumni association.

Once you have found a well-stocked library and a helpful librarian, you need to conduct a computer search of the literature. Occasionally, it may be necessary to search printed indices and catalogs, especially if the topic is of an historical nature. In this case, enlist the help of a health information professional or librarian in locating the best sources of evidence.

The next step is to search the online databases and electronic references on your topic. These may include the following:

- Electronic card catalog and reference books
- U.S. government documents
- Online databases that index journal articles and other materials relevant to your topic
- Healthcare databases such as CINAHL (Cumulative Index to Nursing and Allied Health Literature) and PubMed
- Health profession-specific resources within the library's database or in the general media

The Electronic Catalog and Reference Books

There is a record (or computerized entry) in the library catalog for every item housed in the library, except for individual journal articles. There are three main types of entries for each item: author's last name, title, and subject(s). If you are aware of leading authorities in your topic area, such as A. Jean Ayres in the area of sensory integrative techniques or Singe Brunnstrom in kinesiology, you can search for those authors' names and review titles to find appropriate books. If you are not aware of experts in the field, the subject index and database can be used to find appropriate books or journals. Unfortunately, searching for books by subject can be somewhat frustrating if you are not aware of how the subject terms are chosen. An important point to keep in mind is that the catalog or database makes use of a specialized vocabulary, sometimes in contrast to the terms used in everyday language. A specialized vocabulary list may be referred to as a thesaurus, medical subject headings, descriptors, or subjects, depending on the database searched. See Table 3-1.

U.S. Government Documents

Select libraries around the country are depositories for U.S. government publications. This collection is arranged by the Superintendent of Documents' classification scheme and is updated monthly. It lists publications issued by all branches of the U.S. government, including congressional, department, and bureau publications. Issues are indexed in separate volumes for authors, titles and key words, subjects, and series or report titles. The types of documents

Table 3-1 ■ Specialized Vocabulary List	
Everyday Language	**Health-Based Catalog or Database Language**
Injury	Fracture, Open Wound
Massage	Craniosacral, Myofascial Release
Dressing	Donning, Doffing

likely to be useful to therapists include amendments to Medicare, Americans with Disabilities Act (ADA), Individuals with Disabilities Education Act (IDEA), Equal Educational Opportunities, and the Report of the President's Commission on Mental Health.

Health Professional Databases, Indexes, and Abstracts

To use health profession-based online databases, indexes, and abstracts, you must identify appropriate subject terms or know the authors of specific articles. It is necessary to define the subject being researched carefully in order to locate relevant articles because terminology can be specific to the field and can vary from field to field (e.g., one index may use the term *adolescent*, whereas another uses *teen* or *teenager*). There are user guidelines and tips for all of the following commonly used health profession databases, indexes, and abstracts.

The Cumulative Index to Nursing and Allied Health Literature (CINAHL)

This resource indexes more than 3,000 journals on topics like occupational, physical, and speech therapy, as well as 12 other rehabilitation disciplines. Therapy students and practitioners find this an extremely well-organized and useful database. It includes related books, book chapters, conference proceedings, audiovisuals, and educational software. Enhanced versions of CINAHL provide access to online full-text versions of a large host of journals and books. Identify your subject terms by utilizing the "CINAHL Headings" search function. These headings include both CINAHL subject terms and MeSH (Medical Subject Headings).

ProQuest Dissertations

This online database of dissertations and theses from around the world dating from 1861 to the present can be accessed from ProQuest. Most of the dissertations and theses indexed can be purchased in electronic, hard copy, or microform formats through companies listed in the database. The price varies according to the format. Many of the dissertations and theses can be ordered through interlibrary loan from an academic or public library. However, the database includes comprehensive abstracts of the studies, which may be sufficient for your purposes.

PubMed

PubMed contains more than 21 million citations to biomedical research articles dating from 1948 and includes worldwide coverage. Consult the MeSH (Medical Subject Headings) to identify the most appropriate subject headings pertaining to your topic.

OT Search, the Occupational Therapy Bibliographic System (formerly OT BibSys)

OT Search is a comprehensive database of literature and audiovisual material related to occupational therapy along with information directly related to literature in rehabilitation, education, psychiatry, psychology, healthcare delivery, and administration. The actual material is contained in The Wilma L. West Library of the American Occupational Therapy Association in Bethesda, Maryland. Items indexed date from the 1890s to the present.

ERIC

A database sponsored by the U.S. Department of Education indexes education-related material, including journal articles, conference proceedings, government documents, and more.

PsycINFO

This database, produced by the American Psychological Association, uses a content classification scheme that divides the field of psychology into 16 major categories and 64 subcategories. It is well-organized, containing more than 3.3 million citations, primarily to peer-reviewed journal articles and books pertaining to behavioral sciences and mental health. Coverage begins in 1597, but primarily focuses on the 1880s to the present. A well-developed thesaurus of psychology terms used to index citations is available through the database.

Additional Indexes

- Resources in Education (RIE)
- Current Index to Journals in Education (CUE)
- Exceptional Child Educational Resource (ECER)

The RIE abstracts educational research reports (from 1975) by subject, author, and institution, and most reports are available on microfilm. The CUE and ECER abstract articles in education and education-related journals by subject, author, and journal content and are companions to the RIE. A thesaurus of terms accompanies these indexes.

Searching and Selecting Databases

Give careful consideration to how far in the past you want to review your topic. If the subject is rapidly developing or changing a great deal, or is currently being written about (e.g., autism, occupational health systems, surgical procedures in orthopedics), then 2 to 5 years may be sufficient to give you a great deal of material on the most up-to-date thinking. If the subject has been developed over many years (topics such as the development of personal values or carpal tunnel syndrome) and has remained fairly stable in content since the original work, it may be wise to go back to the time of most plentiful writing on that topic, sometimes as many as 20 or 30 years, to find the classic works. If one or two articles or books are constantly referred to in more recent works, they are probably the classic and important writings related to that topic; therefore, it would be worthwhile to read them for a more thorough understanding of the topic.

When beginning a computerized search of any database, the user should have a well-developed research question and official subject terms (usually called subjects, descriptors, or MeSH headings) identified. The terms come from the thesaurus that accompanies each index (Box 3-4). If you cannot find the topic under one heading, try finding a similar or related term. Look for broader or narrower terms than the original one used for searching. It is more efficient

---

BOX 3-4 ■ Specialized Terms to Use When Searching a Database

In a study on recruitment and retention issues for occupational therapists in mental health practice (Scanlan, Still, Stewart, & Croaker, 2010), the researchers identified terms such as *job satisfaction*, *attitude of occupational therapists*, *career mobility*, *career planning*, *employee attitudes*, *retention*, and *occupational stress*. These terms were found in the thesauruses of PubMed, PsycINFO, and OT Search. As mentioned previously, different indexes and abstracts use different terms to identify similar subjects. For example, one index used the term *occupational therapy personnel*, whereas another used *occupational therapists*.

---

to look through the list of terms in the accompanying thesaurus than ponder alternative words.

Selecting the database to be searched (e.g., PubMed or ERIC) will depend on which field you think will contain material relevant to your project, such as medicine, sociology, or education. Once the terms are entered, the computer will scan all the material in that database for literature keyed in with those words for as far back as you wish or is available in the database. Terms can be combined with one another using the connector AND so that you receive only those articles keyed in with both terms (e.g., arthritis AND joint protection). You can search for three or four terms to be listed for each literature source, but likely you will get very few responses when being this specific. Synonymous terms should be searched using the OR connector. It is often simpler and more cost-effective to print titles out at first, so that the items that appear most promising can be selected before purchasing or obtaining the full-text artifact (i.e., book, article, dissertation).

Locating Articles and Books

Once a list of artifacts has been generated from a search, the abstracts need to be reviewed to see if they appear relevant to the study. Numerous books and articles are available in full-text online. The cost of obtaining copies depends on many factors, including publishers' willingness to offer free access and your own affiliation with libraries that might own items or subscribe to databases. For print copies, you must go to the book stacks, the periodical room, or the government documents depository to find the items. If an article is only peripherally related to your topic, you can jot down the relevant points together with the complete reference while you are in the library. However, it will probably be preferable to make copies of the most pertinent articles or to borrow the most relevant books, so that it is possible to study them at your leisure.

Organizing the Material

Some people feel comfortable organizing the literature directly on their computers or handheld devices, whereas others still prefer hard copy methods. There is an endless choice of programs that make this a simpler task. However, some still find index cards useful in keeping information manageable and retrievable. You may find that a combination of filling out index cards and keeping data on your handheld device works best. Whatever method you use, devise a system early on that will help you organize the large amount of information you will gather while engaged in a research study or an evidence-based practice experience.

Again, as committee members for hundreds of research and evidence-based agendas, we have found that, given the sheer volume of material that a student collects, the student must have an organizational plan early on in the process. Those who prefer to organize the information from their literature search directly on the computer may choose to use a simple coding program to cross-reference materials. Software programs are readily available to help the researcher organize and annotate citations. It is wise to enlist the help of a friend, peer, or the student learning center at the institution you are attending to review the various options available to you. All of these programs provide an efficient way to organize material because a single file or a collection of files can eventually be used to construct the actual literature review section of the article.

As soon as you have read and prepared cards or computerized notes on all the artifacts, you are ready to write the review. Start by reviewing the subject headings and putting them in a logical sequence (Box 3-5). In this way, the reader is carried through a progression of topics pertinent to the study or evidence-based practice experience. By the end of the literature review, the reader should understand why the project was being undertaken.

Next, concentrate on one grouping of the literature base at a time. Look for common themes that run through the various authors' research, and make a note of the themes. If a sole author makes a point you would like to include, mark it. Now look at these themes and important points. Do they fall into a logical sequence? Do they flow from one to the other, making the progression of ideas you want to convey to the reader? Write these ideas down in sequence and see if any steps are missing. If so, add them in your own words. When you are satisfied that you have stated the important issues about this topic in a clear, concise manner, add the authors' names whose ideas you have cited, together with the year of publication, in parentheses, after each idea. You are now ready to move on to the next major subject area of your literature review and to repeat the process.

It is a true challenge to write a literature review well. Try to avoid starting every sentence with "Smith

---

BOX 3-5 ■ Logical Sequence of Information

If you were writing a review of the study concerning prostheses mentioned earlier, it would be logical to order the literature review in the following way:

1. Causes and incidence of amputation in elderly people
2. Decision to fit the elderly patient with a prosthesis
3. Types of prostheses
4. Costs versus benefits
5. Physical limitations and motivation
6. Training procedures
7. Functional outcomes

(2012) says . . ." or "Brown (2013) feels that. . . ." Read through some literature sections in published articles to get some ideas for imaginative ways to start sentences and ways to incorporate several authors' ideas and findings in one or two sentences. There are space constraints in journals, so you will not be able to devote many paragraphs to the literature summary. In fact, you will probably read many more articles and books than you will be able to include. Restrict yourself to the most important and convincing work on the points you wish to make. Do a search to find three to four well-written literature reviews and use them as a guide, incorporating the best of each into your own work. Also, remember that the format used to cite references in the literature review is very specific, so try to find literature reviews that are cited and written in the format that you need to write in. Styles will be addressed in detail in Chapter 14, which will address publishing your work.

How Long Should the Literature Review Be?

We are asked this question a great deal, and the bottom line is that your literature review needs to be expansive enough so you and the reader have a clear understanding of what has informed the research project or evidence-based practice project you are about to embark upon. The length of a literature review varies greatly depending on the type of document being produced. For the student writing a thesis, the literature review should be comprehensive and demonstrate that a great deal of literature relevant to the study has been examined to assure the reader that the most important material has been analyzed. A large amount of literature should be examined that explains the issue, suggests why your study is appropriate to it, describes your study's capability for informing the issue, and relates to any other studies or evidence-based interventions that have attempted to solve the issue.

The literature review for a journal article, on the other hand, tends to be brief and to the point. This is because space constraints are imposed by journal editors and there is often a requirement that an entire article be kept within five to seven printed pages.

The *Publication Manual of the American Psychological Association* (2010) offers helpful guidelines for what to include in the background or literature review section of your work.

At this juncture you know that completing the literature review is a major step in the right direction. It does not have to be written in final form at this stage of the project, of course, but it is certainly a potential hurdle and it is a good idea to get the writing accomplished as soon as possible. You are now ready to refine your research or evidence-based practice question and to develop the background material for your study based on what you have read.

Points to Remember When Writing the Literature Review

Although it is important to discuss the literature, you do not need to include an exhaustive historical review of your topic. Assume that the reader has knowledge in the field for which you are writing and does not require a complete digest. A scholarly review of earlier work provides an appropriate history and recognizes the priority of others' work. Citation of and specific credit to relevant earlier works is part of the author's scientific and scholarly responsibility. Although it is essential for the growth of cumulative science, cite and reference only works pertinent to the specific issue and not works of tangential or general significance. If you summarize earlier works, avoid nonessential details; instead, emphasize pertinent findings, relevant methodological issues, and major conclusions. Refer the reader to general surveys or reviews of the topic if they are available.

Demonstrate the logical continuity between previous and present work. Develop the question with enough breadth and clarity to make it generally understood by as wide a professional audience as possible. Do not let the goal of brevity mislead you into writing a statement intelligible to only an expert in the field.

Chapter Summary

This chapter explores the task of conducting a literature review to inform the path of an inquiry. Before any inquiry is initiated there is a need to explore the dialogue that has or has not occurred in relation to the subject matter that is going to be addressed. Furthermore, it explores the process of approaching and undertaking an investigation of the literature that is pertinent to the inquiry. Collectively, the bodies of literature create the background for in-depth understanding of the issues related to the topic of inquiry. The chapter highlights the fact that the analysis of the literature acknowledges and brings to the forefront the limitations of existing research, pro-viding justification of an inquiry and its research methodology. Lastly, it identifies potential resources to facilitate the literature review process.

SKILL-BUILDING TIPS

■ By documenting all points of the reference informa-tion immediately as you prepare your hardcopy or computer-based source index, you will save yourself time and trouble when you are ready to organize the reference list. When organizing the reference list, you may find that you have:

- Lost the article
- Returned the book
- Loaned the article to someone else
- Spilled coffee on the volume number

■ When you are immersed in piles of journals, books, computer files, or copies, it is common to lose sight of the primary topic and to get sidetracked into other interesting areas. We find it helpful to have a sticky note in front of us containing our research or evidence-based question and a list of the major areas for which we are searching. When we feel as if we may be straying too far from the original intent of our inquiry or have forgotten the major issues (which does happen when you are reviewing 2,000–3,000 pages of information), we glance at the sticky note and it gets us back on track.

■ If during a computer search you cannot find any sources or very few sources relevant to your topic, there are several possibilities for what may be happening:

- Your topic does not make sense. No one has writ-ten in this area because it is not logical and there is nothing there to research.
- You are looking in the wrong database (e.g., you are looking in medicine and should be looking in vocational services).
- You have chosen new territory; research has not been conducted in your area. This is very exciting—go ahead!

■ Because many people find writing literature reviews a tiresome task and one that they put off as long as possible, promptness is definitely the best policy and possibly the only policy that will ensure the completion of your work. Besides, it is easier to write a review with the material fresh in your mind and while inspiration is still present. Sometimes your only stumbling block is active engagement in conducting the literature review. It is easy to do all the reading and take all the notes, but sometimes it is difficult to get around to synthesizing and writing the literature review. It is a difficult and time-consuming task, but stay focused and you will be successful.

● LEARNING ACTIVITIES

1. Locate a local library or visit the institutional library to which you are connected. Spend some time in the library and familiarize your-self with the following:
   - Online catalog
   - Reference librarian
   - Interlibrary loan services
   - Online databases
   - Reference section
   - Periodical room
   - List of periodicals and journals stocked by that library
   - Location of copying machines
   - Location of nearest depository of government documents

2. Complete an online catalog and database search for a topic of interest.

Decide on the database most appropriate for your subjects (discuss with the librarian) and peruse the thesaurus for terms.

Database: Database:
Terms: Terms:

When the search has been completed, review the list of titles and abstracts generated by the computer and check off those you wish to locate.

Find books, articles, or dissertation abstracts and complete index cards on peripheral subjects at the library.

3. Write a rough outline for your literature review.

4. Locate at least four literature reviews that can inform your work and are well-written.

5. Develop an online database for your topic and catalog articles on your computer.

DavisPlus | For additional materials, please visit **http://davisplus.fadavis.com, key word: Hissong.**

REFERENCES

American Psychological Association. (2012). *Publication manual of the American Psychological Association* (6th ed.). Washington, DC: Author.

McCrory, B. J. (2012). *Improving health care quality and safety: The development and assessment of laparoscopic surgery instrumentation, practices and procedures.* The University of Nebraska–Lincoln. *ProQuest Dissertations and Theses,* 127. Retrieved from http://search.proquest.com/docview/1010422327?accountid=13158

Scanlan, J. N., Still, M., Stewart, K., & Croaker, J. (2010). Recruitment and retention issues for occupational therapists in mental health: Balancing the pull and the push. *Australian Occupational Therapy Journal, 57,* 102–110.

Chapter 4

Refining the Topic of Interest and Developing the Background Story

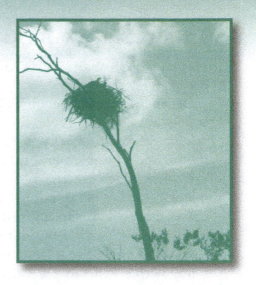

When you go out on a limb, that's when you really know you're living.
—*Robin Quivers*

LEARNING OUTCOMES

The information provided in this chapter will assist the reader to:

- Understand the initial phases of the research process.
- Consider all the facets of a problem statement.
- Identify the background, purpose, and significance of a research study.

Refine the Question and Develop the Background

As a way of refining the research question and developing the background, it is helpful to start writing about the project at this juncture. Information from the literature search is still fresh in your mind, and most of the literature findings will be incorporated into the early parts of the research manuscript. Writing the initial sections makes preparation for publication easier when that time comes.

Problem

The heart of the study is the problem statement, from which all other elements will flow. This is the reason for undertaking the study; it is the problem or question that caught your interest in the first place—the issue you wanted to solve in your clinical practice. After reviewing what has been written about the topic, you should be able to write about the problem comprehensively. At this point stop and ponder this thought, "Is it a problem for many healthcare professionals?" or "Am I going to write from a space I have been having difficulty with over the years or an area I want to know more about?" Have others identified the problem and tried to do something about it? Were their attempts successful or unsuccessful? What will you do differently in your attempt to solve the problem? Or are you merely trying to gather more data about it? (See Box 4-1.)

The research is usually driven by an action, such as carrying out research by identifying something that is wrong or something that needs attention, or by old

27

BOX 4-1 ■ Statement of Study Problem

Phipps and Roberts state the **underlying problem** for their study:

Because of the challenging clinical presentation in children, adolescents, and young adults with cerebral palsy (CP), occupational therapy practitioners and other health care providers must use the best available evidence to optimize functional outcomes for these clients. Yet, the base of evidence for predicting self-care, mobility, and social function is limited to a few research studies, many with small sample sizes. The current study includes 2,768 children, adolescents, and young adults ages 0–19 yr to provide needed evidence for optimal therapy treatment planning, caregiver education, and clinical resource allocation. (Phipps & Roberts, 2012, pp. 422–423)

BOX 4-2 ■ Statement of Study Problem

Wideman and Sullivan state **the problem** for their study in the following sentence:

This study was conducted to determine whether the level of risk for problematic recovery following work-related injuries is associated with the number of elevated psychosocial factors.

They elaborate on the study's objective through two more concise sentences:

Psychosocial variables such as fear of movement, depression, and pain catastrophizing have been shown to be important prognostic factors for a wide range of pain-related outcomes. The potential for a cumulative relationship between different elevated psychosocial factors and problematic recovery following physical therapy has not been fully explored. (Wideman & Sullivan, 2012, p. 58)

---

ideas or methods that are no longer adequate. The paragraph stating the problem should be brief and to the point. Tell the reader what is wrong, what has failed, what is missing, what current ideas are presumed true that you wish to challenge, or what program needs to be scrutinized. Write two or three sentences about the problem and read them to a colleague. If he or she misses the point, try again. Listen to yourself as you read. Is this really the problem you want to do something about? See another example in Box 4-2.

Background

Once you are satisfied with the wording of the problem, you are ready to address the background of your study. The background answers the questions, "Why is this problem of concern?" "Why is it of theoretical interest?" Based on your reading, you should mention why other people think the problem is important and needs work, but most important is background material and your extensive literature review of the topic which supports the study you are going to embark upon. As noted, opinion as well as fact can be given

in the background material when it relates to the importance of the problem (e.g., a leader of your national association may believe that a certain stance on the issue you are researching is of primary importance; therefore, you can quote her or him if it lends credence to your problem statement).

In preparing this section of your research for publication, try to make it interesting to readers. It should capture their attention and leave them agreeing that the problem is important and worthy of investigation. If readers are not captivated by this section, they may not read any further.

If, during your literature search in government publications, you found general statistics related to your topic, now is the time to use them. More often than not, these types of data offer additional background information about the problem but do not have direct bearing on the specific clinical situation under investigation. For example, if the central problem concerns insufficient subsidized health care for persons living in rural America, statistics on how many people are without health care in the United States, and the dollar amount of the rural poverty line as defined by the government, may be included in the background. However, the study itself might be concerned specifically with access as a partial solution to the problem. In another example, you might be studying the specific issue of falls experienced by elderly persons that result in femur fractures. In this case, it would be useful to mention the number of falls by elderly persons each year, the cost of medical treatment for these traumatic events, and the percentage of elders who are unable to return to their homes as a result of the fall. See the expanded example in Box 4-3.

Purpose of the Study

A clear statement of the study's purpose should follow the background material. Some advisors prefer that the purpose be nearer the beginning of the research manuscript, in which case you can insert it immediately after the problem statement and before the background. The purpose should tell the reader what you hope to accomplish regarding the problem by carrying out your study. Be clear about this by starting the sentence, "The purpose of the research was . . . ." Then describe your intentions. The purposes of various studies are illustrated in Boxes 4-4 through 4-6. At this point in your manuscript, the reader should be able to understand what you intend to accomplish within your research and will later judge whether your methodology is likely to achieve it.

Importance of the Study

Another section of the manuscript that can be written as a result of the literature review is the importance of the study. The significance elaborates on what

---

BOX 4-3 ■ Statement of Background of Study

In their 2011 research article entitled *Stability of Measurement Outcomes for Voluntary Task Performance in Participants With Chronic Ankle Instability and Healthy Participants,* Van Deun et al. described the following:

Background: Ankle sprains are among the most common injuries seen in daily life and sport activities. Approximately 40% of the patients who have a lateral ankle sprain develop chronic ankle instability (CAI). In the literature, little attention was paid to the stability of measurements of electromyography (EMG) for the ankle region.

Context: Acceptable measurement stability during data collections was critically important to research. The purpose was to interpret differences in measurement outcomes among participants or changes within participants after an intervention program. We need to know whether the measurement is stable and consistent.

Setting: Musculoskeletal laboratory.

(Van Deun, Stappaerts, Levin, Janssens, & Staes, 2011, p. 366)

BOX 4-4 ■ Statement of How the Problem of the Study Will Be Addressed

The **purpose** of the study is to describe three measures of incidence used in sports injury epidemiology.

BOX 4-5 ■ Statement of How the Problem of the Study Will Be Addressed

The **purpose** of this study is to assess if the inclusion of the additional x-ray projections altered the sensitivity of bony injury detection.

BOX 4-6 ■ Statement of How the Problem of the Study Will Be Addressed

The **purpose** of the study is to determine when (in minutes) a client can identify the mind, body, and spiritual benefits after a 90-minute bamboo massage.

your study will do to affect the problem and why your study is important. It tells what makes your purpose worth pursuing. There are many ways to address a problem—for example, why did you choose your particular purpose? This section will justify your search. For example, there may be other studies addressing the issue, but you have a different purpose in mind (e.g., a group of individuals may have been overlooked by other studies, and you wish to address their needs). The significance paragraph says that your study is appropriate for the research problem and that some important benefits will occur if you do it. This is the answer to the question, "So what?" It gives you the chance to provide a persuasive, rational response (Box 4-7).

In writing these four sections—the problem, background, purpose, and significance—you have engaged in expansive thinking, using global and far-reaching ideas. Now is a good time to pull back into microscopic thinking and ask yourself, "How would I go about achieving all this? Is it feasible?" This will give you a glimpse at methodology, the reality of how you will accomplish your purpose. Different methods for conducting studies are discussed in later chapters.

Research Question

As a result of the writing that has been done so far, the original research question should have become clearer. *This is the time to refine and reshape it.* For example, what may have started out as the global question, "What causes physician assistants to leave suburban practices?" now becomes, "Physician assistants are leaving their suburban practices because they want to move to urban or rural areas to expand their practice interests and enhance their level of advancement." Rework your research question until it contains all the variables you wish to study and puts them in a relationship with one another that is supported by the literature. They may have a cause-and-effect relationship; that is, one variable causes something else to happen. Or they may merely be correlated; that is, if one happens, the other is more (or less) likely to happen in its presence.

In a directional research question, you are predicting that by manipulating or adding a variable there will be a negative or positive outcome. On the other hand, for a nondirectional research question, you are not going to be able to state or predetermine if the outcome will be positive or negative. Whether you choose to pose your research question in the directional or nondirectional format will depend on your clinical experience, what you want to investigate, and the outcome of the literature review. If most of the literature leaned in a specific direction, it would be appropriate to frame your question in that direction. If the material was noncommittal, it would be appropriate to form a nondirectional question. Alternately, sometimes there is no-minimal literature regarding a question that a researcher wants to investigate. In this case, the research question should be framed and written according to what you want to investigate, identify, or prove.

When you feel pleased with your research question, go back to Chapter 2 and review the items that make a question realistic and researchable to be sure that yours still meets the criteria. Perhaps you will find that you now need different resources or a more refined selection of participants.

BOX 4-7 ■ Statement of the Importance of the Study

Ried and Chiu note the **importance** of conducting occupational therapy research with culturally diverse mothers of premature infants:

Researchers need to be sensitized to the Western cultural values upon which most research designs and instrumentation are constructed. Involvement of a culturally diverse research team, openness to feedback, adaptability, and critical reflection on what is important to the cultural groups are among the suggestions for researchers planning home-based occupational therapy research with culturally diverse populations. Furthermore, the objective of the research was to share lessons learned in conducting home-based occupational therapy research with Canadian, immigrant South Asian, and Chinese mothers of premature infants in a large Canadian city.

(Reid & Chiu, 2011, p. 173)

Chapter Summary

It is quite common for you, as the researcher, to confuse the problem, purpose, and significance of a study. Remember:

- The **problem** is the larger issue.
- The **purpose** is what you hope to accomplish as a result of your contribution to the larger problem.
- The **significance** is the importance of your particular study and what it will do to help solve the larger problem. It is the "So what?" part of the study.

These sections of your research manuscript may change several times, so do not get anxious or upset about a particular component of the process. Remember, this is a learning process. There may be steps of the research study that do not go as planned. You must simply document these steps as you go along in order to make an accurate and honest account of events. This allows you to go back and determine the factors that led to your change in plans. There will come a point when everything is as perfect as it can get. Just remember that when pieces begin to blur together, it is very helpful to stay focused on your question and come back to it as often as needed as your guide. *Advice: Put your question on post-it notes and place them throughout your home, work, and daily agendas for several months to ensure every minute you are doing research your focus is on THE question.*

SKILL-BUILDING TIPS

- Find at least 10 topic-related abstracts before writing your own. The abstracts typically list the problem, background, purpose, and significance of the research study and can be invaluable in helping you focus on your own work. Abstracts from other studies are a quick way to get a handle on what was done in a study and they are helpful in guiding you through your own inquiry without the burden of reading the entire research manuscript.
- Don't feel pressured to write everything perfectly the first time. Also, try different ways to get your ideas to print: type on the computer, use notecards, buy a nice notebook and divide it into chapters. When you come up with a thought for a chapter, go to that section and write down your thoughts.
- Enlist a peer. Tell the peer your problem statement. Did the peer understand it? Ask the peer if it makes sense to research this issue and do something about it.
- Remember that the question you think you are starting with will most likely evolve into something else. The concepts will stay the same, but the question may look different. Write down many versions of the same question and just sit with them to see where the literature leads you.

LEARNING ACTIVITIES

1. Write down your original research question.
2. State the general topic area of your project. What is the specific problem you plan to address?
   - Is there something wrong?
   - Does something need attention?
   - Who is the individual, group, or community that will engage in the study?
   - Is something missing?
   - Do old ideas need to be revisited?
3. Practice writing your question several different ways to expand or limit the options of your research.
4. Give at least three reasons why your research agenda is important and valid to you, to society, and to your profession. Why is your study important?
   - What can happen that will be beneficial if the study is done?
   - What is the benefit of this study? Who benefits from the findings?
   - What might happen if the study is not done?
   - Write a significance statement.
5. State what you hope to accomplish regarding the research you are going to engage in.

6. What do you hope to accomplish regarding the problem by carrying out your research agenda?
   - Who are the individuals, groups, or community members this research will impact in a positive way?
   - Will you change something?
   - Will you understand something?
   - Will you interpret something differently?

DavisPlus | For additional materials, please visit **http://davisplus.fadavis.com, key word: Hissong.**

REFERENCES

Phipps, S., & Roberts, P. (2012). Predicting the effects of cerebral palsy severity on self-care, mobility, and social function. *American Journal of Occupational Therapy, 66*, 422–429. http://dx.doi.org/10.5014/ajot.2012.003921

Reid, D. T., & Chiu, T. M. L. (2011). Research lessons learned: Occupational therapy with culturally diverse mothers of premature infants. *Canadian Journal of Occupational Therapy, 78*, 173–179. doi: 10.2182/cjot.2011.78.3.5

Van Deun, S., Stappaerts, K., Levin, O., Janssens, L., & Staes, F. (2011). Stability of measurement outcomes for voluntary task performance in participants with chronic ankle instability and healthy participants. *Journal of Athletic Training, 46*(4), 366–375.

Wideman, T. H., & Sullivan, M. J. L. (2012). Development of a cumulative psychosocial factor index for problematic recovery following work related musculoskeletal injuries. *Physical Therapy, 92*, 58–68.

Research Methodologies and Designs

Chapter 5

Getting Started in the Research Process

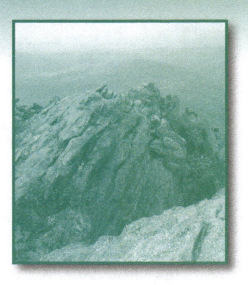

LEARNING OUTCOMES

The information provided in this chapter will assist the reader to:

- Differentiate between quantitative, qualitative, and mixed methods research designs.
- Construct operational definitions of key study terms.
- Examine assumptions made related to the study population, testing measures, and procedures.
- Select an appropriate conceptual framework to guide the study and adequately define the scope of the study.
- Discern conceptual and procedural limitations within a study and their impact on the results.

Research Methodologies

After you have committed to the research process, identified a topic of interest, refined your research question, and explored the background literature, you are ready to consider the research methodology that will be used to investigate your research question. Some questions are best answered with quantitative research designs, whereas others are more appropriate for qualitative ones. Moreover, some questions may be answered using both of these methods simultaneously, which is referred to as a mixed methods design. In order to decide on a study design, the features of each type of research are considered.

Comparison of Quantitative and Qualitative Research

Purpose

The purpose of quantitative research is theory-testing: to establish facts, show causal relationships between variables, allow prediction of outcomes, and strive for generalizability. Conversely, the purpose of qualitative research is to cultivate an understanding of cultures, environments, or groups of people; to develop grounded theory; and to describe views, experiences, and beliefs.

Designs

Quantitative research designs, which are explored in detail in Chapter 6, are predetermined and structured, and do not change during the course of the study; the plan is formal and objective. Qualitative research designs, which are discussed in Chapter 8, fall at the other end of the spectrum. The procedures are more general in nature and tend to evolve throughout the study. They also guide progression of the study and can be modified as necessary.

Subjects

In quantitative studies, the subjects are typically recruited based upon specific inclusion and exclusion criteria, and then randomly selected and randomly assigned to study groups. Subject samples tend to be large in an effort to accurately represent the larger population of interest from which the sample was drawn. In their most simplistic form, quantitative studies usually include at least two study groups—an experimental group and a control or comparison group, with the control or comparison group serving to control for extraneous variables that could impact study results. Other variations of this design are discussed in Chapter 6. In qualitative studies, the subject sample is small and may be non-representative of the larger population. Subjects are also selected based upon their roles, culture, or environment, depending on the purpose of the study, and there is no need for randomization or a control or comparison group.

Researcher's Relationship With Subjects

Quantitative researchers typically have limited contact with the subjects on a short-term basis. They are detached and distant, keeping the roles of researcher and subject distinct. The researcher's role is to observe and measure; as the researcher must be objective, care is taken to prevent the researcher from influencing the data through personal involvement with the research subjects. In contrast, during a qualitative study, researchers usually have intense contact with subjects over an extended period of time. There is an emphasis on trust. The subjects are viewed as participants in an egalitarian relationship, and the researcher may empathize with the subjects and their situations.

Data Collection

Data collection tools and techniques used in quantitative and qualitative research vary greatly. In quantitative research, data collection methods can include structured observation, interviews, surveys, record review, hardware and equipment use, or standardized and nonstandardized assessments and tests. Techniques used in qualitative research can include observation, review of documents and artifacts, open-ended interviews, and focus groups. In a qualitative study, the researchers are often the only "tool" for data collection. Credibility is determined by the researcher's skill, competence, and rigor. He or she may use guiding questions to elicit responses during an interview, as well as audio or video recorders, translators, and transcribers to document responses for later analysis. Using more than one data collection method within a research design, referred to as **triangulation**, can help the researcher confirm the validity of the results.

Data Generated

The data gathered in quantitative research designs are quantifiable and statistical, using counts and measures. Data are collected and managed according to very specific procedures developed before initiation of the study. Data gathered in qualitative designs are descriptive and deal with qualities. They may consist of field notes, artifacts, people's own words, personal records, recordings, or official documents. Qualitative data are extensive and can be difficult to manage. As noted in the following section, specific procedures are used to process qualitative data.

Data Analysis

Perhaps the greatest difference in the two styles of research is in how the data are analyzed. Data analysis occurs at the conclusion of data collection in a quantitative study. It tends to be deductive and uses statistical manipulation as planned in the study design phase. It is a straightforward operation that is often completed rather speedily. On the other hand, data analysis is ongoing throughout qualitative studies, using a constant comparison method. Data are analyzed as they are gathered, then reanalyzed in light of new information, in a recursive manner. Qualitative data analysis is inductive in nature and addresses models, themes, and concepts. Techniques such as coding, memoing, event listing, pattern-matching, charting, matrices, and triangulation may be used.

Outcomes

The outcomes of quantitative and qualitative research can be quite different. Quantitative research studies answer specific research questions by producing statistical evidence to prove or disprove hypotheses that were developed before the study. Although the researcher can certainly discuss the findings, there is a common saying that the data, meaning the statistical outcomes, speak for themselves. The outcome of qualitative research, more often than not, is a lengthy descriptive document, presenting the data in words rather than numbers. The report is rich, textural, anecdotal, and full of thick description in narrative form. The final analysis provides either verification of an existing theory or new grounded theory, together with well-formulated research questions that now need to be investigated.

Potential Issues

Although each type of research has definitive advantages, issues may be encountered in conducting either type. Problems in quantitative studies could include:

- Difficulty isolating or controlling variables that will affect the study
- Difficulty recruiting an adequate number of appropriate subjects
- Questionable validity of the study, as some critics feel that highly controlled experimental studies have little relevance to real life
- Obtrusiveness of the researcher and data collection methods that may affect the subjects or environment
- Ethical concerns regarding provision of experimental treatments on human subjects

  Problems in qualitative research include:

- Nonstandardization of procedures
- Difficulty of managing large amounts of data and data reduction methods
- Extremely time-consuming nature of the whole process
- Difficulty of using naturalistic methods to study large populations
- Difficulty generalizing results to the larger population of interest

Mixed Methods Designs

Although the two styles of research are presented as if they were mutually exclusive, in reality, the designs may be integrated and many research projects employ a combination of both designs, often referred to as a **mixed methods design**. Some of the reasons to use a mixed methods design are:

- To investigate a research question that cannot be effectively answered by quantitative or qualitative methods alone
- To strengthen a study so that methods complement each other and increase confidence in the findings
- To gain a comprehensive understanding of a phenomenon by uncovering different dimensions with different techniques
- To compensate for the weaknesses of one design with the strengths of another
- To achieve triangulation. **Triangulation** is a technique that involves the use of two or more separate research methods or data collection techniques to confirm study results. When similar results are obtained via multiple methods or techniques, the researchers have increased confidence that their findings are valid.

Box 5-1 provides an example to further distinguish between quantitative, qualitative, and mixed methods approaches.

It is important to understand the basic tenets that define quantitative and qualitative research including their purpose, methodologies, and outcomes. The goal of quantitative research is to answer a specific research question via use of statistical evidence, whereas qualitative research aims to verify or generate descriptive theory. To achieve these goals, the researchers approach the study in very different ways. The quantitative researcher begins the study with a theory and very specific hypotheses that address one defined issue, whereas the qualitative researcher begins with multiple vague research questions on a broad topic. The questions may change throughout the qualitative study process, and the project ends by posing some specific hypotheses and grounded theory. In both cases, the methodologies to achieve these outcomes are significantly different, with quantitative designs employing rigorous formalized procedures, and qualitative designs using more general evolving ones. When the principles and activities of both methods are fully grasped, the researcher can become adept at using the methods independently or together. For

BOX 5-1 ■ Example to Highlight Quantitative, Qualitative, and Mixed Methods Designs

Three groups of researchers were asked to design a study that would investigate the research question: Are healthcare practitioners increasing their use of evidence-based approaches in daily practice? Teaching of evidence-based practice has become commonplace in educational programs because of changes in education standards. Many disciplines have committees and publications devoted specifically to evidence-based practice, and patients and third-party payers are beginning to demand it. But have all these factors led to actual changes in the healthcare practice? This question can be addressed in several ways.

The first group of researchers felt that an answer could be found by asking experienced practitioners to complete a quantitative survey in which they reported the percentage of time spent on evidence-based practice activities, such as searching for evidence or participating in a journal club, each day. Fifty practitioners were asked to quantify the percentage of time in the work day that they engaged in the outlined evidence-based practice activities 5 years ago and then in their current practice. The researchers set out to answer the research question quantitatively, by comparing numerical data indicative of practice 5 years ago and at the present time.

A second group elected to garner opinions from practitioners regarding the topic of evidence-based practice and its use within their specific discipline from a qualitative perspective. These individuals felt it was important to investigate the whole notion of evidence-based practice in order to make some substantiated guesses about whether evidence-based practice was gaining momentum in recent years. The researchers interviewed 35 practitioners from a variety of practice settings to assess their opinions on evidence-based practice. Questions included:

- How do you feel about engaging in evidence-based practice activities?
- What value do you place on the use of evidence-based practice related to your daily work?
- How prepared do you feel to engage in evidence-based practice activities?

This group of qualitative researchers felt that gathering sufficient data on the general topic to propose hypotheses was more important than answering the assigned research question.

The third group chose a mixed approach, which involved asking 45 practitioners to quantify the percentage of time that they engaged in evidence-based practice activities over the last month. However, the researchers also chose to interview a subset of this group, which included 20 practitioners, to supplement the numerical data with additional qualitative data. Interview questions included:

- Why do you engage in evidence-based practice activities?
- What barriers have you encountered when engaging or attempting to engage in evidence-based practice?
- How has your practice changed related to the evidence-based practice movement?

This group felt it was ineffective to look at the time spent engaging in evidence-based practice activities without investigating the motivations and barriers to engagement. Using both quantitative and qualitative methods gave them a more comprehensive picture of the phenomenon than either of these methods used alone.

this reason, quantitative and qualitative research methods are treated separately in the next chapters.

General Considerations for Any Research Study

Regardless of the research method that you choose, in order to enable others to understand and apply your research, you will need to consider and identify the following:

- Definitions and operationalization of all key terms if the meanings are not obvious
- Assumptions about underlying principles of the study
- Conceptual or theoretical framework used to guide the study
- Scope of the study (how it fits into the scheme of existing professional literature)
- Limitations that are likely to influence results or their interpretation

Each of these topics will be covered in greater depth here.

Defining and Operationalizing Terms

Some of the terms in the study need to be defined, whereas others need to be operationalized. In both cases, the specific meanings of the terms in your study need to be made clear to the reader. First, let's consider the simple definitions.

People who read your study may come from a variety of professional backgrounds and may not be familiar with terms specific to your discipline or specialty. Defining your terms will help the reader know their precise meaning in the context of the study. Some terms that need defining include those specific to your field or which have everyday language counterparts with which they might be confused. One example is the word *grounded*, which has a meaning in ethnography that is quite different from its nautical or electrical meanings. Another is the term *occupation*, which is used frequently in the occupational therapy literature to refer to all of life's meaningful activities including self-care, productive work, and leisure. Those outside the discipline associate this term with paid employment. It is especially important to define terms that occur in

the problem statement, the purpose of the study, and the research questions or hypotheses because a misunderstanding here could threaten the reader's grasp of the entire study. Definitions may come from sources such as dictionaries, medical textbooks, lists of synonyms, and glossaries, and may range from just a few words to elaborate explanations several paragraphs long. Researchers may also use existing definitions from authorities and cite the authors.

When beginning a research project, some terms may also need to be operationalized. **Operationalizing** involves strictly defining concepts in terms of how they are measured so that their meaning cannot be misinterpreted. For example, researchers interested in studying the effect of a multisensory treatment environment on negative behaviors in clients with dementia would need to operationally define *multisensory treatment environment, negative behaviors,* and *dementia.* Clearly describing the treatment environment allows the reader to fully understand the intervention being provided. Negative behaviors could include aggression, agitation, or lethargy, to name a few. How will these behaviors be quantified and documented? Furthermore, several types of dementia exist and the severity can be rated on a number of scales. Is the researcher interested in presenile dementia, multi-infarct dementia, or Alzheimer's dementia, for example? Specifying these aspects will facilitate appropriate application of the study results as well as replication in future studies. Operational definitions may apply not only to measurable items, such as degrees of flexion or percentage of oral intake, but also to more abstract concepts, such as independence or self-esteem. See Box 5-2 for an example of defining and operationalizing study terms and concepts.

Assumptions

Next, you need to consider your own assumptions regarding the study and the premises upon which the study is designed. **Assumptions** are underlying principles that the researcher believes or accepts but that are difficult to prove in any concrete way. They are frequently untested and untestable hypotheses, basic values, or views about the world. They include such values as the notion that people are basically good or

---

BOX 5-2 ■ Example of Defining and Operationalizing Study Terms and Concepts

In an occupational therapy study, Chippendale and Bear-Lehman (2012) explored the impact of life review via therapeutic writing on reported symptoms of depression for adults in senior living communities. They provided the following definition of therapeutic writing in their article:

> *Therapeutic writing,* a form of expressive therapy that uses the act of writing and processing the written word, can take several forms. *Emotional disclosure* includes writing about emotional or traumatic life events without additional prompts, whereas *guided autobiography,* or life review through writing, includes written or verbal prompts to encourage writing about one's life in a systematic, chronological way irrespective of emotional content. (p. 439)

They go on to describe the 90-minute writing sessions conducted in the study, including the prompts and additional questions raised to participants.

Next, they defined depressive symptoms in terms of their impact on quality of life and functional independence in the aging population. A review of current literature provides the rationale for this study; therefore, depressive symptoms must be operationalized in order to determine the effect, if any, life review writing has on these symptoms. The authors resolved to measure depressive symptoms with the 30-item *Geriatric Depression Scale* (Lelito, Palumbo, & Hanley, 2001), which has been recognized as a valid and reliable tool with the chosen population.

---

that people want to function independently in their day-to-day activities. These ideas would be very difficult to prove with the population at large or even with a small research group.

Two kinds of assumptions need to be examined: first, assumptions about the ideological principles upon which the study is based, and second, assumptions that are made concerning the procedures used in the study. We all adhere to certain ingrained principles that will affect the way we approach situations and therefore the way we design research studies.

For example, in following their ideological principles, a client-centered researcher and a financially-oriented researcher might approach Chippendale and Bear-Lehman's (2012) study about the use of therapeutic writing with adults in senior living communities from quite different viewpoints. The client-centered researcher might hold the assumption that as adults age, everything should be done to preserve their quality of life and to minimize depressive symptoms. Therapeutic writing might be one tool to accomplish this. The money-conscious administrative researcher might feel that therapeutic writing contributes to improved mental well-being and that

regular participation may reduce the cost of medical care for adults in subsidized housing and on government medical plans.

The two researchers are likely to adopt different study methods when addressing the impact of therapeutic writing on depressive symptoms in adults in senior living communities. The client-centered researcher would probably investigate the impact of the therapeutic writing on the well-being and quality of life of the subjects, whereas the financially-oriented researcher might investigate the results of the therapeutic writing on the health status and resulting healthcare costs of the subjects.

The second type of assumption relates to the procedures used during the research study. Usually these pertain to the instruments used and the willingness of subjects to participate in the study. For instance, researchers are often obliged to assume that the measuring instrument being used is valid and reliable because, at least in human subject research, it is often difficult to prove validity and reliability conclusively. The most notoriously unreliable instruments (in experimental research when replication is desirable) are interviews and questionnaires, yet it is sometimes impossible to conduct a quantitative study without them.

There are other basic assumptions associated with the use of measuring instruments, such as assuming that the subjects will answer questions honestly and respond to tests of skill to the best of their abilities. In designing study procedures, the researcher must consider, in advance, events that may occur during the study and must try to control for those events to avoid having to make procedural assumptions about them. For example, in some studies in which performance of a skill is being measured, it is imperative for the study that subjects try as hard as they can on the test. To ensure this, some researchers have devised reward systems to compensate subjects according to their motivation level. When these types of strategies are used, assumptions need to be made less frequently and only for items beyond the researcher's control and ingenuity. Making your assumptions known is important so that readers know where you stand on issues related to the research and where they should keep a critical eye on procedures.

To further clarify, people often make the mistake of including in their assumptions those notions that can be proven; in other words, ideas that are referenced in scientific literature. If an idea can be proven scientifically, it need not be presented as an assumption but rather should be presented in the literature review as part of the reason for conducting the study in a certain manner. Only beliefs that are difficult to prove concretely, those that are untested or untestable, or those assimilated from a variety of sources should be included in the assumptions section.

Researchers routinely examine their assumptions carefully and state them to the reader near the beginning of the study. Readers need not agree with the assumptions put forth by the researcher but they should be able to follow the logic of the propositions and understand why the researchers approached the study as they did. Box 5-3 illustrates how one author clearly discussed important assumptions in her doctoral project.

BOX 5-3 ■ Example of Assumptions in Research

For her doctoral thesis, Trickey-Rokenbrod (2011) studied the driving skills of community-living elderly adults. Being employed in an outpatient setting, she was specifically concerned with what clinic-based interventions would be most effective for improving driving subskills and self-awareness of driving performance in this population. She clearly and concisely articulated her assumptions in designing her intervention as follows:

> Before conducting a literature review the author of this project had a general assumption that all elderly drivers want to continue to drive. This impression comes from experience working and interacting with elderly clients as well as older family members that drive. Another assumption is that clients in the outpatient OT clinic will want to work on driving as a part of therapy, and will put forth significant effort both during clinic treatment time and in following through outside of therapy to make progress toward the established goals related to driving. This assumption is partly based on confidence in the skill the author has in establishing therapeutic rapport with new clients.
>
> A major assumption underlying this project is that driving performance can be influenced by in-clinic remediation of subskills and increased older-driver self-awareness. While there have been indications of this [outcome] (Sivak et al., 1984; Caragata et al., 2009; Marottoli et al., 2007) many studies have been inconclusive or have limitations in size, population or methodology that limits generalization to the proposed setting. A last assumption is that without an on-road assessment method, the proposed assessment tools will be sensitive enough to pick up progress made toward driving-related goals. (pp. 60–61)

Scope of the Study and Guiding Conceptual Framework

The **scope of a study** includes a clear explanation of the study's area of focus, purpose, and relationship to existing literature. **Conceptual frameworks**, also known as models of practice, are theoretical explanations of functioning that can guide practitioners in their treatment approach with clients or researchers in their approach to a study. Some examples of these frameworks include a behavioral approach, a biomechanical model, a sensory processing model, or a model of change. These models can be individualized to specific disciplines or applied across disciplines.

In some cases, the description of the scope is elaborate and meticulously presented, perhaps in instances when the researchers are presenting a new treatment choice for a particular client population. Detailed explanations of the background and the guiding framework may be necessary for the reader to fully grasp the logic and meaning behind the study. In another study, where the purpose and approach are more easily understood, it might be appropriate to explain the scope and conceptual framework within one paragraph.

For example, the purpose of Carnaby-Mann and Crary's (2008) study was to determine the effect of adjunctive neuromuscular electrical stimulation on the treatment of pharyngeal dysphagia, or difficulty swallowing. Although other techniques—such as thermal stimulation and oral motor exercises—may improve swallowing function, these interventions were beyond the scope of the study. The researchers reviewed the existing literature on use of neuromuscular electrical stimulation, noting 11 other studies completed thus far with affirming results; however, they also noted that this approach to treatment was still not well-defined. In order to expound on this prior research, the authors made it clear to readers that they were applying the first of Robey's five-phase model for clinical-outcome research (Robey, 2004). This model, typically used to comprehensively describe a therapeutic intervention and evaluate its outcomes, usually involves case study, case series, or retrospective designs. Thus, Carnaby-Mann and Crary (2008) chose a prospective case series design, defined their population precisely, and explained the rationale for the study.

The scope tells the reader the study's focus, what will be covered in the project, and what will not be included. For instance, if a sensory integrative approach will be taken in a study, it is unreasonable to expect the researcher to cover the possibilities of what might happen to subjects if a behavioral approach had been used. Informing the reader of the background and any guiding principles puts the study in context within the work that was previously accomplished on the topic. In this way, it is immediately apparent to readers how the current study can add to the existing body of literature on the subject.

Limitations of the Study

In setting forth your study's limitations, you should include conceptual and methodological shortcomings that cannot be overcome in the study design. Limitations in experimental research may include the inability to randomly select the subjects, or to include a control group, or the lack of a standardized instrument to measure variables. Nonexperimental research may have insurmountable methodological problems, such as lack of an appropriate mailing list of the people you want to poll in an attitude survey, which could force you to make do with an over-inclusive or under-inclusive list. Conceptual limitations could include such problems as an underlying principle of the study not being widely accepted outside your professional specialty.

Naturally, listing a study's limitations does not excuse you from making all possible attempts to overcome the problems. After all possible improvements in study design have been made, pointing out the remaining limitations shows that you are aware of them and will consider them when discussing the results. Although some researchers may be tempted to give litanies of limitations, doing so may discount the fact that the research may still prove useful in advancing knowledge in the area of study. There is a middle ground to be achieved between listing every conceivable problem and quirk in a study and being fair with the reader and presenting those things that could truly bias the results. Knowledgeable readers will pick up obvious limitations but will respect an author who acknowledges problems and considers them in the interpretation of the findings. Box 5-4 of-fers an example of how a group of physical therapists made clear the important limitations in their study.

BOX 5-4 ■ **Example of Study Limitations**

A group of physical therapists from Loma Linda University in California studied the effects of virtual reality gaming on dynamic balance and strength in older adults (Rendon et al., 2012). Because of the increased inci-dence of falls in this population, finding in-terventions that effectively improve mobility and balance was critical. Although the study supports the use of virtual reality gaming in this endeavor, these findings must be applied with consideration of the study's limitations as reported:

> There were several limitations in this investi-gation. No participant was able to complete the entire series of exercises without the use of the assistive devices at least one time. This fact is cause for concern for potential injury in regard to independent practice devoid of supervision.
>
> Also, the sample pool from which the par-ticipants were selected from is a limiting fac-tor in terms of generalising [sic] the outcome measures. All participants were veterans or spouses of veterans from the US military, which created a specific mindset of account-ability of appointment keeping and exercise rigour [sic], which is possibly higher than the average population. Another potential limi-tation is that this intervention was not com-pared with any other form of traditional physical therapy balance training program. Additionally, we did not have the control group perform the warm-up and cool-down exercises and therefore cannot say with cer-tainty that the intervention group benefits were not due to the warm-up/cool-down routines. (Rendon et al., 2012, pp. 551–552)

Chapter Summary

In this chapter, you were provided with foundational knowledge regarding research methodologies, and you may now have some early ideas about which type of design might be suitable for your research question. Considering your research question, cir-cumstances, and objectives is the first step in making this decision. Chapters 6 and 7 provide additional information and support for conducting quantitative research, and the corresponding information on qual-itative designs can be found in Chapters 8 and 9.

SKILL-BUILDING TIPS

■ Consider a quantitative study if you:
  ■ Want to support a hypothesis
  ■ Want to look for the effect of one variable upon another
  ■ Are interested in the relationship between two or more variables
  ■ Want to find out some specific facts about a large group of people
  ■ Have access to a large group of people who meet your criteria

Review Chapters 6 and 7 for more details if you feel a quantitative design may fit your goals.

■ Consider a qualitative study if you:
  ■ Want to generate a new theory
  ■ Want to generate new hypotheses to be tested later
  ■ Are interested in exploring the thoughts, feelings, and beliefs of a small group of people
  ■ Want to gather data in a naturalistic setting
  ■ Have access to a natural setting and the ability to spend large amounts of time there gathering data from individuals, groups, and records

Review Chapters 8 and 9 for more details if you feel a qualitative design may fit your goals.

■ Mixed methods designs may require advanced knowledge, skills, and time, and more in-depth ex-planation is beyond the scope of this text. If you feel this approach may suit your purposes, be sure to seek assistance from a research advisor at your facility or institution, or review some of the additional resources provided at the end of this chapter.

■ Once you have decided upon a methodology, find three studies in the literature that employed this methodology. Reviewing these studies will help you to determine if your topic and goals will be supported by the chosen method.

■ Choose a topic that you have some experience with and feel passionate about. Without these two criteria, you will spend much time establishing baseline knowledge to formulate a research question, and your motivation for the project may fade quickly.

■ Review the conceptual or theoretical frameworks commonly used within your discipline. Determining an appropriate framework can help you to gain a perspective on your study and to shape its design.

■ Do not be discouraged if your study topic and design change multiple times. Remember that research is a process and these features typically evolve over time as you delve deeper into the topic.

LEARNING ACTIVITIES

1. Consider the example in Box 5-1, then reflect on your proposed topic. Could your topic be explored via quantitative, qualitative, or mixed methods designs? Draw up a simplified plan to explore your topic with each of these research designs.

2. Make a list of key terms for your study. Then operationalize each term. Don't forget terms associated with defining your subjects, measuring the variables and phenomena in question, and any treatments or interventions provided.

3. What assumptions have you made in contemplating your study? Make a list of assumptions regarding your population, testing instruments and procedures, and the study environment, as well as your rationale for assuming these things.

4. What is the underlying framework or scope of your study?

5. What conceptual and procedural limitations can you anticipate for your study in this early phase of development?

REFERENCES

Carnaby-Mann, G. D., & Crary, M. A. (2008). Adjunctive neuromuscular electrical stimulation for treatment-refractory dysphagia. *Annals of Otology, Rhinology & Laryngology, 117*(4), 279–287.

Chippendale, T., & Bear-Lehman, J. (2012). Effect of life review writing on depressive symptoms in older adults: A randomized controlled trial. *American Journal of Occupational Therapy, 66,* 438–446. http://dx.doi.org/10.5014/ajot.2012.004291

Lelito, R. H., Palumbo, L. O., & Hanley, M. (2001). Psychometric evaluation of a brief geriatric depression screen. *Aging and Mental Health, 5,* 387–393. http://doi.org/10.1080/13607860120080350

Rendon, A. A., Lohman, E. B., Thorpe, D., Johnson, E. G., Medina, E., & Bradley, B. (2012). The effect of virtual reality gaming on dynamic balance in older adults. *Age and Aging, 41,* 549–552. doi:10.1093/ageing/afs053

Robey, R. R. (2004). A five-phase model for clinical-outcome research. *Journal of Communication Disorders, 37,* 401–411.

Trickey-Rokenbrod, D. (2011). *Improving driving subskills and self-awareness in older drivers in an outpatient setting.* Unpublished manuscript, Department of Occupational Therapy, Chatham University, Pittsburgh, PA.

RESOURCES FOR MIXED METHODS RESEARCH DESIGNS

Creswell, J. W. (2013). *Research design: Qualitative, quantitative, and mixed methods approaches* (4th ed.). Thousand Oaks, CA: SAGE Publications, Inc.

Hesse-Biber, S. N. (2010). *Mixed methods research: Merging theory with practice.* New York, NY: The Guilford Press.

DavisPlus | For additional materials, please visit **http://davisplus.fadavis.com, key word: Hissong.**

Chapter 6

Quantitative Research Methodology and Design

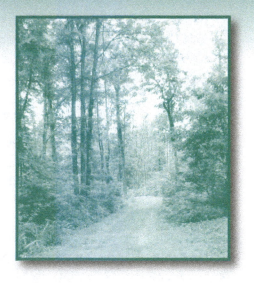

Success is a journey, not a destination.
—*Arthur Ashe*

LEARNING OUTCOMES

The information provided in this chapter will assist the reader to:

- Identify features of quantitative research, including manipulation, control, and randomization.
- Understand basic quantitative research designs.
- Explain how aspects of internal and external validity can impact outcomes of quantitative research.
- Describe how reliability can influence outcomes of quantitative research.

"Quantitative research is a formal, objective, systematic process in which numerical data are used to obtain information about the world" (Burns & Grove, 2009, p. 22). Quantitative research designs are most often employed "to describe variables, examine relationships among variables, and determine cause-and-effect interactions between variables" (Burns & Grove, 2009, p. 22). In this chapter, some of the major quantitative research designs will be described and their advantages and disadvantages discussed. Of course, there are many more designs than those presented here, but beginning researchers should be able to find a design to fit their needs when starting the research process. Broad categories of research designs discussed here include experimental designs, quasi-experimental designs, and nonexperimental designs.

Features of Quantitative Research

Before choosing a quantitative research design, it is important to consider several features that can affect experimental rigor. These three concepts will be explored:

1. Manipulation
2. Control
3. Randomization

Manipulation

Manipulation merely means doing something to one or more variables in the study. A variable is anything that can vary or change and therefore can be measured. For example, if the researcher offers a group of patients with schizophrenia a daily program of self-care activities to determine whether their appearance can be improved, manipulation is provided in the form of daily self-care activities. Generally, any treatment or intervention offered to subjects in the hope that they will show improvement can be called manipulation. Changing the environment or the timing of an intervention can also be considered manipulation.

In other words, the researcher is manipulating one or more variables in connection with the subjects. In the foregoing example, the variable of self-care is being manipulated or given as treatment to determine whether it will have an effect on another variable, namely, the patient's appearance.

Dependent and Independent Variables

It is important to understand the difference between variables in a quantitative study. The **independent variable** is the variable that is being manipulated, which could affect the outcome (or dependent variable). Conversely, the **dependent variable** is typically the variable being measured. In the previous example, the independent variable (self-care) is manipulated to determine the effect on the dependent variable (the patients' appearance). The independent variable is sometimes called the experimental or treatment variable. The dependent variable (appearance) determines the effectiveness of the manipulation or treatment and is the outcome observed and measured at the beginning and end of the study.

Manipulation must be part of the methodology if the study is to qualify as a true experimental design. Thus, if the researcher does not actually manipulate a variable pertaining to the subjects, a study cannot be termed *experimental*. For example, a study in which subjects are asked to complete a questionnaire and the researcher merely examines answers or variables after the fact is not experimental.

Control

The second concept that needs defining in order to understand quantitative research designs is control. **Control** refers to the researcher's ability to control or eliminate interfering and irrelevant influences in a study's design. This will allow the researcher to say that the results are because of manipulation of the variables and not because of chance interferences of other variables. In the earlier example, if there were no control, it is possible that instead of the program of self-care skills, some other event in the patients' lives (such as a volunteer taking the patients to the store to buy new clothes) might have caused improvement in their appearance.

The researcher may be able to control some variables such as:

- Environmental influences (e.g., the amount of noise or the aesthetics of the surroundings)
- Change of healthcare practitioner providing the treatment (it might be important to the study that the same practitioner be used so that patients become accustomed to him or her, or it might be equally important that different practitioners be used to eliminate the influence of certain practitioners' styles)
- Certain events in the patients' lives (such as obtaining a physician's cooperation in maintaining patients' medications during the period of the study)

However, it is not possible to control all variables that may affect the study results. Thus, it is important to have a control group of subjects who experience the same day-to-day occurrences and influences as the experimental group yet do not receive the study treatment. By including a control group, the researcher is attempting to ensure that any helpful or detrimental event influencing the amount of change in the dependent variable (the one being measured) will happen to both groups of subjects. At the end of the study, when the dependent variable is measured for both groups, if there is greater improvement in the experimental group, the researcher can say that this was likely because of the manipulation or treatment.

In certain situations, it is not ethical to withhold treatment from a group of patients in order for them to serve as a control group. There are generally three ways to deal with these circumstances. For example, a researcher might like to know if a new form of treatment is more effective for a certain condition than the traditional treatment for that condition. One option to test this question is to have the control group receive the traditional treatment and the experimental group receive the new treatment, holding all other conditions constant. This design satisfies the need for a control group as well as the ethical concern. Another option might involve collecting data on the experimental group before initiation of the new treatment. By comparing data before and after the new treatment, the experimental group functions as its own control. A third option is to use two distinct groups—an experimental and a control group, with the control group being offered the experimental treatment following the initial phase of the study. This allows the researcher to draw conclusions regarding the experimental treatment and to satisfy ethical concerns by permitting both groups to undergo the same treatment. The concept of control embraces elements of the third concept to be discussed—that of randomization.

Randomization

Systematic bias refers to inherent flaws in a study's design that can influence or skew results. Randomization is used to reduce the risk of this bias creeping into the study. In addition, randomization increases the study's *external validity*, which is the chance that the results found in the subjects can be generalized to others who are similar. It also increases the study's *internal validity*, which is the chance that observed changes are because of the intervention or treatment being provided and not because of other possible causes. Randomization involves two components—random selection and random assignment.

Random selection means that every subject in the population being studied has an equal chance of being selected for the study sample. Researchers carefully consider who they wish to study and then set criteria for the subjects. For example, inclusion criteria might consist of people diagnosed with chronic schizophrenia who had multiple admissions to hospitals totaling at least 5 years and who have one or more family members available for support. For the same study, the researchers might determine exclusion criteria as patients younger than 18 years of age, and those living more than 25 miles from the research center. Once the inclusion and exclusion criteria are determined, the researchers must choose a method to select a group of individuals (sample) to be in the study from among those who meet the criteria.

In research, the population of interest refers to the entire group of people or items that meet the subject inclusion criteria set by the researcher. The population consists of all such subjects, whereas the subpopulation is a researcher-defined subgroup of

the population. A sample is selected from the population or the subpopulation (Box 6-1). A population does not necessarily refer to people; it may also refer to things such as records or events that are being studied (Box 6-2).

For true random selection, every subject in the population of interest must have an equal opportunity of being selected. Therefore, merely using patients who come through your door or client records that happen to land on your desk would mean that not all subjects had the same chance of inclusion in the study, because all those who did not walk through your door or whose records did not land on your desk had no chance of being selected. Instead, a complete

---

BOX 6-1 ■ **Example of Subject Selection**

In Walach, Güthlin, and König's 2003 study of the effects of massage therapy on chronic pain, the population of interest included all the patients with chronic pain, namely noninflammatory rheumatic conditions and headache, although the subpopulation included all the patients with these symptoms residing in a locale in Germany. The sample for the study was selected from this subpopulation. Subjects were randomly assigned to the experimental group, who received the massage therapy treatments, or to the control group, who received standard medical care for their condition.

BOX 6-2 ■ **Example of Study of Records or Events as Population**

In studying the comprehensiveness of physical therapy documentation, Leerar et al. (2007) reviewed medical records in six private practice clinics in Tacoma, Washington. Their subpopulation was comprised of all patient records containing medical codes related to low back pain. From this subpopulation, 160 records were randomly selected for review.

list of people or items in the population or subpopulation of interest must be available to the researcher and a random selection made from that list. In the study by Walach et al. (2003) (see Box 6-1), they would have needed a complete list of all the patients in Germany who met the research criteria, namely all those with noninflammatory rheumatic pain. They then could have placed all the names in a hat and picked out the required number for the study, or assigned a number to each patient and used a random number chart to select patients for the study sample. Either one is an acceptable method of random selection, but the latter is probably more practical. Although true random selection is the ideal, the ability to access and randomly choose subjects from everyone that meets your subject inclusion criteria within an entire population is not usually realistic.

A random number chart, which may be found in a statistics book, lists numbers that have been generated by a computer in true random fashion. The chart may be read in any direction (up or down, side to side, diagonally), starting at any point, to produce a list of random numbers. This method is commonly used when researchers mail questionnaires and have access to a complete mailing list of potential subjects who meet their criteria—a population. It is simple enough to assign a number to each name, then to pick a series of numbers from the chart and to include the people with corresponding numbers in the study. For a list of names that has already been entered into a computer file, many programs and online tools are available that will assist with random selection, saving the researcher a great deal of time. Some examples include *Research Randomizer* (Urbaniak & Plous, 2012), *HotBits* (Walker, 2006), or *Microsoft Excel* (Microsoft, 2010). For more information on types of randomization or other online programs, see Suresh's (2011) article, "An Overview of Randomization Techniques: An Unbiased Assessment of Outcome in Clinical Research."

To further clarify, random selection ensures that the sample is as much like the larger population from which it was drawn as possible, and will therefore improve external validity—that is, that similar findings are likely if another portion of this population of interest is studied. Thus, the results of your study can be more readily generalized to the entire population of interest and are more useful to other healthcare practitioners who would like to use your treatment method with similar patients. Remember, if random selection has not been used, the results of a study may not be easily generalized to other people in the population of interest.

Random assignment, the second component of randomization, means that those in the selected sample each have an equal chance of being assigned to either the experimental group or the control group. A complete subject sample should be selected first, and then a similar process is used to assign subjects randomly to the two groups. Random assignment is done primarily to ensure that the candidates in each group will be as alike (or as unalike) as possible; it also ensures that the researcher will not be tempted to assign a "good" candidate to the experimental group because it looks as if he or she will show a lot of improvement. This technique helps to minimize researcher bias, which can impact study results. Random assignment will improve internal validity and specifically help to ensure that the experimental treatment made a difference rather than something else within the study design. It will also "even out" the effect on the study of such things as attrition (subjects dropping out of the study), developmental maturation (changes or improvements as a result of natural aging or development), practice effects (changes because of new learning or repeated testing and training), or regression (patients getting sicker over time).

The point of randomization is to ensure that the sample is as representative of the population of interest as possible and that the experimental and control groups are as similar to each other as possible. This enables the researcher to state more confidently that the results are because of the treatment given rather than to a difference in characteristics between the two groups. It also minimizes the chance that the sample members were not typical of the population and improved because of some uncontrolled trait they held in common. It is important to remember that some variations in samples are usually expected and preferred, for eliminating all variation among a sample would greatly decrease external validity, or limit the ability to generalize results to groups with dissimilar attributes. For example, the results of a study examining the effects of an afterschool recreation program on Caucasian female kindergartners with obesity in the rural Midwestern United States might not be easily generalized to older children, males, those of other ethnicities, or those residing in urban communities. Although the study may yield beneficial information for this select group, application beyond the original study is limited.

Randomization is not perfect. It is based on the laws of probability; however, every once in a while the improbable will happen and a source of bias will appear in a study. For example, one group may end up being composed of patients who are sicker or older than those in the other group. Also, methods must be used correctly for random selection to be effective (Box 6-3).

Keeping the concepts of manipulation, control, and randomization in mind, we can review three categories of quantitative research designs: true experimental designs, quasi-experimental designs, and nonexperimental designs.

Experimental Designs

True experimental research designs involve manipulation of at least one independent variable, control of a variety of other phenomena in the methodology, and random selection and assignment of subjects to study groups. These designs are prospective in nature, meaning the plans for the study are laid out well in advance, and the subjects are followed moving forward in time, as opposed to retrospective studies where subjects or phenomena are examined backwards in time in relation to an outcome that has already occurred. Experimental designs are most commonly used to determine cause-and-effect relationships, thus denoting a strong chance that the manipulation of the independent variable caused a change in the dependent variable. This method allows the researcher to compare different types of treatment and to determine which type is likely to be the most effective.

Basic Experimental Design

In a classic experimental design, the researcher deliberately manipulates the independent variable in the experimental group, but not in the control group, and then looks for the results of those differences on the dependent variable. For example, with the rise in the aging population and the increased incidence of Alzheimer's disease, a researcher might be interested in studying the effects of a formal caregiver training program on the stress level of caregivers of Alzheimer's patients. Caregivers can be randomly selected and assigned to one of two groups—an experimental group that will be provided with formal education on how to care for individuals with Alzheimer's disease, and a control group that will not receive this training. The dependent variable, caregiver stress level, is measured for both groups before and after treatment so that comparisons can be made on the same group; comparisons between groups can also be made by measuring both "after" tests. The before and after tests are called pretests and posttests.

A variation of the basic research design, a **randomized controlled trial** (RCT) is the most rigorous design, as it has high internal validity and is regarded as the "gold standard" for clinical research (Portney & Watkins, 2009, p. 22). Internal validity can be further improved if the study is single- or double-blinded. In a **double-blinded** RCT, the researchers and the subjects are unaware of the hypothesis being tested

---

BOX 6-3 ■ Example of Poor Randomization

A classic example of poor methodology occurred in the 1969 selection of men who were to be drafted into the army. A slip of paper with the name and month of birth for each man were put into an urn and drawn out, but the slips were not well mixed. The last slips put into the urn were of men whose birthdays fell in October, November, and December, and disproportionately more of these men's names were drawn than others. This was a case in which poor methodology had serious consequences.

or the assignment of subjects to experimental and control groups. This lack of awareness prevents changes in subject performance because of their knowledge of treatment or the researcher's expectations. In a **single-blinded** RCT, only one group, either the subjects or the researchers, are blinded to the treatment. Blindness can also be preserved by having different individuals responsible for study design, implementation, data collection, and statistical analysis (Portney & Watkins, 2009).

For ease of communication with other researchers and to permit the researcher to sketch out designs quickly, a system of shorthand known as research notation was developed by Campbell and Stanley (1969). An O represents the observations or measurements that occur at pretesting and posttesting; an R represents random assignment; and an X represents manipulation or treatment. Each study group is written or represented on a separate line, and time periods are aligned vertically. In research notion, a design consisting of two randomly assigned groups, one with treatment and one without, and both with pretesting and posttesting, would be illustrated as follows:

R	O	X	O
R	O		O

Using this design, the resulting data from the pretests will enable the researcher to see whether or not the two groups were truly similar to begin with. In some circumstances, the pretest may be necessary to assist with subject selection. For example, subject inclusion criteria might require participants to be able to remember and follow a short sequence of directions. Pretesting might include a brief cognitive screen to determine that subjects fit the study's inclusion criteria. At the conclusion of the study, posttest scores can be compared to see which group shows the greatest change in the dependent variable. Finally, the pretest and posttest of each group can be compared to see how much change occurred for the experimental versus the control group.

If circumstances dictate, the random assignment to groups can be performed after the pretest; however, the assignment should not be influenced by the results of the pretest. Following random assignment, equivalency between the two groups may be assumed; however, performing a pretest provides a further check on equivalency. This double check is particularly useful in dealing with small samples (Portney & Watkins, 2009). Nevertheless, attrition (loss of participants), particularly that which differs between experimental and control groups, is a continuing concern.

Pretest–Posttest Design With Follow-Up

If you want to determine whether or not the effect of an intervention is long-lasting, the design may be further improved by adding a follow-up observation or posttest (O_2 and O_4), as shown here:

R	O	X	O_1	O_2
R	O		O_3	O_4

This will enable you to see if any improvement following the treatment has been maintained over time. Box 6-4 illustrates the point with a follow-up occurring 26 weeks after the posttest.

Posttest-only Design

Sometimes, the results of the treatment may be influenced by the fact that a pretest has been administered. For example, subjects may benefit from practicing a task used in the pretest, thus diminishing the effect of the intervention. In this case, the pretest might be omitted as long as subjects have been randomly selected and assigned to groups. In other cases, the pretest may be excluded when administration is deemed too time-consuming to support its use. A disadvantage of this study design is that the researcher has no way of confirming if the two study groups are equivalent before the intervention, which can impact the ability to draw conclusions about the effectiveness of the intervention being provided (Thomas &

BOX 6-4 ■ Example of a Pretest–Posttest Design With Follow-Up

A 2010 study compared the effectiveness of therapeutic massage, thermotherapy (control group), and a relaxing room therapy for individuals with generalized anxiety disorder. The 68 subjects were randomly assigned to the three groups and received the assigned "treatment" for 10 sessions over a period of 12 weeks. An anxiety rating scale was administered pre-intervention, post-intervention (12 weeks), and for follow-up at 26 weeks. All groups demonstrated improvements in anxiety level following the intervention, and there was no significant difference among the groups (Sherman et al., 2010). This design could be notated as follows:

R	O	X_1	O	O
R	O	X_2	O	O
R	O	X_3	O	O

can eliminate this design flaw, but it requires many subjects and a great deal of researcher time. It is constructed as follows:

Group 1	R	O	X	O_1
Group 2	R	O		O_2
Group 3	R		X	O_3
Group 4	R			O_4

There is random assignment to four groups—two experimental and two control groups:

- Group 1 receives the pretest, the experimental treatment, and then the posttest.
- Group 2 is given the pretest and the posttest, but undergoes no treatment.
- Group 3 is not given a pretest but receives the experimental treatment and the posttest.
- Group 4 only receives the posttest.

In comparing the posttest results, the researcher is able to test not only for differences between experimental and control groups but for any interaction between the pretest and experimental treatment by comparing groups 1 and 3 (on O_1 and O_3) and groups 2 and 4 (on O_2 and O_4). An example of this study design can be found in Box 6-5.

Factorial Designs

The experimental designs mentioned so far are designed to cope with one independent variable only; however, researchers may be concerned with more than one variable in the same study. Factorial designs may be used to investigate two or more independent variables and their interaction with the dependent variable. These designs allow the researcher to use the same subjects to study the effects of the independent variables on the dependent variable as well as any joint effect or interaction effect. In factorial designs, each independent variable is called a factor.

For example, a study by two occupational therapists provides insight into how visual acuity and age affect performance on cognitive assessments. Hunt

Hersen, 2011). Using research notation, this design appears as follows:

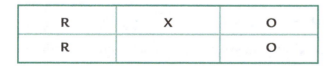

R	X		O
R			O

Solomon Four-Group Design

In cases where the researcher is unsure whether or not the pretest has an effect, or knows that it has an effect but feels that it provides crucial information, the Solomon four-group design can be employed. Use of some pretests could impact outcomes by allowing the subjects to practice or learn skills being tested or by raising awareness of elements being investigated (Wludyka, 2012). The Solomon four-group design is a powerful research design that

---

BOX 6-5 ■ Example of Solomon Four-Group Design

Garvin and Damson (2008) used the Solomon four-group design to determine the effect of viewing ideal fitness images in the media on physiological affect in male and female college students. Subjects were randomly assigned to one of two experimental groups (who viewed fitness magazines) or to one of two control groups (who viewed *National Geographic* magazines). Only one experimental group and one control group underwent pretesting, and all four groups completed posttesting. Results indicate that the completion of the pretest did not impact overall study outcomes, but without use of this study design, researchers would have been unable to confirm this.

Table 6-1 ■ Depiction of Hunt and Bassi's 2010 Factorial Design Study

Visual Acuity	Young Adult	Older Adult
20/30	Group 1	Group 4
20/50	Group 2	Group 5
20/100	Group 3	Group 6

If age were expanded to contain a third category, such as middle-aged adult, it would be a 3 X 3 design; this is shown in Table 6-2.

In a different variation, a third variable or factor, such as gender, might be added to the original design, with two levels for the gender factor, making it a 3 X 2 X 2 design as depicted in Table 6-3. Age and gender are actually pseudo-independent variables because they are not being manipulated by the researcher; they are already occurring attributes of the subjects. However, in factorial designs, pseudo-independent variables are often treated in the same manner as true independent variables.

As more variables are added, both the complexity of the design and the number of subjects required increases. Specific statistical procedures are used to analyze these designs, and usually the services of a statistician or a statistical software package are required.

and Bassi (2010) assessed 124 community-dwelling adults, and divided them into six groups as follows:

1. Young adults tested with 20/30 or better visual acuity (control group)
2. Young adults tested with 20/50 visual acuity
3. Young adults tested with 20/100 visual acuity
4. Older adults tested with 20/30 or better visual acuity (control group)
5. Older adults tested with 20/50 visual acuity
6. Older adults tested with 20/100 visual acuity

The two independent variables were the level of visual acuity (20/30, which served as the control, 20/50, or 20/100) and the factor of age (young adult, ages 19–30, versus older adults, 65 years of age or older). Therefore, the study was concerned with the effects of these variables on the dependent variable—performance on common cognitive assessments.

This study is charted in Table 6-1. There are three levels for the independent variable or factor of visual acuity (20/30, 20/50, and 20/100), and two levels for the independent variable of age (young adult and older adult). Thus, this is called a 3 X 2 design.

Quasi-Experimental Designs

Similar to true experimental designs, quasi-experimental designs still contain an independent variable that is

---

Table 6-2 ■ Chart Depicting 3 X 3 Factorial Design

Visual Acuity	Young Adult	Middle Age Adult	Older Adult
20/30	Group 1	Group 4	Group 7
20/50	Group 2	Group 5	Group 8
20/100	Group 3	Group 6	Group 9

Table 6-3 ■ **Chart Depicting 3 X 2 X 2 Factorial Design**

Young Adult						Older Adult					
Male			Female			Male			Female		
20/30	20/50	20/100	20/30	20/50	20/100	20/30	20/50	20/100	20/30	20/50	20/100

manipulated in order to determine the effect on a dependent variable; however, they typically lack a control group or random selection and assignment of subjects, or both. The resulting designs are still very useful to practitioners looking for validation of treatment methods and techniques. When researchers want to study naturally occurring real world situations, or when there are ethical concerns with use of a control group or withholding treatment from a particular group, quasi-experimental designs are most appropriate. In some cases, time and financial constraints might also support use of a quasi-experimental design. Regardless, caution should be used in generalizing study results if random-

ization is lacking or a control group was not employed. Box 6-6 includes an example of a study without random selection or a control group.

Quasi-Experimental Design Lacking Control

As noted previously, sometimes researchers use subjects as their own control. There is no second group of subjects who are without treatment; rather, the subjects in the experimental group double as the control group. They receive the treatment, but they also experience a period of no treatment, which is considered the control period. Sometimes data can be collected before the treatment, for a period of time equal

---

BOX 6-6 ■ **Example of a Study Lacking Random Selection and a Control Group**

In studying the effects of two treatment approaches on plantar heel pain, Cleland et al. (2009) recruited patients from two outpatient orthopedic clinics—one in New Hampshire, United States, and one in New Zealand. Subjects were randomly assigned to one of the two groups, and results of pretesting indicate that the groups were analogous. If they had been found to be substantially different at the pretest stage, the researchers could have either abandoned the groups and started the study over or used statistical techniques to take into account the differences.

In this study, one group received a series of modalities and an exercise regimen, whereas the other group received manual physical therapy and an exercise regimen. The design looked like this:

Even though the two groups were found to be equivalent on pretesting, caution must be taken in generalizing results because subjects were not randomly selected. Subjects were recruited from only two clinics; therefore, they may not represent the broader population of all individuals with plantar heel pain. Outcomes indicate increased success with use of the manual physical therapy and exercise program versus the program of modalities and exercise. Yet, one must consider that without a control group (for example, a group that received only the exercise regimen), it is difficult to determine if it was the combination of these approaches that helped the patients or the manual therapy and modalities alone.

R	O	X_1	O
R	O	X_2	O

to the treatment period, and then later compared to outcomes following the treatment. This can be referred to as a **one-group pretest–posttest design**. For example, data on handwriting legibility for second graders might be collected during one semester, and then compared to data on handwriting legibility from this same group obtained during the next semester when students participate in a structured multisensory handwriting curriculum. By comparing handwriting legibility in these two semesters, conclusions can be drawn about the effectiveness of the multisensory handwriting curriculum in comparison to the traditional handwriting program.

Quasi-Experimental Design Lacking Randomization

In some situations, random selection or assignment of subjects may be unrealistic or unethical. Convenience sampling is the most popular type of sampling because it is the easiest and least expensive of all sampling techniques, and it is utilized when it is impractical to randomly sample the entire population of interest. Major differences are likely to occur when the two groups are convenience samples (i.e., groups that are already formed by some event preceding the research study). They may be groups of patients in two different wards of the same hospital, two different nursing homes, or two day-care centers, for example. Box 6-7 illustrates the use of convenience samples. Additional sampling techniques will be reviewed in Chapter 7.

Some criticize the use of convenience samples, maintaining that it is impossible to make reasonable comparisons between such groups. Because subjects are chosen based upon availability, one cannot assume that the sample will accurately represent the population or subpopulation of interest. Yet, others suggest that using convenience samples provides a practical solution to a very real problem and that valuable information can still be gained as long as this bias is considered when interpreting and applying results. The crucial question to ask is whether the two study groups truly come from the same population. The researcher may match subjects in the study groups so that there are commonalities in such items as socioeconomic status, gender, age, diagnosis, or

> ### BOX 6-7 ■ Example of Convenience Sampling
>
> In a study aimed at determining the effectiveness of discharge planning among pairs of stroke survivors and their caregivers, the subjects were recruited from four neurological wards in a hospital in Taiwan. Even though the sample was one of convenience, the researchers took additional steps to decrease bias. Two wards were randomly selected to serve as the experimental groups, and two as the control groups. All four wards consisted of the same physical arrangement and number of beds, admitted patients with similar diagnoses, and were staffed by the same neurologists, nurses, therapists, social workers, and doctors, thereby mitigating the effects of staff behaviors and environmental conditions (Shyu, Chen, Chen, Wang, & Shao, 2008).

other attributes considered important to the study. Rubin (2006) offers a plethora of foundational articles on matching in research designs, and explains the methodology of matching subjects. An example of matching is shown in Box 6-8.

Nonequivalent study groups are less likely to occur if the subjects have been randomly assigned, even though they were not randomly selected from the population of interest. This obviously cannot be achieved if convenience samples are taken from different locations, but can be achieved with a convenience sample taken entirely from one facility. Random assignment may ensure that the two groups are similar in characteristics, even though they may not be representative of the population.

Cohort Designs

Cohort designs involve specific groups, or cohorts, of subjects that are followed over time. When using cohort designs, a control group is again used to assess the changes made in the experimental group, but this time the groups are not observed at the same time. The groups follow each other through a

---

BOX 6-8 ■ Example of Subject Matching

Classen et al. (2011) used matched controls in their study to determine what screening tests could be used by driving rehabilitation specialists and neurologists to predict actual driving performance in patients with Parkinson's disease. A convenience sample of 41 individuals with Parkinson's disease was age-matched with a group of 41 community-dwelling adults. Matching the sample by age allowed the researchers to attribute differences in performance on the screening tests to Parkinson's symptoms rather than age alone. This, in turn, led to conclusions about which screening tools are most predictive of actual driving performance.

BOX 6-9 ■ Example of How History Can Impact a Study

In studying the impact of depression on self-care management in a group of hospitalized depressed patients, a therapist reported that the death of President John F. Kennedy, which occurred partway into the study, had a profound impact on the patients (Clark, 1964). She surmised that this historically tragic event compounded the results of her study.

---

setting such as classes of students moving through a therapist training program or groups of trainees entering a sheltered workshop for a training period. One group is selected as the experimental group and subjected to a unique experience, whereas another group acts as the control group and experiences the usual events of the setting. The subjects in these groups are obviously not randomly chosen, because the groups are naturally occurring. Nonetheless, the two groups may be considered somewhat similar in that they both meet the setting's admission requirements. The design may be depicted as follows, where Time 1 and Time 2 represent two distinct differences in time:

Time 1			Time 2		
O	X	O	O		O

There are internal validity problems with this design because of the difference in the time of the observations. History (i.e., some sort of global event that has an effect on all subjects in the sample) may play a part in accounting for the differences in data from the posttests (Box 6-9).

The cohort design can be improved by employing recurrent institutional cycles, using three different cohorts. The design is as follows:

Time 1		Time 2			Time 3
X	O_1	O_2	X	O_3	O_4
	(Posttest)	(Pretest)		(Posttest)	(Pretest)

The first group receives the experimental treatment followed by a posttest; the second group receives the traditional pretest, treatment, and posttest; and the third group receives only a pretest. The ideal pattern of results from this design would be a similarity of responses on pre-tests O_2 and O_4 and on posttests O_1 and O_3. The effect of the treatment would be evident by comparing scores on pretest O_2 and posttest O_3.

Time-Series Designs

Time-series designs are used when the researcher wishes to study the effects of some treatment or condition over time. These studies may also be referred to as case series or longitudinal studies, and they can involve multiple measurements (pre- and posttests) before and after treatment. The amount of time from the study's beginning to conclusion can range from several weeks to decades. For example, Herman, Hopman, and Craig (2010) were interested in determining the effect of childhood body mass index (BMI) and physical activity on adult health-related quality of life. Data obtained from a fitness survey in 1981 of 310 subjects ages 7 to 18 years was compared to data obtained on follow-up assessments 22 years later.

Time-series designs have no control group, and the subjects in the experimental group act as their own control. In the single-group time-series design, subjects are given a pretest, followed by experimental treatment and a posttest. Then a period of time is allowed to elapse, typically equivalent to the amount of the experimental treatment time, and then another posttest follows. Periods of treatment and nontreatment are alternated with tests. During the treatment periods, the subjects in the group comprise an experimental group, and during the nontreatment periods they act as a control group. The design is notated as follows:

O	X	O		O	X	O		O	X	O

The group may be randomly selected to increase the likelihood of its being representative of the population of interest. Of course, the issue of random assignment to groups is a moot point because there is only one group. Overall, this design provides a high degree of internal validity, meaning that one can be fairly sure that any changes that occur in the dependent variable at posttests are because of the experimental treatment.

In a variation of the time-series design, a researcher may wish to assess the permanence of change in the dependent variable and may do so by administering several posttests after the intervention, thus:

O	X	O_1	O_2	O_3	O_4

However, this design does have a flaw, in that it is difficult to know if improvement at the first posttest (O_1) was because of the intervention or because of something else, such as:

- Some other event that occurred concurrently
- Something special that occurred with the procedure, instrument, or researcher

- A learning effect (i.e., changes because of education, repeated exposure to testing, or other information)
- An inherent characteristic in the subject such as a seasonal improvement

There is no subsequent treatment period to use as a test for these possibilities.

A third possible variation of the time-series design can control for some of these flaws:

O	O	O	O	X	O	O	O	O

The multiple pretests will give a more accurate picture of how subjects score on the dependent variable before the experimental treatment, will control for seasonal or cyclical changes in abilities, and will eliminate the effect of history. An even more preferable design would be:

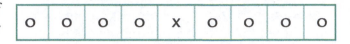

O	O	O	X	O_1	X	O_2	X	O_3	O_4	O_5

Here, history is controlled for and the effects of experimental treatment can be viewed on more than one occasion (at O_1, O_2, and O_3), and the permanence of the effect can be measured (O_3 through O_5). The disadvantages of this design are that it is often impractical to wait long enough to administer several pretests before treating the patient and that the entire study becomes lengthy (Box 6-10).

Despite the fact that these are quasi-experimental designs, they are effective and can be quite practical for the clinical researcher. It is sometimes easier to gain permission to recruit patients for quasi-experimental studies than it is for experimental studies; for example, it is difficult to deny treatment to patients in control groups. Finally, the fact that these designs are carried out in clinical settings, with all the concomitant interferences and lack of control inherent in such settings, makes them more likely to be generalizable to other clinical settings. It is, after all, in day-to-day clinical practice that we wish to put the results of research into effect.

BOX 6-10 ■ Example of Time-Series Design

Curran, Sharpe, Flynn, and Button (2010) used a time-series design to study the attitudes of undergraduate healthcare students in regard to interprofessional education and teamwork. Students from pharmacy, medical, nursing, and social work programs participated in a series of interprofessional learning modules over a period of 3 years. Multiple assessments, designed to measure student attitudes and satisfaction about their experiences, were administered as students progressed through their education. Results of these assessments were then compared to determine if differences existed among professions or if attitudes changed as they progressed through the program.

Nonexperimental Designs

Nonexperimental designs are frequently used to describe or characterize phenomena, to examine relationships among variables, or to determine the reliability and validity of evaluations, tests, or equipment. They may also be referred to as preexperimental designs because they often serve as precursors to later experimental or quasi-experimental studies. Nonexperimental designs are commonly used in health care, where research often focuses on various forms of disability or illness, and the researchers only have access to subjects after they have acquired the disability or illness. In these cases, causal relationships cannot be assumed, but insight into the condition and the response to treatments can be explored. These designs are also said to be retrospective because the dependent variable (disability or illness) has already occurred. The most common nonexperimental designs are reviewed here.

Correlational Research

Many nonexperimental studies in health care fall into the correlational category, and may serve as precursors to later experimental studies. Correlational research is similar to experimental research in that a hypothesis is being tested; however, it differs in that there is no manipulation of independent variables, and a cause-effect relationship cannot be established. Instead, in correlational research, the researcher is looking for a relationship between variables. Rather than hypothesizing, for instance, that being blind will cause an individual to have heightened tactile sensitivity, one might conjecture that there is simply a relationship between the variables "blindness" and "heightened tactile sensitivity." Blindness has already occurred by the time the researcher is studying it, making this retrospective, nonexperimental research.

The researcher tests a hypothesis, comparing two or more variables by measuring differences and looking for a relationship. The procedure for the correlational research design is similar to that for experimental designs; that is, reviewing the literature, formulating research questions or hypotheses, defining and operationalizing terms, selecting a sample from the population of interest, and selecting data collection and interpretation methods. However, in correlational research, specific statistical tests, which look for an association between two variables, are used. This association is known as a correlation coefficient and yields a value between -1 and $+1$, where 0 indicates no relationship and the two extremes indicate a perfect negative (or inverse) relationship (indicated by -1) or a perfect positive (or direct) relationship (indicated by $+1$) (Box 6-11).

Because this is nonexperimental research and, therefore, is not subjected to the stringent rules of experimental research, similar results should be replicated in many studies before healthcare practitioners can claim relationships between variables concerning their patients.

Survey Research

"Survey research is a method of inquiry characterized by collecting data using structured questions to elicit self-reported information from a sample of people" (Forsyth & Kviz, 2006).

Surveys are cross sectional in the sense that they generally describe the group at one point in time, and they are most commonly used to determine the prevalence or distribution of disease or disability, to evaluate circumstances or needs of a population, or to describe interrelationships (Kielhofner & Fossey, 2006). Information collected in survey research covers

BOX 6-11 ■ Example of Correlational Study Design

A correlational study was conducted by Tawashy, Eng, Lin, Tang, and Hung (2009) to see if there was a relationship between the physical activity level of individuals with spinal cord injury and their levels of pain, fatigue, and depression. High intensity physical activity was strongly correlated with less fatigue ($r = -0.767$) and pain ($r = -0.612$), and increased self-efficacy ($r = 0.656$). Moreover, mild physical activity was correlated with fewer symptoms of depression ($r = -0.565$) (p. 304). For negative r values, the two attributes were inversely proportional, whereas for positive r values, the two attributes are directly proportional.

a vast array of topics and may include items ranging from attitudes, values, opinions, and motives, to more concrete information such as the respondents' work situation, environment, living situation, and behaviors.

To qualify as research, the survey must be carefully crafted to answer a well-defined set of questions that have been grounded in a literature review and have significance and relevance. The manner of analysis and interpretation of the data also make this a research design rather than solely a survey to elicit some facts about a particular group. The method of analysis needs to be chosen and applied judiciously; interpretations and application to the population of interest must be made with care. Information may be collected directly through a face-to-face interview or telephone interview, or indirectly through the mail, e-mail, or various web-based survey sites.

It is crucial that the relevant population be defined clearly and that its characteristics and limits are described. Random sampling is most commonly used to ensure that the conclusions of the survey can be generalized to the larger population of interest. If you are not confident that the sample is representative of the population, the resulting discussion will be invalid for the larger group about whom you are

generalizing. Methods of sampling as well as designing effective survey questions are critically important in survey research and these topics are addressed in greater detail in Chapter 7. Several other texts also provide additional information on these topics (Fowler, 2009; Groves et al., 2009; Salant & Dillman, 1994). Box 6-12 offers an example of survey research.

Quantitative Case Study Research

In quantitative case study research, an individual, group, unit, community, institution, or event is studied in great depth over time—anywhere from a few weeks to several years. Thus, it is a longitudinal study, rather than a cross-sectional study like the survey design discussed previously. Quantitative case studies are often referred to as single-subject, single-case, multiple-case, case series (more than one case), or small-N studies in other publications. This design is used to examine unique cases or situations where the subject or intervention in question is unusual, little understood, or impractical to study under experimental conditions (Berg & Latin, 2008). The number of variables is usually very large. Data is generally gathered by one researcher at various points throughout the life of the case and may occur in a natural setting,

BOX 6-12 ■ Example of Survey Research

In Fuller's 2010 study, she wanted to investigate the practice of speech therapists (type of treatment, trainings, interdisciplinary services, locations of treatment) working in the United Kingdom's Sure Start program. Sure Start was a governmental program to provide multidisciplinary services to children up to 5 years of age from disadvantaged situations. She recruited speech therapists by contacting all Sure Start program sites and inviting the speech therapists employed there to complete her survey. Of 501 sites contacted, 113 speech therapists completed the survey, consisting of both closed and open-ended questions, via e-mail. This yielded a response rate of 23%. Please refer to Fowler's text (2009) for further details on adequate response rates.

such as the home, but more often in a clinical setting, such as a hospital.

Case studies often fall into the category of exploratory studies, in which the goal is hypothesis generation for further study under experimental conditions. Information obtained can be generalized to theoretical propositions, rather than to populations in the way that experimental results are. The researcher's goal is to expand and generalize theories, such as how a phenomenon occurs, changes, or is sustained over time, rather than to enumerate the frequency or prevalence of the phenomena. An abundance of case studies can be found in the rehabilitation and healthcare literature, which provide accounts of treatment techniques and procedures that have helped practitioners to be more effective in the direct care of clients.

When trying to decide whether to use a case study rather than another type of exploratory study such as a survey, it is useful to bear in mind that "how" and "why" questions are best answered by case studies. For example, Nwora and Gee (2009) asked, "How can sound-based interventions be used to improve sensory processing and language skills in a child with pervasive developmental disorder?" Healthcare practitioners often ask how and why a particular adaptive aid or treatment procedure worked with a particular patient. In the current example, the researchers wished to generate ideas about the role of a therapeutic sound program in improving sensory processing and language skills in children with pervasive developmental disorders, rather than just enumerating the times or the degree to which the child was able to respond more appropriately. Their hope was that other occupational therapists would try this idea with similar patients, testing the hypotheses and elaborating on the theory. More details about this example are included in Box 6-13.

BOX 6-13 ■ Example of Case Study Research

In a case report in *Occupational Therapy International*, Nwora and Gee (2009) recount the story of John, a 5-year-old boy diagnosed with pervasive developmental disorder–not otherwise specified. He was currently receiving traditional occupational therapy services because of decreased attention, aggressiveness toward siblings and peers, and decreased tolerance to touch and sound. John's deficits were similar to those of other children diagnosed with various autism spectrum disorders, and the researchers were interested in how a therapeutic sound program might impact these deficits. Research dating back to the early 1950s supports use of sound-based clinical interventions with this population, but testing on current therapeutic listening programs that involve use of "psycho-acoustically modified music" in the client's own home has been very limited.

During the intervention, John participated in the therapeutic listening program two times per day, for 15 minutes each time, for a total of 20 weeks. At the conclusion, posttesting revealed improvements in receptive and expressive language, attention, tolerance to touch and sound, and the ability to regulate his behaviors in classroom situations. A video of his in-classroom performance confirmed the results of these administered assessments. Functionally, he was able to participate in classroom games and songs, interact more effectively with his peers and siblings, and respond appropriately to directives and questions from his teacher and his parents.

In the discussion, the authors argue that although John was not diagnosed with an auditory processing disorder, progress in this area led to improvements in social and behavioral symptoms. They also suggest that because children with disorders on the autism spectrum each present with symptoms that vary in nature and severity, alternative treatments should be explored to ensure the most success. Therefore, more research is needed to validate the use of sound-based interventions with this population.

Once you have determined that a case study design is most appropriate for your purposes, you will need to decide if you will use a single-case study or multiple-case study. Single-case studies are often easier to manage for researchers who have difficulty gathering groups of homogeneous patients to form experimental groups. Furthermore, group studies are usually concerned with comparing the average change between two groups; however, researchers may not be as interested in the average changes of a group as they are in changes in individuals. They are interested not only in the patient's overall change by the end of the study, but also in the course of that clinical change over time. Single-subject studies allow the researcher an opportunity for continuous assessment of a client's progress at various points during treatment. The researcher can not only monitor changes throughout treatment, but can also alter the intervention based on the study data, should this be indicated. This is not usually possible with group study designs. Data can be collected during the intervention period and compared with data collected when the intervention is not being provided (the process of using subjects as their own control that was described earlier). For these reasons, researchers tend to find single-case studies manageable and desirable in the clinical setting, whereas readers find them relevant to their own practice.

Multiple-case study designs are more appropriate when numerous similar cases are present, and when the aim is to substantiate theoretical constructs. In this scenario, replicating the same experiment with multiple cases can increase the strength of the evidence generated. If you get very different findings among the cases, you need to rethink the original theory for the study.

Moreover, multiple-case designs typically do not involve critical, unusual, or revelatory cases (Yin, 2009). If you chose the multiple-case study approach, how many cases should you use? If there are not too many variables under study, use two or three cases; if there are many variables, increase to five or six cases. It is also appropriate to use a pilot case study to explore your choice of subject, data collection methods, and data analysis techniques before conducting a multiple-case study. Table 6-4 further differentiates the reasons to select a single-case study versus a multiple-case study.

In quantitative case study research, the investigator is often designing and testing a specific treatment protocol, splint, or piece of adaptive equipment for a client with a particular disability. In the earlier example (Box 6-13), the researchers were studying a specific treatment—therapeutic listening (Nwora & Gee, 2009). In these types of studies, the researcher

Table 6-4 ■ Differences Between Single-Case and Multiple-Case Designs

Single-Case Designs Are Appropriate When:	Multiple-Case Designs Are Appropriate When:
■ You can identify *the* critical case that illustrates all the theoretical propositions of the study. ■ One case is extreme or unique. ■ You have a typical or representative case that can capture information on common scenarios or situations. ■ A revelatory case is available that exposes a previously inaccessible phenomenon. ■ A case is available over time, and you are interested in looking at changes, transitions, and causation over that period. ■ You have one case that will likely be used as a pilot study for a future multiple-case study.	■ Your aim is to build theory across cases, thus presenting a stronger outcome. ■ You have two or more cases available to you (thus, cases are not critical, unique, or revelatory) ■ Single-case studies were previously completed on the topic, and replication can corroborate earlier findings.

gathers baseline data on the client's condition in order to test whether the program or device has had the desired effect. This is similar to the classic experimental design in that a pretest, intervention, and posttest are conducted; however, the case study is carried out with an individual rather than a group.

Data for the quantitative case study are likely gathered in several ways: observing and counting such things as behaviors that are targeted for change, using hardware to measure such things as joint flexion and extension or muscle strength, or using a formal index to evaluate some portion of self-care activities or pain. These data will provide the baseline information that will be measured against data from later collection periods, usually conducted at various points throughout the study. Baseline data are often supplemented by documentary evidence such as information in patients' charts, reports from case conferences, and previous assessments or progress reports. Although providing the researcher with a rich source of data for comparison, these data also "flesh out" a picture of the subject for the reader. In the example of the therapeutic listening program (Box 6-13), John's medical record was reviewed; several standardized assessments were completed, and his in-class performance was videotaped pre- and post-intervention, so that conclusions could be drawn about the effect of the listening program (Nwora & Gee, 2009).

It may be appropriate to use statistical data analyses for a quantitative case study if you have sufficient data. For example, if you have collected data after various phases of treatment, and perhaps at several follow-up points after treatment has ended, this could yield a dozen or more groups of data that could be tallied and otherwise statistically manipulated in order to show change over time. A pictorial presentation, such as a graph, is often an informative way to indicate changes that have occurred. See Chapter 12 for details on visually displaying data.

Case studies are a useful and fascinating way for practitioners and new researchers to learn the investigation process and to contribute to the body of research in their profession. Most practitioners likely have at least one client whose progress and style of learning could benefit others, whereas the case study process itself requires discipline and is thought-provoking.

Methodological Research

For many years, healthcare practitioners have been interested in developing and fabricating their own adaptive aids, equipment, tests, and other instruments for use in the evaluation and treatment of their patients. Methodological research can be used to test and improve the validity and reliability of such materials, and to develop, validate, and produce standardized testing measures. If the instruments used in clinical research are reliable and valid, the researcher can have more confidence in the results of the research, and results can be compared across studies.

The precise set of procedures used in standardizing measures is described by Benson and Clark (1982) in their article, "A Guide for Instrument Development and Validation." The stages include:

1. Deciding on the purpose of the measure and the population of concern (Why is the measure needed? What group of individuals will it be used on? Considerations could include age, gender, diagnoses, symptomatology, place of residence, vocational goals, or psychological attributes, to name a few.)
2. Elucidating the content of the measure by using personal experience, review of relevant literature, and opinions of experts in the field
3. Organizing and compiling the content into a logical and meaningful sequence
4. Testing the resulting measure on a large sample of the population of interest
5. Subjecting the results to statistical tests for reliability and validity
6. Improving the design and content of the measure based on the findings
7. Retesting the measure
8. Repeating the last four steps several times until you are satisfied with the results
9. Writing an accompanying manual outlining the research process used, the population for whom the measure is intended, the results of the tests for reliability and validity, and exact procedures for using the measure

As you can readily see from this list, the procedure to develop a standardized measure is quite labor intensive and rigorous. As a result, we often use self-made instruments in research studies without showing sufficient concern or caution in interpreting data produced by these nonstandardized measures. In quantitative research designs, measures are usually selected as a way to objectively quantify some phenomenon, and to compare results before and after the study or intervention, to determine the impact of the experimental intervention. In clinical settings, these measures are used to document patient progress, which is often required by regulatory agencies and insurance companies in order to continue treatment or to receive payment for services rendered. The development, testing, and refinement of sound standardized measures are critical to producing quality research that can be generalized to broader populations. An example of methodological research appears in Box 6-14.

Evaluation Research

Evaluation research is designed to determine the need for new programs and to assess existing programs for possible quality improvement. Thus, the results of evaluation research will provide answers to the questions "What should we do?" and "How well are we doing?" This type of research can be referred to by a variety of other terms including *audits, outcome analysis, cost-benefit analysis,* or *impact analysis.* Regardless of the term that is used, the goals include assessing the potential for new programs, practices, or policies, or to determine the success of existing ones.

Evaluation research involves two strategies—formative research and summative research. **Formative research** involves collecting data or opinions that can be used to form a policy upon which to design a new program, whereas **summative research** entails assessment of an existing program and its policies. In formative research, data is typically collected from potential users and providers of the proposed program, and then it is analyzed to determine the appropriateness and feasibility of actually initiating the program.

In summative research, the existing program goals are examined and data is collected to determine whether the goals are being met. Goals for all programs should be written in objective and measurable terms while keeping them aligned with the program's mission, so that they can later be used to evaluate the program's effectiveness. Data can be gathered from many sources including past and present consumers of a program, providers of a program, written policies and procedures, client records, and the physical plant and its equipment. Often large quantities of data need to be organized and applied to each of the program's stated goals. The researcher then must make judgments as to whether or not the goals are being met.

This type of research is often conducted by a program evaluator from outside the program, who is more likely to be objective about the program's good and bad points and is free of the burden of implementing recommended changes. If evaluators knew that they would have to make the required changes at the end of an evaluation, they might be biased in the type of changes being recommended. The negative side of having an outside evaluator is that it takes time for the outsider to be accepted by program staff. Also, staff members have been known to sabotage evaluations by not cooperating or by being dishonest with the outside evaluator. Box 6-15 provides an example of evaluation research.

Validity and Reliability of Quantitative Research

In order to prove the value of their studies, researchers need to address the credibility of their study's methodology and tools. In order to do so, the principles of study validity and reliability need to be understood. Validity is concerned with the accuracy of scientific findings, whereas reliability is concerned with the replicability of scientific findings.

BOX 6-14 ■ Example of Methodological Research

Lach, Ball, and Birge (2012) conducted a methodological study to determine the reliability and validity of *The Nursing Home Falls Self-efficacy Scale*. They noted lower self-efficacy in patients with decreased functional mobility and cognition, as well as those with increased fall risk and fear of falling. The study provides initial support for use of this scale, which could impact future research and nursing home practices.

Validity

A study is valid only if researchers are truly addressing the constructs they set out to study and measure. Validity needs to be addressed from two points of view. First, internal validity—are researchers actually observing and measuring what they think they are observing and measuring? And, second, external validity—to what extent are the ideas generated or tested by the researchers applicable to other similar groups or situations?

Internal Validity

The effects of history (the events that have happened throughout the study), maturation of the subjects during the study, testing of the subjects, instrumentation used in the study, subject selection, and subject attrition (why and how many subjects were lost before completion of the study) can all have an impact on the study's internal validity. These situations will be discussed in some detail.

1. **History.** Historical contamination occurs when something happens to the subjects or the environment that was not planned in the study design, such as a subject having an injury or losing interest in the study and not making an effort during treatment sessions. Measurement scores can be impacted by such events and internal validity is compromised. Historical contamination can be prevented by careful sampling and by controlling subjects' activities during the study.

2. **Maturation.** Maturation refers to the subjects' growth, development, or changes that occur naturally over time, which may influence pretest and posttest measurements. For example, it might be difficult to determine if a year-long remedial writing program has resulted in improvement in a child's handwriting, or if that improvement would have occurred anyway with the passage of time.

3. **Testing.** If the same test is being used several times throughout the study, it is possible that subjects will experience a practice effect and score higher simply because they have been able to practice the test. Additionally, if the test involves performing an activity to demonstrate strength or endurance, it is possible that performing the test itself will increase the subjects' skills and level of performance.

4. **Instrumentation.** The condition of the instruments themselves may influence measurements. For example, an instrument may not be calibrated accurately or it may be old, worn out, or in poor condition and not give accurate readings. Mailed surveys or attitude surveys may include cultural, racial, intelligence, or language bias that would influence the results.

5. **Subject Selection.** Subjects who volunteer for a study are likely to be different from those who are selected to participate. However, there is an element of volunteerism for all subjects because of the consent process. This can be controlled by using more than one study group and by randomly assigning subjects to the groups.

6. **Subject Attrition or Mortality.** However well a study is designed, it is difficult to prevent subject attrition because of such things as illness, a geographic move, or death. Extra subjects should be recruited into the study to account for these losses. This is particularly important in a case study.

External Validity

External validity refers to the extent that research findings can be generalized and applied to "real-world" situations and clinical cases. Researchers must balance the concepts of internal and external validity, as many of the controls that increase internal validity (rigorous methodology, highly controlled study environments, strict testing procedures, and randomization of subjects) can compromise the relevancy and application of research findings to real life clinical situations. Some of the most common threats to external validity are mentioned here.

1. **Hawthorne Effect.** If subjects perform better on the study task simply because they are being observed, and not necessarily because of the treatment they are receiving, then subjects are said to exhibit the Hawthorne effect. This situation is named after a series of experiments that were completed with factory workers at the Hawthorne Works, an electric company in Illinois, in the early 1900s. In these experiments, worker productivity increased regardless of manipulation of environmental and psychological variables; this increase was attributed to the extra attention the workers received from the researchers (Franke & Kaul, 1978).

2. **Replication.** When researchers report on their studies, they must describe their methods in sufficient detail that others may replicate the studies. If you cannot be assured that the same methods have been followed in replicated studies, then findings cannot be generalized confidently, thereby threatening external validity.

3. **Generalizability.** Generalizability refers to the extent that the results found in the study sample will also be found in the larger population from which the sample was drawn. Is the smaller sample being studied truly representative of those in the larger population? Randomly selecting the sample from the population of interest is a sound way to increase the likelihood that results of the study can be applied to the larger population.

4. **Multiple Treatments.** In a study in which subjects are given more than one treatment as the independent variable, the results cannot be generalized to other settings in which only one of those treatments is used. Effects of more than one treatment must be viewed as cumulative and intermingled. Studies that use a single treatment as the independent variable and a single measure for the dependent variable have greater external validity.

5. **Researcher Bias.** Sometimes subjects react to the study in a certain way because of their relationship with the researcher, whether it is positive or negative. Similarly, the researchers may unintentionally alter their interactions with subjects, based upon their perceptions or feelings. These are particularly important considerations if the dependent variable has to do with interpersonal relationships or emotion-laden topics.

Reliability

A study is considered reliable if, when it is repeated, similar findings are produced. Dependability of procedures is indicated whenever equivalent results are obtained during repetitions of the same study. Whenever close agreement occurs among several measures of the same phenomenon, the reliability of the procedure, instrument, or research will be high and consumers may have confidence in that portion of the study. In addition, reliability can refer to the extent to which an instrument agrees with itself, and four types of reliability pertaining to test instruments will be described in Chapter 7: test-retest reliability, split-half reliability, intra-rater reliability, and inter-rater reliability.

Some problems confounding the reliability of the study itself, rather than instruments used, need to be discussed. In the following cases, the study instrument might be reliable but the study itself will not be if these items are not considered.

1. **Subject Fatigue.** This can be a problem when subjects are expected to perform physical or mental tasks repeatedly, and are tired toward the end of the testing procedures. As a consequence, they do not perform to the best of their abilities and results are affected. Physiological abilities can change in response to diurnal or circadian rhythms, which may result in different results at different times for the same person. Scheduling testing and other performance tasks with adequate breaks can decrease subject fatigue.

2. **Subject Motivation.** Subjects are not always interested in the study and may not perform at their best because of lack of motivation or decreased mood. They may even dislike participating in the study, which would certainly influence the effort they put forth in testing procedures. In this case, test results will be varied and will not be reliable indicators of the subjects' abilities. Recruiting subjects who have a vested interest in the study's purpose and results can combat this issue.

3. **Subject Learning.** If there are repeated tests using the same instrument within the study, subjects are likely to achieve some learning. They may perform better on later tests simply because they have learned the material on the test rather than because of an experimental intervention. Considering use of a variety of assessment methods can decrease the impact of subject learning.

4. **Subject Ability.** Subjects' ability to respond to certain questions or tasks will vary according to their skill level or knowledge of the topic. Responses may vary for the same subject, if he or she chooses to create a response to appease the examiner or to make himself or herself look better. This might be especially true if a relationship already exists between the subject and researcher or if a sensitive or embarrassing subject is being investigated. Preserving a distinct researcher-subject relationship and handling sensitive topics appropriately can minimize this concern.

5. **Tester Skill.** If a tester does not administer the study instruments in exactly the same manner each time, responses for each subject may not be accurate. Training of those assigned to administer assessments can increase the reliability of results, and is discussed further in Chapter 7.

6. **Different Testers.** People administering the test differ in such things as their degree of enthusiasm, delivery of instructions, voice, personality, and ability to handle the situation. The same subject may score differently on the test depending on who administers it. Again, adequate training of test administrators can reduce this issue.

7. **Test Environment.** Changes in the environment from test to test can influence a subject's responses. Distractions such as noise or interruptions are particularly intrusive on test results. Controlling the study environment so that subjects are tested under the same conditions each time can minimize environmental influences.

Once you have decided on the research method you will employ in your study, you will want to make an effort to control for as many of these threats to validity and reliability as possible. Comparing this list of threats against your proposed study design can help you to identify potential issues early on. You likely will be unable to control for all threats to validity and reliability, but being aware of these limitations is necessary when interpreting your results.

Chapter Summary

Some design examples have been provided that may be employed in the three categories of quantitative research: experimental, quasi-experimental, and nonexperimental. Naturally, there are many more types of quantitative research designs than have been mentioned here. In particular, there are many variations of the basic themes presented in the experimental and quasi-experimental categories. Additionally, although quantitative and qualitative designs offer distinct features, advantages, and disadvantages, use of a mixed methods design (multimethodology) may offer the best of both worlds by allowing the researcher to address multiple aspects simultaneously, holistically, and with greater detail (Johnson, Onwuegbuzie, & Turner, 2007; Teddlie & Tashakkori, 2008). Mixed methods designs include both quantitative and qualitative measures, and are appropriate when some phenomena can be quantified and others warrant rich description. These designs bear mentioning because they can be commonly found in healthcare literature; however, detailed explanations are beyond the scope of this text because mixed methods designs can be quite complex and are best undertaken by experienced researchers. Careful reading of such texts such as Portney and Watkins' (2009) *Foundations of Clinical Research: Applications to Practice* and Creswell's (2008) *Research Design: Qualitative, Quantitative, and Mixed Methods Approaches* will guide researchers toward the best design for their particular sets of circumstances.

SKILL-BUILDING TIPS

■ When choosing a study topic and design, be sure to read a variety of existing studies on your topic. This can help you formulate your question and choose an appropriate design. After all, most research builds on previously completed studies.

■ Start small. Students and professional researchers often have lofty goals, but considering your skills, financial resources, time constraints, and other supports can help you keep the project in perspective. The research need not be a large-scale randomized controlled trial to effectively contribute to the body of knowledge in your area of interest.

■ Review current research on your topic with a critical eye. Can you redo an existing study that included one or more serious design flaws by correcting for these errors? Also, consulting the *Conclusions* or *Future Research* sections of published studies can spark ideas.

■ Realize that no research is without flaws or bias. Taking steps to minimize these problems to the greatest extent possible, and considering the impact of them on your conclusions, is all that you can do. Acknowledging these issues is respectable and lets others know that you are aware of the shortcomings.

■ Once you have narrowed your focus a bit, discuss your ideas and possible study design with others interested in your topic. Collective brainstorming is an essential part of honing your ideas and identifying potential roadblocks to the process and design early on.

🔵 LEARNING ACTIVITIES

1. What advantages and disadvantages do quantitative research designs offer?

2. Can you identify the independent and dependent variable(s) that you are interested in studying?

3. Does your setting or situation lend itself more to one type of design versus another?

4. What ideas do you have for increasing your study's validity and reliability?

REFERENCES

Benson, J., & Clark, F. (1982). A guide for instrument development and validation. *American Journal of Occupational Therapy, 36*(12), 789–800.

Berg, K. E., & Latin, R. W. (2008). *Essentials of research methods in health, physical education, exercise science, and recreation* (3rd ed.). Baltimore, MD: Lippincott Williams & Wilkins.

Burns, N., & Grove, S. K. (2009). *The practice of nursing research: Appraisal, synthesis, and generation of evidence* (6th ed.). St. Louis, MO: Saunders Elsevier.

Campbell, D. T., & Stanley, J. C. (1969). *Experimental and quasi-experimental designs for research.* Chicago, IL: Rand McNally.

Clark, M. (1964). The effect of depression on self-care management (unpublished paper).

Classen, S., Witter, D. P., Lanford, D. N., Okun, M. S., Rodriguez, R. L., Romrell, J., . . . Fernandez, H. H. (2011). Usefulness of screening tools for predicting driving performance in people with Parkinson's disease. *American Journal of Occupational Therapy, 65,* 579–588. doi:10.5014/ajot.2011.001073

Cleland, J. A., Abbott, J. H., Kidd, M. O., Stockwell, S., Cheney, S., Gerrard, D. F., & Flynn, T. W. (2009). Manual physical therapy & exercise versus electrophysical agents and exercise in the management of plantar heel pain: A multicenter randomized clinical trial. *Journal of Orthopaedic and Sports Physical Therapy, 39*(8), 573–585.

Creswell, J. W. (2008). *Research design: Qualitative, quantitative, and mixed methods approaches* (3rd ed.). Thousand Oaks, CA: SAGE Publications, Inc.

Curran, V. R., Sharpe, D., Flynn, K., & Button, P. (2010). A longitudinal study of the effect of an interprofessional education curriculum on student satisfaction and attitudes towards interprofessional teamwork and education. *Journal of Interprofessional Care, 24,* 41–52. doi:10.3109/13561820903011927

Forsyth, K., & Kviz, F. (2006). Survey research design. In G. Kielhofner (Ed.), *Research in occupational therapy: Methods of inquiry for enhancing practice* (pp. 91–109). Philadelphia, PA: F.A. Davis.

Fowler, F. J. (2009). *Survey research methods* (4th ed.). Thousand Oaks, CA: SAGE Publications, Inc.

Franke, R. H., & Kaul, J. D. (1978). The Hawthorne experiments: First statistical interpretation. *American Sociological Review, 43,* 623–643.

Fuller, A. (2010). Speech and language therapy in sure start local programmes: A survey-based analysis of practice and innovation. *International Journal of Language & Communication Disorders, 45*(2), 182–203. doi:10.3109/13682820902836286

Garvin, A., & Damson, C. (2008). The effects of idealized fitness images on anxiety, depression and global mood states in college age males and females. *Journal of Health Psychology, 13*(3), 433–437.

Groves, R. M., Fowler, F. J., Couper, M. P., Lepkowski, J. M., Singer, E., & Tourangeau, R. (2009). *Survey methodology* (2nd ed.). Hoboken, NJ: John Wiley & Sons, Inc.

Herman, K. M., Hopman, W. M., & Craig, C. L. (2010). Are youth BMI and physical activity associated with better or worse than expected health-related quality of life in adulthood? The physical activity longitudinal study. *Quality of Life Research, 19*(3), 339–349. doi:10.1007/s11136-010-9586-8

Hunt, L. A., & Bassi, C. J. (2010). Near-vision acuity levels and performance on neuropsychological assessments used in occupational therapy. *American Journal of Occupational Therapy, 64*(1), 105–113.

Johnson, R. B., Onwuegbuzie, A. J., & Turner, L. A. (2007). Toward a definition of mixed methods research. *Journal of Mixed Methods Research, 1*(2), 112–133.

Kielhofner, G., & Fossey, E. (2006). The range of research. In G. Kielhofner (Ed.), *Research in occupational therapy: Methods of inquiry for enhancing practice* (pp. 91–109). Philadelphia, PA: F.A. Davis.

Lach, H. W., Ball, L. J., & Birge, S. J. (2012). The nursing home falls self-efficacy scale: Development and testing. *Clinical Nursing Research, 21*(1), 79–91. doi:10.1177/1054773811426927

Leerar, P., Boissonnault, W., Domholdt, E., & Roddey, T. (2007). Documentation of red flags by physical therapists for patients with low back pain. *The Journal of Manual & Manipulative Therapy, 15*(1), 42–49.

Microsoft. (2010). Microsoft Excel [computer software]. Redmond, WA: Author.

Nwora, A. J., & Gee, B. M. (2009). A case study of a five-year-old child with pervasive developmental disorder–not otherwise specified using sound-based interventions. *Occupational Therapy International, 16*(1), 25–43. doi:10.1002/oti.263

O'Neil, M. E., Fragala-Pinkham, M., Ideishi, R. I., & Ideishi, S. K. (2012). Community-based programs for children and youth: Our experiences in design, implementation, & evaluation. *Physical & Occupational Therapy in Pediatrics, 32*(2), 111–119.

Portney, L. G., & Watkins, M. P. (2009). *Foundations of clinical research: Applications to practice* (3rd ed.). Upper Saddle River, NJ: Pearson Education, Inc.

Rubin, D. B. (2006). *Matched sampling for causal effects.* New York, NY: Cambridge University Press.

Salant, P., & Dillman, D. (1994). *How to conduct your own survey: Leading professionals give you techniques for getting the reliable results.* New York: John Wiley & Sons, Inc.

Sherman, K., Ludman, E., Cook, A., Hawkes, R., Roy-Byrne, P., Bentley, S., . . . Cherkin, D. (2010). Effectiveness of therapeutic massage for generalized anxiety disorder: A randomized controlled trial. *Depression and Anxiety, 27,* 441–450.

Shyu, Y., Chen, M., Chen, S., Wang, H., & Shao, J. (2008). A family caregiver-oriented discharge planning program for older stroke patients and their family caregivers. *Journal of Clinical Nursing, 17,* 2497–2508. doi:10.1111/j.1365-2702.2008.02450.x

Suresh, K. P. (2011). An overview of randomization techniques: An unbiased assessment of outcome in clinical research. *Journal of Human Reproductive Sciences, 4*(1), 8–11.

Tawashy, A., Eng, J., Lin, K., Tang, P., & Hung, C. (2009). Physical activity is related to lower levels of pain, fatigue and depression in individuals with spinal-cord injury: A correlational study. *Spinal Cord, 47*(4), 301–306. doi:10.1038/sc.2008.120

Teddlie, C., & Tashakkori, A. (Eds.). (2008). *Foundations of mixed methods research: Integrating quantitative and qualitative approaches in the social and behavioral sciences.* Thousand Oaks, CA: SAGE Publications, Inc.

Thomas, J., & Hersen, M. (2011). *Understanding research in clinical and counseling psychology* (2nd ed.). New York, NY: Routledge.

Urbaniak, G. C., & Plous, S. (2012). *Research randomizer.* Social Psychology Network. http://www.randomizer.org/

Walach, H., Güthlin, C., & König, M. (2003). Efficacy of massage therapy in chronic pain: A pragmatic randomized trial. *Journal of Alternative & Complementary Medicine, 9*(6), 837–846.

Walker, J. (2006). *HotBits: Genuine random numbers, generated by radioactive decay.* http://www.fourmilab.ch/hotbits/

Wludyka, P. (2012). Study designs and their outcomes. In K. Macha & J. P. McDonough (Eds.), *Epidemiology for advanced nursing practice* (pp. 81–114). Sudbury, MA: Jones & Barlett Learning, LLC.

Yin, R. K. (2009). *Case study research: Design and methods* (4th ed.). Thousand Oaks, CA: Sage Publications, Inc.

DavisPlus | For additional materials, please visit **http://davisplus.fadavis.com, key word: Hissong.**

Chapter 7

Technical Aspects of Quantitative Research

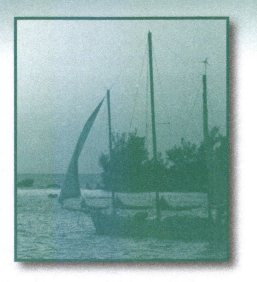

> *To reach a port, we must sail—Sail, not tie at anchor—Sail, not drift.*
>
> —*Franklin Roosevelt*

LEARNING OUTCOMES

The information provided in this chapter will assist the reader to:

- Establish proper inclusion and exclusion criteria for research subjects.
- Consider subject recruitment and select the most appropriate sampling technique.
- Choose a suitable method for data collection from those reviewed (observation, interviews, surveys, record review, equipment use, assessments, or tests).
- Understand the complexities of survey construction and where to locate additional resources to assist in this endeavor.
- Examine the validity and reliability of proposed testing instruments before electing their use.
- Comprehend differences between descriptive and inferential statistics used in data analysis.
- Identify appropriate resources for statistical analysis.
- Report results and synthesize them with existing literature to effectively draw conclusions.

Considerations in Quantitative Research

To enable others to understand and apply your quantitative research, you will need to consider and identify the following: subject inclusion and exclusion criteria, recruitment and sampling methods, data collection techniques, and data analysis. Each of these topics will be covered in greater depth here.

Subject Inclusion and Exclusion Criteria

Subject inclusion and exclusion criteria are specific conditions set forth by the researchers that must be met for eligibility to participate in their study. The population of interest refers to the entire group of individuals, events, documents, or records that meet these criteria. Although the subjects in healthcare research are frequently individuals, they can also include records or events. (See Boxes 6-1 and 6-2 for examples.) In either case, those deemed eligible for participation in a study must meet a specific set of characteristics that have been established by the researcher before initiation of the study.

 Subject inclusion criteria consist of characteristics or traits that subjects must have to qualify for participation in the study. For example, you might be interested in studying adults diagnosed with multiple sclerosis in the United States who are 40 to 60 years old and who are employed full time. If so, demographic data is collected before the study begins to ensure all participants meet these criteria. **Subject exclusion criteria** take into account undesirable features for participants. These could include subjects residing more than 50 miles from the research center, those who only work one or more part-time jobs, or those with impaired cognitive abilities that might influence performance on study measures, for instance.

Inclusion and exclusion criteria are determined based upon the literature review and goals for the study, and they typically evolve as the assumptions and theoretical base of the study unfold. Therefore, these criteria are established well in advance of the study's beginning. It is important to identify all applicable criteria, so that readers have a clear understanding of the population being investigated.

Subject Recruitment

Once the inclusion and exclusion criteria have been established, the researcher must decide where the subjects will come from. This decision can be made only after consideration of the goals, geographic location, funding, and other logistics of the study. Recruitment for studies in community-based settings such as fitness centers, day cares, and senior centers typically rely on advertisements, directories, and mailings to solicit subjects. Clinical research that occurs in hospitals, rehabilitation clinics, or other medical centers often relies on recruitment of actual patients via word of mouth by the practitioner or researcher.

Sampling

After identification of the population of interest and recruitment of subjects, the researcher must determine the sampling method to be used. **Sampling** involves selection of a smaller subset of the population of interest to participate in the study. This technique is often employed when it is impractical to study the entire population of interest because of time constraints, financial concerns, or other logistics such as geographic location or transportation issues. For example, a population of interest might consist of 713 individuals who underwent rotator cuff repair surgery at one university

hospital system; 200 of those individuals (a sample) would be selected to participate in a study. There are two basic sampling methods—nonprobability sampling and probability sampling.

Nonprobability Sampling

In **nonprobability sampling**, the subjects are not selected randomly, but rather on the basis of some other phenomena such as location or convenient access. This means that not all members of the population of interest have an equal chance of being selected for the sample. Recall the earlier discussion in Chapter 6 on **convenience sampling**, which involves the use of subjects simply because they are readily available. Although convenience sampling is the least expensive and easiest of the sampling techniques, it may decrease the generalizability of results. In health care, researchers frequently conduct their studies on patients they already have on their caseloads or those who are readily available in their facility. Using volunteers is also a common convenience sampling technique. Although use of convenience samples can pose challenges, it is an effective way for novice researchers to get started in the research process. See Box 6-7 for an example of convenience sampling. Other types of nonprobability sampling include quota sampling, purposive sampling, and snowball sampling.

Quota sampling refers to the process of dividing the population of interest into two or more subgroups based upon some characteristic. The researcher then draws adequate samples from each subgroup to represent the proportion of this characteristic occurring naturally in the population of interest. This technique ensures that the characteristic in question is equally represented in the population and the chosen sample. For example, a researcher interested in studying ambulation in seniors residing in a skilled nursing facility would likely want a greater number of female subjects than male subjects, because census information reveals a greater number of females residing in these facilities. The researcher determines the desired quota for each subgroup and selects subjects until the quotas are reached.

Purposive sampling, or judgment sampling, involves hand selection of subjects based upon specific attributes. Subjects might be selected based upon their diagnoses, motivational level, or perceived compliance, for example. The purpose of the research can dictate selection of a very specific sample, hence the name of this technique. Finally, **snowballing sampling**, also known as referral sampling or chain sampling, involves selection of a small number of subjects who meet study criteria; these subjects then refer others who also meet the same criteria. The process continues until a sufficient sample has been tested. This technique is useful to identify subjects who might otherwise be inaccessible to the researchers. Examples include subjects with a rare disease, those involved in illicit activity, or members of distinct networks or social groups.

Probability Sampling

Probability sampling is a method of sampling that ensures all members of the population of interest have an equal chance of being selected for the study sample. **Random sampling**, also known as simple random sampling (described in Chapter 6), is one of the most popular types of probability sampling. Random sampling involves compiling an exhaustive list of subjects that meet the study's inclusion criteria, and then randomly selecting the study's sample from this list. This can be accomplished by placing all names in a hat and drawing names until an adequate number of subjects have been selected. In reality, most researchers find the use of a random numbers table (found in a statistical text) or a statistical software package to randomly select subjects to be a more practical method. Random sampling increases the likelihood that the study results will be similar to results that would have been found if the entire population had been studied.

Other types of probability sampling include stratified random sampling, systematic random sampling, and cluster sampling. **Stratified random sampling** involves dividing the population into homogeneous subgroups, and then randomly sampling each subgroup. This technique ensures that each subgroup is adequately represented in the sample. This type of sampling is similar to the quota sampling discussed earlier in that each technique involves dividing the population based on a particular attribute. However, in stratified random sampling the sample from each subgroup is drawn randomly, but in quota sampling they are not. **Systematic random sampling** involves randomly ordering all possible subjects and then selecting every nth one for participation. You must consider the total number of subjects needed for your study (for example, 25) divided by the available subjects in your population (say 100). This means you need 25% of the population for your sample. Selecting every fourth subject in the random list of the 100-subject population will accomplish your goal.

Cluster sampling is useful when your population is spread out geographically. In this case, it is beneficial to divide the population into smaller clusters, which will then be randomly sampled. This is especially useful if the researcher needs to be physically present to conduct assessments or interventions with the subjects. Finally, **multistage sampling** involves a combination of probability sampling methods. For more details on the probability sampling techniques presented here or other types, because this discussion is very basic, please see Portney and Watkins' (2009) *Foundations of Clinical Research: Applications to Practice*. In general, keep in mind that your sample should represent the larger population of interest as closely as possible.

Sample Size

The question regarding sample size is not one that is easily answered. Just how many subjects will you need for your proposed study? Ideally, the sample should accurately represent the larger population of interest from which it was drawn, thereby allowing the researcher to generalize the results found in the sample to the population. If the sample is too small, or was not randomly chosen or assigned, the sample may not be reflective of the larger population.

Depending on the purpose of a study, it may not be necessary to draw a sample; instead, all subjects meeting the criteria can be included. For example, studies exploring the efficacy of practices and policies within a specific health system or facility could use as subjects all individuals treated there. Although these results may not be generalizable to other health systems, this is not a disadvantage because the researchers are only looking to gain knowledge on the practices in one facility or system.

In quantitative research, two concepts related to statistical analysis also factor into determining the appropriate sample size—the confidence interval and the confidence level. The **confidence interval**, or margin of error, represents a range of values that likely includes the scores or responses of the population. For example, if the margin of error is 5, and 50% of a study sample responds favorably to a new treatment, the researchers can have confidence that if they tested the entire population of interest, 45% to 55% would also respond favorably. The **confidence level** represents the certainty the researchers have that the scores or responses of the population would fall within this range. Confidence levels of 95% or 99% are typically chosen, indicating that the researchers are either 95% or 99% confident that the scores or responses will fall within the margin of error. Once you have determined the size of your population, the confidence interval, and the confidence level, a statistical program, a web-based calculator, or a statistician can be used to help you determine the appropriate sample size.

Although studies conducted with smaller samples may face criticism, using larger samples does not necessarily translate into more accurate results. How the subjects are recruited, sampled, and assigned to study groups must also be considered. Smaller samples may be appropriate depending on the study's goals, and they are often employed in pilot studies or by novice researchers. Sample size is often dictated by financial and logistical circumstances, and as noted previously, convenience samples are common in healthcare research.

Data Collection Techniques

Sometimes the research method dictates data collection techniques, and at other times the researcher has a wide array of choices. To illuminate the choices, data collection techniques will be categorized and discussed individually. It should be noted that some of these techniques may also be appropriate for use in qualitative research, and they will be discussed further in Chapters 8 and 9. Techniques may be conveniently grouped as follows:

1. Observation
2. Interview
3. Survey
4. Record Review
5. Equipment
6. Tests, Assessments, and Inventories

Observation

This data collection technique may be used with any of the quantitative research designs and is commonly used in conjunction with other techniques. Observations may be made of human subjects, videotape recordings of subjects or events, or nonhuman items such as pieces of equipment. In quantitative research, the observation process is formalized in advance. When observing the frequency or type of events occurring in a quantitative study, a method for recording observations needs to be carefully prepared and the observers should be well trained. Rather than being asked to observe and record subjective items such as *dependence* or *enjoyment*, it is preferable for observers to be given objective criteria believed to represent those subjective items. For example, *dependence* may be represented by the number of times a subject asks for assistance, and *enjoyment* may be represented by the number of smiles, laughs, or verbal statements that would indicate happiness. Observers should be provided with a protocol defining the items to be observed and a method for recording those items, such as noting any occurrence, frequency of occurrence, or length of time between occurrences, on a previously designed form.

Videotapes are useful for training purposes. The observer rates the tapes and the researcher checks the ratings until he or she is satisfied that the observer is making correct and reliable ratings. This procedure ensures **intrarater reliability**, or the degree to which each rater or observer is consistent in his or her ratings. If there is more than one observer or rater, the researcher will probably want to confirm **interrater reliability**, which means the raters are checked against one another, to ensure that the same results are obtained regardless of the rater. Objective measurements and observations are made until all raters score similarly and the researcher has confidence, evidenced by statistics, that all raters will rate consistently well. Consistency between raters is critical to protecting the study's internal validity.

Interview

Interviewing, either face-to-face or via telephone, or through voice-over Internet programs, is one of the techniques used to gather data in survey research. Interviews conducted face-to-face or through videoconferencing methods are more intimate, allowing the interviewer to physically see the interviewee. This direct interaction helps develop rapport and may be important if sensitive issues are being explored. Additionally, the interviewer has a chance to "read" the nonverbal cues given by the interviewee, which may indicate confusion or lack of understanding, so that a question can be rephrased. Nonverbal information may also be an important part of understanding the full response to the question.

The disadvantage of true face-to-face interviews is the amount of effort required to set up the interview, including contacting subjects, arranging mutually convenient times and locations, and traveling. Telephone interviewing eliminates these concerns, but the personal contact and the chance to observe nonverbal cues are lost. Also, it is easier for a subject to refuse an interview on the telephone. Voice-over Internet programs may provide the best of both worlds, but could present technological challenges because both the interviewer and interviewee must have adequate hardware and software and be able to operate both effectively.

In survey research, the interview format may be structured or unstructured, sometimes referred to as formal or informal. In structured interviews, the same questions are always asked, and they are asked in the same order. Although this format may appear stilted and formal, the answers will be easier to compare from one subject to another and frequencies and percentages can be compiled. In unstructured interviews, the volume of material can be difficult to organize and analyze, and often it is not comparable from one subject to the next. For this reason, structured interviews are more common in quantitative research. They are also less difficult for the inexperienced interviewer or beginning researcher, because the data are easily tabulated and analyzed, and interpretations are more likely to be accurate and meaningful. However, unstructured interviews are commonly used in pilot studies to clarify issues on the topic of interest, and for later development of a structured interview for the formal study.

When writing questions, prime consideration should be given to the language style and idiom used by subjects, which may well be different from that used by the researcher. It is especially important to avoid abbreviations, medical terminology (i.e., use *stroke* rather than *cerebrovascular accident*), and vaguely worded questions or those with biased wording or tone (Salant & Dillman, 1994).

One of the problems with data obtained from interviews is that it is difficult to know if subjects are telling the truth or trying to impress the interviewer by saying what they think the interviewer wants to hear. They may also be embarrassed or ashamed to tell the truth on sensitive issues. Experienced interviewers can gain skill in reading nonverbal cues to determine the degree of truthfulness in answers. There is a great deal to be learned about the construction of individual questions and the interview as a whole. Because most of this information on question and interview construction also pertains to surveys, it will be discussed in the following section.

Surveys

There are multiple ways to distribute surveys, also known as written questionnaires. They may be mailed to respondents, e-mailed to respondents, conducted through online survey software such as Survey Monkey® (2012) or SuperSurvey® (Ipathia, 2011), hand delivered to respondents with instructions to mail them back to the researcher, or completed by respondents in the presence of the researcher. If surveys are mailed or e-mailed or left for subjects to complete and return on their own, there are special considerations. First, the questions must be very clear and unambiguous because the researcher will not be present to clarify concerns. This is of particular importance because if a question has been misinterpreted and answered incorrectly, the whole questionnaire must be discarded unless special statistical procedures are followed in analyzing results.

Another concern regarding surveys is whether there will be sufficient responses to justify the study. The **response rate** is defined as the number of surveys returned divided by the total number in the sample. Response rates can vary greatly depending upon the type of survey and method of distribution, but Fowler (2009) cautions that response rates of less than 20% may render little accurate information about the larger population being investigated (p. 51). Actual response rates for most studies fall between 30% to 60%, and response rates above 60% are considered excellent by most researchers (Portney & Watkins, 2009, p. 326). The Office of Management and Budget (2006) of the U.S. federal government requires a response rate of 95% for federally conducted research, as well as justification for lower response rates and plans to address nonresponse bias if this target is not met. In another study, the researchers examined 18 health science journals to explore publication requirements and reporting methods of response rates (Johnson & Owens, 2003). The researchers found that none of the journals specified a minimum response rate and most did not outline standard procedures for reporting it. Thus, it is evident that controversy still exists as to what is an acceptable response rate.

Although the type of survey and method of distribution can affect your response rate, the rate can also be negatively impacted when surveys are returned incomplete and subsequently have to be removed from the sample being analyzed. Conversely, response rates are likely to be higher if the sample has some vested interest in the topic of study and therefore returns the surveys promptly and completely. The *American Association of Public Opinion Research* (n.d.) provides additional information on how to accurately calculate and report your response rate.

It is also important to consider other techniques for improving your response rate. The survey must be attractive and pleasing so that recipients will not discard it without reading the cover letter and initial instructions. The cover letter must be well-written to catch the recipients' attention, and to describe why recipients should be interested in the study and what benefits they can expect from participating (even if the sole benefit is that they will be assisting a student to complete her or his thesis and will thereby be indirectly helping to add one more person to the pool of working healthcare practitioners). Reviewing the goals of the study and other details can capture their interest and increase the likelihood that they will answer the questions.

For mailed surveys, provide a deadline for returning the survey—approximately 2 weeks after it has been received. Research shows that recipients rarely return questionnaires after 2 weeks, and that about 90% of responses for online surveys will be received within the first 3 days of the e-mail invitation (Walonick, 2010). Unless returns are confidential, keep a master list of those to whom you have mailed questionnaires and check off their returns. If you have not heard from recipients in 2 weeks, send them a reminder postcard, e-mail, or text.

Always enclose a stamped, self-addressed envelope if the survey is to be mailed back. This will greatly increase the response rate. Recipients will generally not make the required effort to find an envelope and your address on the cover letter (which has often been destroyed), and may resent having to pay postage for your research project.

Surveys must be short enough to hold the respondents' attention but long enough to obtain the required information. The cost to create and conduct the survey is also a consideration (Fink, 2009). Research reveals that decreased response rates and quality are likely if self-administered surveys take longer than 20 minutes (Cape, 2010). Other sources estimate the time respondents will devote to online surveys is between 7–8 minutes, with respondents abandoning the survey or "satisficing" (speeding) through the survey if it takes longer (Chudoba, 2011). One good rule of thumb is to view your survey as objectively as you can and to ask yourself if you would stick with it and answer all the questions if it was sent to you. In most cases, it is also appropriate and worthwhile to pilot your survey before use in experimental research. This will help to clarify any survey questions that may be confusing to respondents, to increase accuracy of information gained from the survey, and to determine if the method of delivery and completion time are appropriate for your goals.

Question Construction

When constructing questions for surveys and interviews, two types of questions—closed-ended and open-ended—may be used. **Closed-ended questions** are those that require only a simple answer, usually "yes" or "no" or a check mark against a series of options, whereas **open-ended questions** are those that respondents can answer in as many words as they please. Open-ended questions are most useful in dealing with complicated information when slight differences of opinion are important to know. They also provide a good way to elaborate on a closed-ended question, such as:

> Do you teach clinical reasoning skills to your therapy students?   Yes _____ No _____
>   If yes, please explain how and at what point in the curriculum:

Open-ended questions may also be used as a way of finding out which issue in a series of closed-ended questions is the most important or most relevant to the respondent. For example, a series of specific questions about specialty certification may be followed by the question: "What is your opinion of specialty certification?" This technique is useful in that it often makes respondents feel better after having been "boxed in" for possible answers—they can now say what they want to say. You might not use the open-ended piece of information in tabulating results, but it keeps the respondents interested and involved, and increases the likelihood that they will complete the survey.

Open-ended questions are useful in allowing respondents to answer in any style and manner they choose without giving them suggestions. This reduces the chance of their giving what they perceive as socially acceptable answers. Similarly, questions that may be viewed as sensitive or threatening are usually best handled as open-ended questions and may be more honestly answered on an anonymous survey than in a personal interview.

Yet the fact is respondents are often more willing to quickly complete a survey composed of closed-ended questions rather than writing several sentences that they have to think about and compose for questions of the open-ended variety. However, the closed-ended responses may not satisfy the researcher who would prefer more detailed, qualitative, and personal responses. There is a trade-off here, and the choice must be made by the researcher.

In closed-ended questions, response formats should be mutually exclusive and, when ratings are required, there should be a wide array of choices. In the "yes or no" answer, there are differing opinions about whether to include the "don't know," "undecided," or the neutral option. Converse (1970, 1974) first raised this concern, and authors since that time have argued whether it was more beneficial to force respondents into a positive or negative answer, or to give them the option to admit their lack of knowledge or inability to decide (Walonick, 2010). Face-to-face interviews are advantageous as skilled interviewers may be able to elicit clarifying information from interviewees who at first choose one of these neutral responses. Although mailed surveys do not allow additional probing, research on interactive web-based surveys shows that use of additional prompts may combat this problem (DeRouvray & Couper, 2002). The type of question, knowledge-based versus attitude-based, may also dictate the need to include a neutral option.

In addition to simple "yes or no" items, other questions rely on some sort of rating scale, the best known being the semantic differential and the Likert rating scales. The **semantic differential**, developed by Charles Osgood (Osgood, Suci, & Tannenbaum, 1957), is used as a measure of affective meaning. Respondents are given a domain of concern and are asked to rate their affective responses about that domain on a list of bipolar scales. These are seven-point scales with opposing adjectives at the two extremes. Generally, three dimensions exist into which these adjective pairs can be categorized—the evaluative dimension (good or bad), the potency dimension (strong or weak), and the activity dimension (fast or slow). Box 7-1 shows one use of the semantic differential.

In the **Likert scale** (Likert, 1932), a statement is given to respondents to indicate the domain of concern, and the respondents are asked to indicate their level of agreement with that statement on a five-point or seven-point scale. The five-point scale is typically worded as follows: "Strongly agree, Agree, Neutral, Disagree, Strongly disagree." The seven-point scale

BOX 7-1 ■ Example of Semantic Differential

Henry, Nelson, and Duncombe (1984) used the semantic differential to elicit subjects' responses on how they felt about themselves following a choice or no choice situation in an activity group on three affective factors: evaluation, power, and activity. They used Osgood's short-form semantic differential where subjects were asked to assign a rating on a 7-point scale for each of 12 scales. The actual scale looked like this:

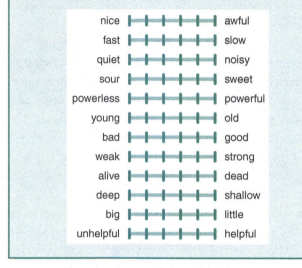

of behavior, or personality traits. A phrase is provided to indicate the domain of concern, and the respondent is asked to complete the sentence. For example:

> My opinion about placing adults with developmental disabilities in group homes is:
> _____.

Multiple-choice items can also be used to elicit opinions or attitudes from respondents. A statement is provided, sometimes in question form, and respondents are asked to select from the list the item that most reflects their opinion, attitude, or even a likely action. For example, if researchers wanted to explore perceptions of common treatment interventions used with stroke patients, the following question might be included in their survey for healthcare professionals working with this population:

> What is the **best** method for decreasing muscle tone following stroke?
> a) Application of moist heat
> b) Gentle massage over the muscle belly
> c) Daily range of motion exercises
> d) Ultrasound
> e) Application of a splint

would add "Very strongly agree" and "Very strongly disagree" at either end. For example, see the box at the bottom of the page.

In other cases, respondents may be asked to fill in the blank or to choose a relevant response from multiple choices—either a rank-ordered or unordered list. Incomplete sentences are sometimes used to find out such things as opinions, attitudes, knowledge, styles

In **rank-ordering items**, a list of items is provided and respondents are asked to place a number beside each, indicating their order of importance. Sometimes only the first two or three items of importance are asked for, and sometimes the whole list must be

Please circle the number that best represents your feelings:					
	Strongly Agree	Agree	Neither Agree Nor Disagree (Neutral)	Disagree	Strongly Disagree
Treatment at this clinic is very client-focused.	5	4	3	2	1

prioritized. It is important to remember that most people find it difficult to prioritize more than about 10 items. Using the previous example, the question would appear as follows:

Please rank the following treatment interventions in order of effectiveness in decreasing muscle tone in stroke patients, starting with "1" for the treatment you believe to be most effective.

	Rank (1 through 5)
Application of moist heat	_____
Gentle massage over the muscle belly	_____
Daily range of motion exercises	_____
Ultrasound	_____
Application of a splint	_____

Survey organization

The survey questions should be sequenced so that they follow one another in a logical order. First, draw subjects in and gain their interest with broad, general questions. Avoid sensitive questions until the respondent is comfortable and, in the case of a face-to-face interview, until rapport has been established. It is a good idea not to give too many questions that require a simple "yes" or "no" or too many requiring a rating at different levels (such as "Rate on a scale of 1 to 5") in a sequence, because respondents lose interest and concentration after a while and may answer without giving the questions much thought. Break up these questions with others written in a different format.

Often researchers add a general open-ended question at the end of a questionnaire, designed to give respondents an opportunity to add any information they did not have a chance to include during the process. On mailed questionnaires, it is quite common for respondents to write notes to the researcher explaining things they think are unclear or adding items they feel are relevant. The final general question gives respondents a legitimate place to do this. Other things to consider in survey organization include the visual layout, including font and spacing, transitions between sections, and adequate pretesting to ensure the information obtained is useful and that the survey is user-friendly and easily understood.

Suffice it to say, much reflection should be given to the type of questions used and the method of presentation. Consideration of your population and the information you hope to gain is critical in making these decisions. The reference list contains a variety of excellent texts that can assist you further in survey construction.

Record Review

Review of written records is an appropriate data collection method in several types of research, including experimental, ethnographic, retrospective or historical, and case study designs. Documents provide both historical and contextual dimensions to your observations and interviews. They enrich what you see and hear by supporting, expanding, and challenging your portrayals and perceptions.

Written documents may include patients' medical records, minutes of meetings and case conferences, letters, speeches, articles, books, diaries, graffiti, notes, membership lists, newsletters, newspapers, and illustrations. Artifacts may include physical materials such as adaptive equipment, adapted clothing, photographs, audio and video recordings, and films. One way to obtain written materials is to ask subjects to keep diaries, journals, or other kinds of records. Collaboration with healthcare practitioners might be necessary so that clinical notes simultaneously meet the needs of the healthcare facility and the research study. For example, if you are interested in patient satisfaction with healthcare services, you might be able to play a role in the design of a patient satisfaction survey that would assist the healthcare facility as well as your study.

Traditionally, records used as research data are divided into primary and secondary sources. **Primary sources** are firsthand accounts about the topic under review, such as autobiographies or eyewitness accounts, and **secondary sources** are accounts written about the topic by others that are not based on personal experience, such as medical records (which are written by clinicians and not by the patients having the experience). Researchers should try to verify both the truth about the writing of the documents (did this person actually write it?), as well as the truth about the content of the documents (did this actually happen?).

Moreover, written materials may be used to corroborate researchers' observations or what they find out in interviews. Records can raise useful questions about the study and shape new directions for observations and interviews. They can provide historical, demographic, and sometimes personal information that is unavailable from other sources.

In summarizing and interpreting the data gathered, the researcher must use logical analysis and be as objective as possible. In a retrospective study, where examination of records is often the only form of data gathering possible, the researcher usually cannot confirm that one event in the past caused another to occur. In this case, the researcher must make assumptions or draw inferences that assign causality. The more information that is uncovered about an event, the more likely the cause of the event may be determined. Researchers must be careful to restrict interpretations about causes and generalizability of the evidence gathered. Box 6-2 provides an example of use of medical records for data collection.

Equipment Used in Research

Many studies performed by healthcare professionals employ physical measures of such functions as joint range, muscle strength, or galvanic skin response. Physical or mechanical instruments that provide a valid and reliable measurement are usually more desirable in experimental research than the subjective feedback given by subjects. However, before relying on a piece of equipment as a measuring instrument in a research study, the researcher should make sure that it is reliable and valid. The use of equipment for measuring is also desirable in research because it provides a simple method for operationally defining and measuring dependent variables. Box 7-2 provides an example.

In these days of sophisticated equipment, many choices are available for objectively measuring dependent variables. Healthcare practitioners use instruments,

---

> **BOX 7-2 ■ Use of Physical Equipment to Operationalize Study Variables**
>
> In a study measuring posttreatment elbow range of motion in patients with hemiplegia, range of motion at the elbow can be operationally defined as the number of degrees registered on a goniometer placed on the joint angle while in extension and in flexion.

---

such as cable tensiometers, spirometers, electroencephalographs, goniometers, dynamometers, pinch meters, pedometers, heart rate monitors, digital calipers, volumeters, scales, pulse oximeters, and ultrasound imaging, to name a few. When utilizing these types of devices, it is important to obtain information from the manufacturer on specifications and settings, and to ensure that the device is adequately calibrated and in good working order. Unfortunately, many variables cannot be measured with hardware, and other means must be found to define and quantify them. These other means are generally written tests and measures, which will be discussed in the next section.

Tests, Assessments, and Inventories

A great deal of research data used by health professionals is gathered via written tests, assessments, and inventories. A plethora of standardized assessments exist to measure variables including psychological factors, functional performance of daily tasks, cognitive abilities, perceptual motor skills, child developmental stages, prevocational skills, vocational interests, personality factors, attitudes, and values, to name a few.

Some of the better-known tests have been gathered and critiqued in such bibliographic texts as Asher's (2007) book on tests used in the practice of occupational therapy, Fischer and Corcoran's (2007) two-volume set of clinical instruments and scales used by a variety of allied health professions, and Burlingame and Blaschko's (2009) collection of assessments for recreational therapy and related fields. Professional organizations representing each discipline often have resources that list applicable assessments to a particular practice area, summarize the purpose of available tools, or provide links to research testing the usefulness, reliability, and validity of assessments. One example is the American Physical Therapy Association's (2005) *List of Assessment Tools Used in Pediatric Physical Therapy*. Other sources for tests are the catalogs from the major test publishers.

If you find that there is no existing test to gather exactly the type of information you are interested in, you will probably need to design your own test. In order for your test to be valid and useful, you should follow accepted test construction techniques. You are referred to Benson and Clark's (1982) article "A Guide for Instrument Development and Validation" for a step-by-step description of the procedure for test construction.

Validity and Reliability of Test Instruments

Tests, measures, and inventories can be standardized or nonstandardized. Standardized tests have been subjected to a process called normalizing, which establishes a level of validity and reliability in relation to the "normal" population, whereas nonstandardized measures have not undergone such rigorous testing.

Validity

A valid test is one that measures what it claims to measure; for example, an intelligence test truly measures a child's intelligence rather than his or her school performance, concentration, or motivation. Yet, "validity is not a property of the test itself. Instead, validity is the extent to which the interpretations of the results of a test are warranted" (Kimberlin & Winterstein, 2008, p. 2278). In the health sciences, researchers are often interested in studying abstract concepts that cannot be directly measured. These might include safety, feelings of self-efficacy, quality of life, collaboration, or satisfaction, to name a few. Thus, the ability to operationalize these terms is critical in being able to provide an accurate system of measurement.

Reliability

A test is reliable if the same results occur during repeated administrations over time. For example, a reliable intelligence test will give the same intelligence quotient (IQ) score for the same individual time after time, all else being equal.

Four types of reliability pertaining to test instruments are important to understand:

1. **Test–retest reliability** is concerned with the consistency of scores over time. More specifically, if subjects are measured regarding some characteristic now, and then re-measured on the same characteristic at a later point in time, the scores should be similar, assuming that the conditions and the characteristic being measured are stable.

2. **Split-half reliability** concerns the extent to which different parts of an instrument measure the same thing. For instance, are two different items on a test for self-esteem both actually measuring components of self-esteem? If not, the whole test may be suspect, and the compiled score may not truly represent the subject's self-esteem score. To assess this type of reliability, the test is divided into two parts and subjects' scores on the two groups of items are compared. The two scores should be similar in order for the test to be considered reliable, and a high correlation between sets of items indicates a higher degree of internal consistency (Kimberlin & Winterstein, 2008).

3. **Intrarater reliability** is the degree to which each rater or observer is consistent in his or her ratings. Multiple repetitions of the same test by one rater should yield consistently similar results, thus ensuring consistent administration and testing procedures by that rater.

4. **Interrater reliability**, or interobserver agreement, is the extent to which different raters or observers perceive the same person or characteristic similarly. To obtain reliable study results, ratings should be similar regardless of the rater. In other words, if two different raters administer an assessment on the same study subject, the scores should be relatively similar. Both intrarater and interrater reliability can be increased by clearly operationalizing all study variables and by conducting formalized training in administering treatments and conducting assessments.

The manual that accompanies a standardized test should include information about the process by which norms were established, details of the population used as normative groups, and the actual degree of validity and reliability achieved for the test. You should review this information to see if the test is rigorous enough for the purpose of your study. It is important that you use the test only on the type of subjects described in the manual. The researcher must learn the test administration procedures, and the test should be given exactly in the manner described in the manual. The reliability and validity of a test can be ensured only if the test is administered to the prescribed population, under the prescribed conditions, and in the prescribed manner. Once any of these conditions are changed, the researchers cannot claim for their study the degree of reliability and validity listed in the manual. Table 7-1 includes a list of considerations in selecting an existing assessment tool.

Table 7-1 ■ Considerations for Selecting an Existing Assessment Tool

- Consider the construct you wish to measure. Your literature review will help operationalize key concepts and determine possible assessment tools for use.

- Review test items and the manual for any tool you are considering to determine if it aligns with your study's goals.

- What is the reliability and validity of the tool? Has it been used on the population you intend to study?

- Can you locate other studies that attest to the tool's reliability and validity?

- Will you need to purchase or request permission to use the tool, or is it in the public domain?

- Are there costs associated with obtaining the tool or administering it?

- What training procedures will be necessary to ensure administration procedures follow the protocol in the manual?

- Is the tool appropriate for your population? Consider your subjects' age, educational level, setting, and motivation to participate in your study. Each of these attributes could impact their ability to understand the tool and provide worthwhile information.

(Kimberlin & Winterstein, 2008)

After you have determined the best method(s) of data collection, you should consider how you will analyze the data. In quantitative research, data result from variables that can be enumerated in some way so as to be tabulated and subjected to statistical procedures.

Analyzing Quantitative Data

This is the part that many people hate! Researchers must decide what to do with the mass of numbers that have been collected and what statistical tests to use. Some people have such a fear of this part of the research process that they never get beyond it. Although this fear or lack of knowledge is very real, it should not be allowed to stand in the way of conducting meaningful research. Those who are intimidated by data analysis should seek assistance from a statistician.

Consulting a Statistician

The question of when to seek statistical assistance during the research process is worthy of discussion. Generally, a statistician should be consulted in the design stage of the project while the methodology and data collection measures are being determined. Once researchers identify their topic of interest, a statistician can ensure selection of the most appropriate study design for their needs, and can make recommendations regarding sample size, blinding, randomization, structure and timing of the therapeutic interventions, and coding of data (American Statistical Association (ASA), 2003).

Although the researchers will decide on the actual measures used and whether these measures will reliably collect the type of data they desire, the statistician understands how the data will be analyzed and may have some advice concerning the format in which the data are collected. For example, if you wish to compare two groups' performances on pretests and posttests in order to determine which group made the most progress, the statistician may advise that data from a certain measure are not in a format suitable for such comparisons. An unclear response from subjects such as, "I feel somewhat better," does not lend itself to objective comparisons, either for that one subject or among subjects. To further expand on this point, the statistician will understand how data will be entered into statistical software, and can make recommendations of how to organize data for ease of data entry.

Additionally, researchers may unknowingly omit some crucial piece of information concerning subjects from their questionnaire—for example, their ages. If they wish to group people by age for comparisons, this information will of course be important. Although anyone has the ability to spot this type of error, it sometimes takes an objective reader who is accustomed to studying data to notice it.

Finally, a statistician can help to determine which statistical tests will be best suited for data analysis and can advise on how many subjects are needed in order to use the chosen tests. Researchers need this information early in the planning stages of a study so that they can recruit a sample of adequate size. Thus, seeking assistance from a statistician early in the research design process is helpful in ensuring that data will be collected in such a way that they can be manipulated effectively.

Consulting a statistician has a price, but most people who have hired someone feel it is worth the cost. You may be fortunate enough to be connected to a university or other facility that employs a statistician who is willing to help free of charge or for a nominal fee. The *American Statistical Association* (http://www.amstat.org/index.cfm) or the *International Statistics Institute* (http://www.isi-web.org/) can provide additional information about hiring a statistician.

Anything other than basic statistics is beyond the scope of this text. However, a simple explanation of some of the processes involved in organizing and manipulating data will hopefully enable the reader who has a fear of statistics to cope with the material and know when to get help.

Descriptive versus Inferential Statistics

Statistics are divided into two categories: descriptive and inferential statistics. **Descriptive statistics** describe, organize, and summarize data. They include frequencies, percentages, descriptions of central tendency (mean, median, mode), and descriptions of relative position (range, standard deviation).

These procedures allow for the description of all the individual scores in a sample on one variable by using one or two numbers, such as the mean and standard deviation. They can be used to describe each dependent variable, such as the percentage and mean of each item physical therapists checked off on a list of reasons for moving into supervisory positions and their ages when they moved. Descriptive statistics can also be used to give the variation or spread of scores within each group studied, such as the mean and range of scores for experimental and control groups in a study on a new treatment technique for carpal tunnel syndrome.

Inferential statistics, on the other hand, allow researchers to make inferences about the population from the sample findings. Sufficient subjects are needed in the sample to be able to do this; in addition, random selection should be used. The types of statistical tests used in inferential statistics include *t* tests, *F* tests, and tests for *r*. These tests result in probability statements that help one draw conclusions about differences or relationships between groups. For example, if a difference is found between the mean scores of two groups at the end of a study, the researcher must decide whether a similar difference is likely to be found between the same mean scores in the whole population from which the sample groups were drawn. The *t*, *F*, and *r* tests allow the researcher to make this decision.

Both descriptive and inferential statistics are often used in the same research study. Descriptive statistical methods are the same regardless of the type of data being used; however, inferential statistical methods vary according to the type of data used.

Types of Data

Data are classified into four levels or scales of measurement: nominal, ordinal, interval, and ratio. Each data type builds on the characteristics of those previously described.

Nominal Data

Nominal data are the numbers applied to nonnumerical variables; for example, a group of people's disabilities could be coded as follows: right hemiplegia = 1, left hemiplegia = 2, paraplegia = 3, and so on. Each category of data must be mutually exclusive, meaning that no individual or variable can be assigned to more than one group. There is no ordered relationship between categories, meaning that one category cannot be considered to come before or after another category. This type of data is sometimes referred to as *discrete* as opposed to *continuous*. For discrete data there is no limit to the number of categories that can be included, whereas with continuous data there are an infinite number of possible values along a continuum. Because there is no numerical value assigned to categories of nominal data, they cannot be meaningfully added, subtracted, or multiplied, and so forth. One cannot calculate an average (mean) disability, for example.

Examples of categories might include male and female; inpatient, outpatient, and day treatment settings; and patients with schizophrenia, bipolar disease, or depression. A nominal scale may also be used to code "yes or no" responses on a survey.

Ordinal Data

Ordinal data are numbers that are still discrete but are ordered; however, the intervals between the categories are unknown and cannot be assumed to be equal. In contrast to nominal data in which assignment of numbers to categories is arbitrary, numbers assigned to groups of ordinal data signify a rank order or meaningful sequence. For instance, a review committee may rank-order a series of program proposals and assign first, second, and third place, but the top-ranked proposal may be considerably better than the ones ranked second and third, whereas the ones ranked fourth, fifth, and sixth may be similar to each other in quality. These differences among intervals are not reflected in the numerical assignment. Other examples would be ratings on a Likert scale such as "Strongly agree," "Agree," "Neutral," "Disagree," "Strongly disagree," or classifications for client ability such as "Dependent," "Needs partial assistance," "Independent." An ordinal data scale indicates a greater or lesser degree of something, or it may reflect a "precedes" or "superior" concept.

Interval Data

Interval data are also ordered in a logical sequence. However, this time the intervals between the numbers are considered equal and represent actual amounts. These are continuous data. Examples are intelligence scores, degrees of temperature, and magnitude rating scales. Items are ordered on a continuum; however, there is no zero starting point. For example, temperatures can fall below zero or subjects can be asked to rate the magnitude of a particular stimuli on a 1 to 10 scale, where the intervals are assumed to be equal.

Ratio Data

Ratio data are numbers that are also continuous with equal intervals between them. Additionally, ratio data have a meaningful zero point. In other words, the zero point indicates a total absence of whatever ability or property is being measured. For instance, there can legitimately be zero range of motion or visual acuity. Other examples of ratio data include time, weight, and income. Ratio data can be multiplied and divided to reveal proportions. For example, if a goniometer is used to measure elbow extension in a child with cerebral palsy, and the right elbow is measured at 160 degrees of extension, whereas the left elbow is measured at 80 degrees of extension, one could report that the right elbow extends twice as much as the left.

As you can see, each data type builds on the characteristics of those previously described. Nominal data are separated into categories; with ordinal data these categories can be rank-ordered; with interval data the values between categories are equal, but there is no zero starting point; and finally with ratio data, a real zero point exists. In healthcare research, ratio data are the most common type.

Parametric and Nonparametric Data

Interval and ratio data are known as **parametric data**, whereas nominal and ordinal data are **nonparametric data**. It is important to make this distinction so that you will know what kind of statistics can be used to manipulate your data. Although most of the descriptive statistics can be used on both parametric and nonparametric data (the exception being that mean and standard deviations cannot be used on nominal data), different inferential statistics must be used on the two types of data. This is because of the properties of the data, such as the data being ordered or the intervals between numbers being equal. Some tests are not powerful enough to cope with unordered, unequal data, whereas others are. Table 7-2 summarizes the categories of data with their corresponding parametric

Table 7-2 ■ Categories of Data With Corresponding Classifications and Statistical Tests

Category of Data	Classification	Appropriate Descriptive Statistics	Appropriate Inferential Statistics
Nominal (*named categories; unordered*)	Nonparametric	■ Frequencies ■ Percentages ■ Mode	■ Pearson's chi-square ■ Fisher's exact ■ Goodman & Kruskal's tau b
Ordinal (*ordered categories; unequal intervals*)	Nonparametric	■ Frequencies ■ Percentages ■ Mode ■ Median	■ Pearson's chi-square ■ Spearman rho ■ Wilcoxon rank sum ■ Mann-Whitney ■ Kruskal-Wallis ■ Kendall's tau
Interval (*ordered data; equal intervals; no zero starting point*)	Parametric	■ Frequencies ■ Percentages ■ Mean ■ Median ■ Mode ■ Range ■ Standard deviation	■ *t* test ■ Analysis of variance (ANOVA) ■ Analysis of covariance (ANCOVA)
Ratio (*equal intervals with zero point*)	Parametric	■ Frequencies ■ Percentages ■ Mean ■ Median ■ Mode ■ Range ■ Standard deviation	■ *t* test ■ Analysis of variance (ANOVA) ■ Pearson product moment correlation

and nonparametric classifications and types of statistical tests.

Parametric tests are appropriate when:

1. The sample is randomly selected, thereby helping to ensure the sample is representative of the population of interest, and that the variables being measured fall within the normal distribution for that population.
2. Variables are measured in a manner that generates interval or ratio data.
3. Random assignment or matching of study groups is completed, to ensure similarity between the two groups.

Conversely, nonparametric statistics should be used when:

1. Random selection has not occurred, so that the sample is not considered representative of the population of interest and variables are probably not normally distributed.
2. Variables have been measured in a manner that generates nominal or ordinal data.
3. The number of subjects in the sample is small.

Because nonparametric tests have less statistical power, substantial differences must be found between sets of scores before those differences are considered meaningful. Nonparametric statistics are frequently used in healthcare research because pathological human conditions are being studied. The variables of illness or pathology are often not distributed normally in the target population. Also, it is often difficult to locate many subjects with the requisite pathology, so samples tend to be smaller.

Descriptive Statistics

A great deal of quantitative data can be effectively analyzed using descriptive statistics. In fact, if a non-experimental research design is used, almost all of the data can be appropriately analyzed descriptively because of the lack of random selection or use of a control group. It is difficult to make inferences from a sample to a population of interest (the purpose of inferential statistics) if random sampling and control criteria have not been met. The initial description and compilation of data can be achieved using descriptive statistics—that is, providing the frequencies, percentages, and means for all the characteristics under study so that the reader has a thorough understanding of the subjects and variables. It is customary to present percentages alongside the frequencies, both in the text and in illustrative tables.

It is often useful to give the reader the group's average score—that is, their **central tendency.** The three measures of central tendency are the mean, median, and mode. The **mean** is the most common average and is computed by adding all the scores and dividing the total by the number in the group. The **median** is the midpoint among all the scores. Each score must be listed in order from the highest to the lowest, or vice versa, to locate the score that falls in the center. For example, a ranked order of IQ scores might be as follows: 150, 100, 98, 75, and 50. The median would be 98 because that score falls in the middle. For lists consisting of an even number of scores, it is protocol to calculate the mean, or average, of the two middle-most scores. Finally, the **mode** is the most commonly occurring score or answer. For instance, in a study of employment status on quality of life, subjects might be asked to indicate if they were employed full-time, part-time, or if they were unemployed. If the majority of respondents indicated they were employed full-time, this category would be the mode. It is also possible for there to be more than one mode

(bimodal)—say if equal numbers of participants were employed full-time and part-time. Each measure of central tendency has advantages and use is typically dictated by the type of data being analyzed. Salkind (2011) provides some additional guidelines:

- Use the mode when you have nominal data— namely data that are arranged in mutually exclusive categories.
- Use the median when your set of scores includes several outliers that will skew the mean.
- Use the mean when you have interval or ratio data that do not include outliers (p. 30).

The reader also may wish to know the spread or variability of scores. These descriptive statistics, known as **measures of variation**, include the range and standard deviation. The **range** is the simplest and is calculated by subtracting the lowest score in the set from the highest score. In essence, a range will explain the section of the continuum in which the subjects scored, perhaps IQ scores from 90 to 120, resulting in a range of 30. The range could have practical implications as in the following scenario: You are asked to conduct a therapeutic intervention on Monday for a class of 7-year-olds with a mean IQ of 100 whose scores ranged from 90 to 110; on Tuesday, you are scheduled to conduct the same intervention with a group of 7-year-olds with a mean IQ of 100 whose scores ranged from 60 to 120. In the second group, you might need more assistance or have to structure the session differently to meet the needs of children with a wider array of cognitive abilities.

Another way to describe variations is to use the **standard deviation**, referred to as s or SD. The standard deviation indicates how the scores are grouped around the mean. If your standard deviation is small, this is indicative of scores clustered close to the mean, whereas a larger standard deviation denotes a wider spread in scores. The standard deviation is also important when you want to determine consistency of a particular variable; a standard deviation of zero signifies no variability.

Inferential Statistics

Inferential statistics are used to draw conclusions or make inferences about the population of interest from a smaller chosen sample. They also help researchers to determine the probability of phenomena observed in the sample occurring in the larger population from which the sample was taken. If results are statistically significant, a researcher may decide that results can be generalized to the target population. Inferential statistics can be divided into three groups:

1. Those aimed at determining statistical significance
2. Those aimed at determining the correlation or association between two or more variables
3. Those that compare two or more sets of scores to determine the extent to which they vary among each other

Statistical Significance

In this group, the tests assist the researcher in deciding whether the changes in the mean pretest and posttest scores of the experimental group are, in fact, a result of the experimental treatment rather than chance. They allow comparison of results from the sample with that which was hypothesized as normally occurring in the population of interest. The tests can be used with a directional hypothesis or with a two-sided hypothesis. We will use the classic experimental research design as an example:

R	O_1	X	O_2
R	O_3		O_4

Statistical difference tests are applied to the scores from the pretest and posttest results of the experimental group (O_1 and O_2), and to the pretest and posttest scores of the control group (O_3 and O_4), and finally to the posttest scores of the two groups (O_2 and O_4). The first result indicates the degree of change following the experimental treatment; the second, changes following no treatment; and the third, the difference between end conditions of the experimental and control groups. If the difference between the scores on the third test (between O_2 and O_4) were statistically significant, it would indicate that changes can be attributed to the treatment rather than to chance.

Significance testing is based on the laws of probability. It answers the questions: What is the probability that this change occurred because of events in the research study, and what is the probability that this change would have occurred anyway, by chance? The tests that are used to make this determination result in a level of probability, and the researcher must decide whether or not this level is significant. In the social sciences, the usual convention is that 5 out of 100 occurrences of a phenomenon being caused by chance is a reasonable number to accept, and that any result better than that is statistically significant. This result would imply that you are 95% certain that the improvement in posttest scores was caused by the treatment. This probability level (or confidence level) is expressed as p "<" 0.05. Some scientific endeavors require more stringent proof, and a standard of p "<" 0.01, or a 1 in 100 chance that the phenomenon occurred by chance, is set for those studies, otherwise known as a 99% success rate. Ultimately, it is up to the researchers to determine the acceptable significance level for their study. See Box 7-3 for an example of statistical significance in an experimental design.

The tests most commonly used to determine significance levels are Pearson's chi-square test on nonparametric (nominal and ordinal) data and the student's t test on parametric (interval and ratio) data. The chi-square and t tests can be used to compare two groups on only one variable at a time.

Pearson's chi-square

The **Pearson's chi-square test** (X^2) is used to analyze categorical data (e.g., "How many subjects are men and how many are women?" or "How many have right hemiplegia and how many have left hemiplegia?"). Pearson's chi-square test may be used when you wish to know if there are significant differences between pretest and posttest scores for a given group, or if you wish to know if two groups are similar when you intend to use one as an experimental group and one as a control group. It can be used to compare groups on a single variable or on groups of variables, one at a time. This test is useful when the researcher is interested in similarities between groups of subjects. If the researcher can determine the numbers of characteristics such as gender, age, or diagnosis, a chi-square test on the subjects will test whether the sample matches the population. The calculated value for the chi-square formula is evaluated using standardized

BOX 7-3 ■ Example of Statistical Significance in an Experimental Design

Researchers in an outpatient physical therapy stroke center were interested in comparing the effects of the Bobath approach to constraint-induced movement therapy on recovery of functional arm movements in stroke patients (Huseyinsinoglu, Ozdincler, & Krespi, 2012). In their single-blinded randomized controlled trial, 22 patients were randomized into two groups. One group received classic Bobath treatment techniques, whereas the other group received constraint-induced movement therapy. Chi-square tests and Mann-Whitney U-tests were completed initially and revealed no significant differences between the two groups at baseline. A variety of standardized tests were employed in the study to measure motor control, hand function, quality of movement, and functional independence. Following the treatments, both groups demonstrated statistically significant improvements in function, indicating that the improvements could be attributed to the provided treatments. When statistics were used to compare the two groups post-intervention, results indicated that the constraint-induced movement group showed greater improvements in movement quality ($p = 0.01$) and quantity of use ($p = 0.003$).

tables that list critical values. When the chi-square exceeds the table value, the hypothesis is supported. In the case of Huseyinsinoglu et al.'s (2012) study of stroke patients, chi-square tests were used to compare the study groups on the characteristics of age, gender, time since onset, educational level, lesion type, and location and extent of paresis. No significant differences were noted among the groups at baseline, although the constraint-induced movement group contained slightly more individuals with paresis affecting their dominant side. During data analysis, statistics were used to determine if dominant-side paresis significantly affected improvements in quality and quantity of movement. P values ($p = 0.551$ for quantity of use; $p = 0.685$ for movement quality) indicate no effect.

t Tests

There are three different t tests, each of which is used with a different research design, but all compare the mean scores of two groups. The **single sample t test** compares the mean for a sample against a known population mean for a particular variable. This test is rarely used because the mean score for a population is rarely available. The **paired samples (correlated) t test** is used when subjects are compared with themselves (i.e., they serve as their own control) or when groups of individuals are compared after being matched on a particular characteristic. In this case, the pretest and posttest scores are compared for the first group and the two scores from the matched pairs are compared for the second group. In the **independent samples t test**, the pretest and posttest means are compared for the experimental and control groups, and the two posttest scores are compared. This is the most commonly used t test. If you have decided on a direction for your hypothesis, a one-tailed t test should be used to determine the significance of results. If a nondirectional hypothesis has been used, a two-tailed t test should be employed to determine the direction of the significance, if any. The t test is quite powerful and can be used on groups of subjects smaller than 30. Box 7-4 contains an example of a study employing t tests.

Wilcoxon rank tests

Wilcoxon rank tests can compare the degree and direction of differences between two groups and are particularly useful for small sample sizes, usually fewer than 30 subjects (Salkind, 2011). The **Wilcoxon signed rank test** is used on nonparametric data and is equivalent to the paired samples t test. It is performed on paired scores and will determine the significance of the difference between either pretest and posttest scores for individuals or scores on matched pairs of subjects. The **Wilcoxon rank sum test** is the equivalent to the independent samples t test, but is used on nonparametric data. For this test, ranks are assigned to scores for all subjects

---

BOX 7-4 ■ Example of Use of *t* Tests

Leerar et al. (2007) used independent *t* tests to determine if the quality of physical therapy documentation was impacted by four variables: patient diagnosis, patient age, referral source, and medical testing completed on the patient. No significant differences were noted on the *t* tests, leading to the conclusion that therapists likely have a set approach to documentation that they use regardless of specific patient characteristics.

---

in the study, and the ranks for all subjects in each group are summed. The test determines the degree of difference between group total scores. An example of a study utilizing a Wilcoxon rank test is included in Box 7-5.

BOX 7-5 ■ Example of Use of Wilcoxon Rank Test

Several occupational therapists were interested in examining social participation in psychiatric occupational therapy activity groups (Donohue, Hanif, & Berns, 2011). Specifically, they administered the *Social Profile,* a 39-item assessment in which levels of social participation are rated on a 6-point Likert scale, to participants before and after the intervention. Their sample consisted of 31 psychiatric patients who participated in social skills groups for 1 month. A Wilcoxon rank test was used in data analysis because the Likert scale ratings provided ordinal, nonparametric data. This statistical test revealed posttest scores were significantly (p "<" 0.0001) higher than pretest scores. Although this fact supports use of occupational therapy groups to improve social participation in psychiatric patients, the results have to be applied with caution because the sample was relatively small.

Mann-Whitney test

The **Mann-Whitney test** is another alternative to the *t* test for use on nonparametric data. It compares the means of two independent groups and is equivalent to the independent samples *t* test. See Box 7-6 for an example.

Tests for Correlation

Correlational tests determine the relationship between variables or sets of scores. The two sets of scores might be from one group of individuals or from two different groups of individuals. Once it is seen that one score moves up or down, the intent is to find out if the other score moves in a corresponding fashion. The objective is to find out how closely the scores covary; that is, whether they change together in a particular pattern, in a positive or negative way. If both scores increase together, they are said to be positively correlated; for example, height and weight scores for a group of subjects would probably increase together. On the other hand, if scores for ages over 60 years and scores for muscle strength were compared, age scores might increase whereas strength scores would likely decrease. These scores are said to be negatively correlated. The two sets of scores that are being compared in correlation testing can be

---

BOX 7-6 ■ Example of Use of a Mann-Whitney Test

In studying the effects of virtual reality gaming on dynamic balance and strength in older adults, Rendon et al. (2012) employed a Mann-Whitney *U* (P "<" 0.038) test to investigate differences between the control group and virtual reality group at baseline and after the intervention. Outcome measures included the *8-foot Up and Go* test, a balance confidence scale, and the *Geriatric Depression Scale.* These measures provided ordinal data (numerical scales used to rate fall risk, balance confidence, and feelings of depression); therefore, a Mann-Whitney test was appropriate and results revealed significant improvements in the intervention group.

---

entered on a scattergram to show the degree of correlation graphically. A scattergram is a graph on which two variables are plotted. For example, in the previous example, age can be plotted on the vertical axis and strength can be plotted on the horizontal axis to provide a visual representation of how scores are distributed.

Tests for correlation yield a statistic called a correlation coefficient, expressed as r. The r may range from –1 (indicating a perfect negative relationship) to +1 (indicating a perfect positive relationship). A zero indicates that there is no relationship between the two variables. Decimal factors are used to indicate r scores (i.e., 0.87 or –0.66). As with the previous tests, a level of significance can be computed for an r score. A review of some of the most common correlational tests follows.

Pearson product moment correlation

The most common correlation test is the Pearson product moment method, often called the **Pearson r**, which is used on parametric data. This test, which can be used on group scores or individual scores, indicates only systematic disagreements between scores and does not show the odd or occasional disagreement. It is often used to estimate reliability between tests, as in a test-retest situation, or between two raters to indicate interrater reliability. Box 7-7 includes a study that used Pearson correlations to determine the relationship between variables.

Spearman's rank correlation coefficient (Spearman rho)

The **Spearman rho** (denoted as ρ or r_s) is the equivalent to the Pearson r. It is used in descriptive research resulting in nonparametric data when items have been ranked and the researcher wishes to compare two sets of rankings to see if there is any type of relationship between them. Like the Pearson, it results in an r_s value falling between –1 and +1. It is important to remember that a relationship between two sets of scores does not indicate cause-and-effect. The researcher can claim only that a positive or negative relationship between the variables has been found, and no more. For example, researchers studying the effects of hippotherapy, which employs the motor and sensory features of horseback riding into therapeutic sessions, on balance deficits in

> **BOX 7-7** ■ **Example of Use of Pearson Product Moment Correlations**
>
> A correlational study was conducted by Tawashy et al. (2009) to see if there was a relationship between the physical activity level of individuals with spinal cord injury and their levels of pain, fatigue, and depression. Activity level (heavy, moderate, or mild) was measured using the *Physical Activity Recall Assessment* for individuals with spinal cord injury (PARA-SCI). Pearson correlations revealed that heavy intensity physical activity was strongly correlated with less fatigue ($r = -0.767$) and pain ($r = -0.612$), and increased self-efficacy ($r = 0.656$). For negative r values, the two attributes are inversely proportional; whereas, for positive r values, the two attributes are directly proportional. To clarify, it is likely that as physical activity increases, fatigue and pain decrease and self-efficacy increases. The researchers also found that mild physical activity was correlated with fewer symptoms of depression ($r = -0.565$) (p. 304). Although it might be easy to assume a cause-and-effect relationship, one must remember that correlations only define relationships and cannot prove causation.

children with movement disorders wanted to know if changes in balance correlated with functional performance (Silkwood-Sherer, Killian, Long, & Martin, 2012). They used a Spearman rho correlation to determine that a statistical association exists ($r_s = 0.700$); however, there was no correlation between change in balance and change in function ($r_s = 0.13$) (p. 707).

Simple regression analysis

Regression analysis is a technique that can be used after the correlation coefficient has been established. When a relationship is found between two variables, one can attempt to predict future scores for the dependent variable based on the scores on which the correlation coefficient was found.

Comparison of More Than Two Variables

The researcher often wishes to explore more than two variables in the same study. In this case, different statistical tests are needed.

Analysis of variance

Analysis of variance (ANOVA) is a statistical technique that can compare the mean scores of three or more groups in one study. If a study intends to answer multiple questions or is multi-factorial in nature, using the ANOVA may be most appropriate. For example, in a study of the effect of coordination training on tennis skills, the researchers randomized participants into experimental and control groups (Zetou, Vernadakis, Tsetseli, Kampas, & Michalopoulou, 2012). The control group received traditional tennis skills practice, whereas the experimental group received 20 minutes of a tailored coordination program in addition to the traditional practice. Backhand and forehand techniques were assessed via standardized observations before the training, after 8 weeks of training, and then again 1 week after the training ended. A one-way ANOVA was used to compare both the experimental and control groups at baseline; results revealed no significant differences. A two-way repeated measure ANOVA (2 study groups X 3 measures) showed significant interaction between the study groups and backhand or forehand assessments at three separate points in time. Thus, overall differences existed between the means of all the groups, but using analysis of variance alone will not reveal where the differences lie.

Specifically, the ANOVA yields an *F* ratio, which is evaluated using a standardized table to determine whether there is a significant difference between the largest and smallest of the study group means. If you wish to see if there are significant differences between any of the other means, you must use another test, known as a **post hoc comparison**. A variety of these tests exist including Tukey's honestly significant difference method, the Newman-Keuls test, the Scheffé comparison, Duncan's multiple range test, Fisher's Least Significant Difference, and the Bonferroni *t*-test (Portney & Watkins, 2009). Each test has different features, but detailed discussion is beyond the scope of this text. For more information, consult your statistical text or statistician. In the previous example, the Bonferroni post hoc comparison illustrated that the experimental group demonstrated better performance after the intervention (immediately after and 1 week after) than the control group, thereby supporting the hypothesis that coordination training can improve tennis skills.

Analysis of covariance

A similar test is the **analysis of covariance** (ANCOVA), which controls for initial differences between groups. If pretest scores reveal that the dependent variable is substantially different for the groups because of extraneous variables such as age or sex, an ANCOVA can take into account the extraneous variables by treating them as covariates and extracting their effect from the data. If the groups are made more equitable to begin with, the final results can be compared and judged more fairly. In Hunt and Bassi's (2010) factorial design study of the impact of simulated near-visual acuity levels and age on performance on cognitive assessments, they used an ANCOVA to control statistically for differences among the study groups including a range of actual visual acuities and pupil sizes. Without control of these factors, the researchers might have drawn different conclusions.

Kruskal-Wallis one-way analysis of variance

The **Kruskal-Wallis test** is equivalent to the one-way ANOVA and can be used on nonparametric data. Like other nonparametric tests, this test is based on rankings of scores on the dependent measure in which all subjects are put into one group during the ranking procedure and then put back into their original treatment groups for the remaining analysis. In Chiarello et al.'s (2010) study examining family priorities for activity and participation for children with cerebral palsy, the Kruskal-Wallis one-way analysis was one of the statistics employed. Children were grouped according to age ("less than" 6 years, 6–12 years, and 13–21 years), and were rated on gross motor skills. After family priorities were identified, the researchers wanted to determine if different priorities were found related to age and gross motor skills. Because both measurement data and nominal (categorical) data are included, analysis of variance could not be used because it is effective strictly with parametric data.

Multiple regression analysis

Regression analysis is a statistical technique used for making predictions about the study (dependent) variable by understanding the effects of two or more independent variables on the study variable. In essence, how much do the independent variables correlate with the dependent variable? Sometimes this procedure can be used to imply causal relationships; in other instances, it may be used to simply explore relationships. There are multiple types of regression analysis; the most common include **simple regression** (discussed in the previous section), which involves only one independent (predictor) variable, and **multiple regression**, which provides a methodology for determining how two or more independent variables can impact the dependent (study) variable. It is possible to take the procedure a step further by untangling the relative contributions of each of the independent variables. One can then use **stepwise regression** to look at the independent variables in various combinations to see which combination is most useful in predicting the occurrence of the study variable. See Box 7-8 for an example of a study where regression analysis was used.

BOX 7-8 ■ Example of Use of Regression Analysis

The aim of a recent study in sports medicine was to determine if physical activity can prevent age-related brain atrophy in the frontal and temporal lobes (Yuki et al., 2012). Specifically, the researchers wanted to find out if there was any association between the independent variables (individual activity energy expenditure, number of steps, and total energy expenditure) and the dependent variable (brain atrophy). They used multiple logistic regression to establish if any relationships existed among these factors while controlling for other factors including age, body mass index, medical and educational histories, and alcohol and tobacco use. A predictive relationship was noted with physical activity and total energy expenditure foretelling brain atrophy.

Only some of the many possible tests for manipulating data are reviewed here. A statistician will be familiar with other possibilities and will be able to advise you on the appropriate statistical tests based on your specific research design.

Statistical Software

All of the aforementioned tests can be computed by hand, but this is a tedious and time-consuming process and most people use a computer for statistical processing. With the help of a statistician or a computer assistant, researchers can enter the raw data into a computer program. It is also possible for the relative novice to perform the statistical manipulations via use of a statistical software package. Some of the most commonly used statistical software packages designed for the health and social sciences can be found in Table 7-3.

Reporting Data and Drawing Conclusions

In quantitative research, results should be reported in objective terms with no interpretation. Researchers should focus on providing a factual account of what happened during the study and what was actually found. Results can be discussed in narrative format or displayed in tables and figures, with further details provided on the formal written report in Chapter 12.

For experimental, quasi-experimental, or correlational research, the study will yield quantitative data, and inferential statistics can be used to determine if there are meaningful differences or similarities between groups. The probability ratios provide that information and indicate if the hypotheses have been substantiated. At this point, each hypothesis should be reviewed and checked against the statistical results. For each hypothesis, researchers should inform readers if the hypothesis was substantiated, give the probability level, and report the details of the findings. It is customary for results to be reported from the general to the specific. For example, in their study on the effects of virtual reality gaming on dynamic balance and strength in older adults, Rendon et al. (2012) reported "the Mann-Whitney test was used to determine significant differences (P "<" 0.05)

Table 7-3 ■ **Common Statistical Software Packages**

Software	Publisher	Website
Stata	StataCorp, LP 4905 Lakeway Drive College Station, TX 77845-4512	www.stata.com

SAS or STAT	SAS Institute, Inc.
	100 SAS
	    Campus Drive
	Cary, NC
	    27513-2414
		www.sas.com

SPSS	IBM Corporation
	1 New Orchard
	    Road
	Armonk, NY
	    10504-1722
		www.ibm.com

Minitab	Minitab, Inc.
	Quality Plaza
	1829 Pine Hall
	    Road
	State College,
	    PA 1680-3008
		www.mintab.com

NCSS	NCSS, LLC
	329 North
	    1000 East
	Kaysville,
	    UT 54037
		www.ncss.com

between groups at baseline and change in outcome measures over time" (p. 551). Comparison of the statistical results with the chosen probability level reveals that the virtual reality group demonstrated significantly improved balance ($P = 0.038$) and self-confidence with balance ($P = 0.038$) when compared with the control group (Rendon et al., 2012).

For survey, case study, or evaluation research, the study will generate descriptive quantitative data. The data should be reported using frequencies, percentages, ranges, and central tendencies, and can be discussed in narrative or presented in tables and figures.

It is up to the researcher to determine the most effective method for presenting these results.

In a nonexperimental study, data may have been subjected to one or more coding procedures. The results of the coding must be presented as clearly and simply as possible. In this type of presentation, it is the weight of the evidence that will determine if the hypotheses have been substantiated—a judgment the researcher must make because it is not possible to subject the evidence to statistical significance testing. Clearly delineating the coding methods so that they can be replicated and objectively applied allows the reader to have confidence in the study's analysis.

In quantitative research, discussion of statistical results and drawing of conclusions typically follows data analysis. Comparison of results to the literature review situates the current research within the context of previously conducted studies on the topic and allows the researcher to compare and contrast current results with prior ones. Practical implications for the findings, limitations of the study, and suggestions for future research are also considered. These sections provide the "take home message" of the research study, and readers unfamiliar with or intimidated by statistical methods and analysis may skip to these sections in an effort to draw useful information from the study.

Chapter Summary

Choosing an appropriate quantitative study design is but one piece of the research puzzle. Decisions must also be made regarding subject inclusion and exclusion criteria, recruitment of subjects, sampling methods, data collection, and data analysis. Some choices will undoubtedly be made out of convenience or logistical concern, whereas others will be based directly on a study's goals and topic of investigation. Considering all aspects well in advance of a study's beginning and collaborating with others can be keys to successfully conducting quantitative research.

SKILL-BUILDING TIPS

■ When contemplating features of your study's design, jot down your ideas and concerns. Discuss with your peers, advisors, or other professionals in your field for a period of several weeks. This process will help you to work out the bugs and ensure that you have a truly meaningful project that others will be able to understand.

■ Reflect on attrition (loss of subjects over time) when you are determining sample size and study procedures. Keep in mind that if the demands on subjects' time and skills are high or if the study is longitudinal in nature, the rate of attrition may be higher. Keeping demands low and soliciting subjects who have a vested interest in your topic can boost retention, but may have implications for application of results.

■ Pilot your data collection tools. This will help you to identify any glitches and can increase the study's usefulness by ensuring that you get the data you are aiming for. This may also help you to narrow your study's scope if you find that the tool is giving more information than what you are really concerned with.

■ If you are designing a survey, consider a course on the topic or consult one or more of the texts included in the reference list for this chapter. Use language appropriate for your sample; avoid technical jargon or vague terminology; check consistency of items, and be prepared to pilot and revise it several times. The extra effort will be worth it in the end, when you get the exact data you had hoped for.

■ Consider where you will store your study's data. Typically, approval by your school's or facility's Institutional Review Board (IRB) will be necessary before beginning your project. One of the things they will want to know is how you will keep the data private and protect the subjects.

■ Seek assistance with your statistical analysis. The best way to do this is to consult your advisor or a statistician in the design phase of the research. Remember: You need not be an expert in statistics to conduct meaningful research. Soliciting appropriate help is half the battle!

■ Be prepared to deal with criticism—constructive criticism, that is! Throughout the research process, you will be working with a variety of people—peers, advisors, clients, statisticians, professors, administrators, supervisors, and interdisciplinary team members, to name a few. Each one is likely to view your project from a different perspective and will have different suggestions. Bear in mind that everyone's aim is to assist you to strengthen your project and make it the best that it can be.

■ When drawing conclusions about your study, don't forget the difference between results that are clinically significant, or meaningful in "real life," versus those that are statistically significant. Statistical significance is necessary to apply your results to the entire population, but a positive outcome for only a few subjects still carries importance in the clinical world.

■ Finally, a solid research plan, although tedious and time-consuming to develop, will allow you to effectively investigate your topic. Don't rush the process; take time to contemplate your decisions and reward yourself for small successes along the way. Getting there is half the fun!

🔵 LEARNING ACTIVITIES

1. How will your project contribute to the body of knowledge in your chosen area?

2. What environmental, financial, or other situational factors will impact your study design and procedures?

3. Consider the sampling methods discussed in this chapter. Which one seems most appropriate for your topic and situation? Make a list of advantages and disadvantages of your proposed sampling method.

4. Who will support you in designing your research project? Consider financial, social, and physical supports as well as those who might advise you on content, procedures, and statistics.

5. Ponder how you envision your project taking shape—start to finish. Create a bulleted list of your methodology. Review this list with others to help identify any gaps in your plan.

REFERENCES

American Association of Public Opinion Research [AAPOR]. (n.d.). Resources for researchers. Retrieved from http://www.aapor.org/For_Researchers/4683.htm

American Physical Therapy Association [APTA]. (2005). *List of assessment tools used in pediatric physical therapy.* Alexandria, VA: APTA Section on Pediatrics.

American Statistical Association [ASA]. (2003). *When you consult a statistician. . . What to expect.* Alexandria, VA: ASA Section on Statistical Consulting.

Asher, I. E. (2007). *Occupational therapy assessment tools: An annotated index* (3rd ed.). Bethesda, MD: AOTA Press.

Benson, J., & Clark, F. (1982). A guide for instrument development and validation. *American Journal of Occupational Therapy, 36*(12), 789–800.

Burlingame, J., & Blaschko, T. M. (2009). *Assessment tools for recreational therapy and related fields* (4th ed.). Enumclaw, WA: Idyll Arbor.

Cape, P. (2010). *Questionnaire length, fatigue effects and response quality revisited.* Beijing: Survey Sampling International.

Chiarello, L. A., Palisano, R. J., Maggs, J. M., Orlin, M. N., Almasri, N., Kang, L., & Chang, H. (2010). Family priorities for activity and participation of children and youth with cerebral palsy. *Physical Therapy, 90*(9), 1254–1264.

Chudoba, B. (2011, February 14). How much time are respondents willing to spend on your survey? [Blog post]. Retrieved from http://blog.surveymonkey.com/blog/2011/02/14/survey_completion_times/

Converse, P. E. (1970). Attitudes and non-attitudes: Continuation of a dialogue. In E. Tufte (Ed.), *The analysis of social problems* (pp. 168–189). Reading, MA: Addison-Wesley.

Converse, P. E. (1974). Nonattitudes and American public opinion: Comment. The status of nonattitudes. *American Political Science Review, 68,* 650–666.

DeRouvray, C., & Couper, M. P. (2002). Designing a strategy for reducing "no opinion" responses in web-based surveys. *Social Science Computer Review, 20*(1), 3–9.

Donohue, M. V., Hanif, H., & Berns, L. W. (2011). An exploratory study of social participation in occupational therapy groups. *American Occupational Therapy Association Mental Health Special Interest Section Quarterly, 34*(4), 1–3.

Fink, A. (2009). *How to conduct surveys: A step-by-step guide* (4th ed.). Thousand Oaks, CA: SAGE Publications, Inc.

Fischer, J., & Corcoran, K. (2007). *Measures for clinical practice and research: A sourcebook two-volume set* (4th ed.). New York, NY: Oxford University Press, Inc.

Fowler, F. J. (2009). *Survey research methods* (4th ed.). Thousand Oaks, CA: SAGE Publications, Inc.

Henry, A. D., Nelson, D. L., & Duncombe, L. W. (1984). Choice making in group and individual activity. *American Journal of Occupational Therapy, 38*(4), 245–251.

Hunt, L. A., & Bassi, C. J. (2010). Near-vision acuity levels and performance on neuropsychological assessments used in occupational therapy. *American Journal of Occupational Therapy, 64*(1), 105–113.

Huseyinsinoglu, B. E., Ozdincler, A. R., & Krespi, Y. (2012). Bobath concept versus constraint-induced movement therapy to improve arm functional recovery in stroke patients: A randomized controlled trial. *Clinical Rehabilitation, 26*(8), 705–715. doi: 10.1177/0269215511431903

Ipathia, Inc. (2011). SuperSurvey [online computer software]. Longmont, CO: Author.

Johnson, T. P., & Owens, L. (2003). Survey response rate reporting in the professional literature. *American Association for Public Opinion Research—Section on Survey Research Methods,* 127–133.

Kimberlin, C. L., & Winterstein, A. G. (2008). Validity and reliability of measurement instruments used in research. *American Journal of Health-System Pharmacy, 65,* 2279–2284.

Leerar, P., Boissonnault, W., Domholdt, E., & Roddey, T. (2007). Documentation of red flags by physical therapists for patients with low back pain. *The Journal of Manual & Manipulative Therapy, 15*(1), 42–49.

Likert, R. (1932). A technique for the measurement of attitudes. *Archives of Psychology, 52,* 140–145.

Office of Management and Budget [OMB]. (2006). *Standards and guidelines for statistical surveys.* Washington, DC: Author.

Osgood, C., Suci, G., & Tannenbaum, P. (1957). *The measurement of meaning.* Urbana, IL: University of Illinois Press.

Portney, L. G., & Watkins, M. P. (2009). *Foundations of clinical research: Applications to practice* (3rd ed.). Upper Saddle River, NJ: Pearson Education, Inc.

Rendon, A. A., Lohman, E. B., Thorpe, D., Johnson, E. G., Medina, E., & Bradley, B. (2012). The effect of virtual reality gaming on dynamic balance in older adults. *Age and Aging, 41,* 549–552. doi:10.1093/ageing/afs053

Salant, P., & Dillman, D. (1994). *How to conduct your own survey: Leading professionals give you techniques for getting the reliable results.* New York: John Wiley & Sons, Inc.

Salkind, N. J. (2011). *Statistics for people who (think they) hate statistics* (4th ed.). Thousand Oaks, CA: SAGE Publications, Inc.

Silkwood-Sherer, D. J., Killian, C. B., Long, T. M., & Martin, K. S. (2012). Hippotherapy—An intervention to habilitate balance deficits in children with movement disorders: A clinical trial. *Physical Therapy, 92*(5), 707–717.

SurveyMonkey.com, LLC. (2012). SurveyMonkey [online computer software]. Palo Alto, CA: Author.

Tawashy, A., Eng, J., Lin, K., Tang, P., & Hung, C. (2009). Physical activity is related to lower levels of pain, fatigue and depression in individuals with spinal-cord injury: A correlational study. *Spinal Cord, 47*(4), 301–306. doi:10.1038/sc.2008.120

Walonick, D. S. (2010). *Survival statistics.* Bloomington, MN: StatPac, Inc.

Yuki, A., Lee, S., Kim, H., Kozakai, R., Ando, F., & Shimokata, H. (2012). Relationship between physical activity and brain atrophy progression. *Medicine & Science in Sports & Exercise.* Advance online publication. doi:10.1249/MSS.0b013e3182667d1d

Zetou, E., Vernadakis, N., Tsetseli, M., Kampas, A., & Michalopoulou, M. (2012). The effect of coordination training program on learning tennis skills. *Sport Journal, 15*(1), 1.

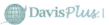 **DavisPlus** | For additional materials, please visit **http://davisplus.fadavis.com,** **key word: Hissong.**

Chapter 8

Qualitative Research Methodology and Design

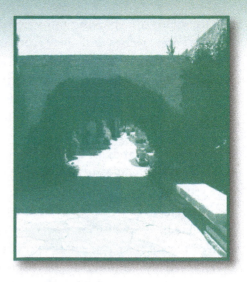

And the end of all our exploring will be to arrive where we started and know the place for the first time.

—T.S. Eliot

LEARNING OBJECTIVES

The information provided in this chapter will assist the reader to:

- Identify the characteristics of qualitative research.
- Explain the qualitative research process.
- Compare and contrast qualitative research theoretical perspectives, as well as designs.

Qualitative Research: Expectations, Potential, and Opportunities

Qualitative researchers are especially concerned with how people develop meaning out of their lived experiences. Qualitative research is the study of people and events in their natural contexts. Denzin and Lincoln (2008) propose that a great majority of topics, if not all of them, are appropriately suited for qualitative inquiry. The promise of the new frontier originates from researchers asking ordinary questions about their current practice and everyday life. Crabtree and Miller (1992) suggest the most efficient means of deciding if a particular topic should be researched from a qualitative perspective is to ask if the topic has a story that needs to be investigated and shared with larger communities of people. Furthermore, Rossman and Rallis (1998) point out the researcher must consistently be aware of the voice utilized in sharing the research with others. This voice is appropriately described as the interaction between the researcher and participant(s).

More specifically, Kliening and Witt (2000) feel that qualitative methodologies should be directed toward any research that is discovery-based. Patton (2002) suggests that qualitative researchers consider the following areas for inquiry: (1) individual experience(s); (2) meanings individuals place on their experiences; (3) individuals studied within their environmental contexts; and (4) a phenomenon for which standardized instruments have not yet been developed. A moderate amount of emphasis is placed on the participant being able to tell the story of his or her lived experience.

Although qualitative research used to be solely the domain of anthropology, history, and political science, in recent years other traditionally "quantitative" fields such as psychology, sociology, education, healthcare administration, and public health policy are utilizing qualitative methodology to investigate areas of strength and needs. In fact, it seems that many fields are "moving more toward phenomeno-logical approaches and away from experimental ap-proaches, thus becoming less precise but more real" (Yerxa, 2000, p. 201). As part of this movement, it has become apparent that qualitative research meth-ods and designs are useful to health professionals. In the 21st century there is a legitimate place in healthcare research for qualitative methods and there are phenomena within health care that can usefully be studied using naturalistic methods. In exploring client-related healthcare experiences with their clients and the process of therapeutic interaction, health-care practitioners' understanding can be significantly increased by conducting research that employs a naturalistic approach (Boxes 8-1, 8-2, and 8-3).

Constructs of Qualitative Research

Certain constructs cross boundaries among different types of naturalistic designs. These are pervasive qual-ities that are common to many qualitative research studies.

BOX 8-2 ■ Qualitative Research in Physician Assistant for the Nurse Practitioner

Tanyi, McKenzie, and Chapek (2009) con-ducted a phenomenological qualitative study to investigate how primary care family prac-titioners incorporate spirituality into their practices in spite of documented barriers. The team utilized semi-structured interviews and engaged 10 participants. Five major themes emerged from the interviews: (1) dis-cerning instances for overt spiritual assess-ment; (2) displaying a genuine and caring attitude; (3) encouraging the use of existing spiritual practices; (4) documenting spiritual care for continuity care; and (5) managing perceived barriers to spiritual care. The out-come of the study provided health profes-sionals with insight to providing spiritual care and options for future research.

BOX 8-1 ■ Qualitative Research in Athletic Training

Pitney (2010) conducted a phenomenological qualitative study to address how work-related demands can challenge an athletic trainer's professional role commitment for an extended period of time while working in a secondary school setting. The set criteria for participants included a minimum of 10 years of experience and a self-identified professional commitment. The study included 17 participants. Data col-lection included interviews, peer debriefing, and member checks. Four themes came from the inquiry: (1) professional responsibility, (2) rewards, (3) respect, and (4) rejuvenation. The conclusion of the inquiry was stated as, "a strong sense of professional responsibility to both students and the athletic training discipline is a central feature of professional commitment" (p. 198).

BOX 8-3 ■ Qualitative Research in Physical Therapy

Self, Driver, Stevens, and Warren (2013) were interested in determining physical activity knowledge, attitudes, intentions, and barriers among individuals with traumatic brain injury (TBI) undergoing outpatient rehabilitation. The qualitative method used was a survey case inquiry. Seventeen participants engaged in group interviews. The themes identified were (1) an inability to differentiate between physical activity and physical therapy; (2) a limited knowledge of physical activity benefits and the relationships to rehabilitation; and (3) an interest in participating in a physical activity-based health promotion program. Implications for practice and future research agendas for physical activity health promo-tion programming were discussed at length as an outcome of the study.

Naturalistic Settings

Qualitative research can be described in general terms as descriptive and naturalistic, with natural settings as the sources of data. Qualitative researchers spend the bulk of their time in the field (at the site of the study), observing and talking to participants, and gathering and analyzing data. They are greatly interested in learning about the participants within the context of the participants' own world. Because understanding the culture is of overriding concern, participants are observed and spoken with in their own environment while going about the usual business of daily life. Qualitative researchers are concerned with the process as well as the outcome of their studies. What happens during the study's data-gathering and analysis phase is crucial to the outcomes that will guide the healthcare professional's future engagement in practice.

Local Groundedness

Local groundedness means that the study is embedded in the participant's local, everyday life. One of the strengths of qualitative research is that the focus on naturally occurring, ordinary events in natural settings gives us a good handle on what "real life" is like for the participants in the study. This confidence in the data is assisted by local groundedness: the data has been collected in proximity to the specific situation under study, rather than through the mail or the telephone. The researcher's emphasis is on a specific case (person, place, event) embedded in its context. Thus underlying, nonobvious issues and local influences can be taken into account.

Phenomenological Perspective

Although many approaches can be grouped under the generic heading of "qualitative research," the phenomenological perspective is central to most qualitative researchers' outlook. The researcher has a primary interest in gathering or knowing more about the meaning of the participants' lived experience—from the participant's point of view. Glesne and Peshkin (1992) define the phenomenological perspective as follows:

> . . . since qualitative researchers deal with multiple, socially constructed realities or "qualities" that are complex and indivisible into discrete variables, they regard their research task as coming to understand and interpret how the various participants in a social setting construct the world around them. (p. 6)

Qualitative data place emphasis on people's lived experience and are thus well suited for identifying and locating the meanings people place on the events, processes, and structures of their lives (Box 8-4). Their perceptions, assumptions, judgments, and suppositions become clear and can be placed in context in the social world around them.

Adopting the phenomenological viewpoint lends itself perfectly to any study in which practitioners are concerned with the patients' perspectives on their own life or environment, or their view of their own particular situation, such as their illness and how they will cope with it.

Data as Thick Description

Geertz (1973) is credited with borrowing the phrase "thick description" when he was discussing a definition for "culture." He stated that culture can be viewed as interwoven systems of symbols and, as such, is a context within which social events, behaviors, institutions, or processes "can be intelligible—that is, thickly—described" (p. 14).

BOX 8-4 ■ **The Phenomenological Perspective**

Anderson (2011) adopted a phenomenological perspective throughout his investigation into the addictive behavior that contributes to, or is a result of, substance abuse. His study shed light on the 10 participants, gaining insight into their lives from their own viewpoint based on a self-management and recovering training program. The study's main outcome was that an internal locus of control contributed significantly to their recovery and the assumptions concerning substance abuse and treatment for the participants were felt to be relatable to other individuals experiencing the same program of recovery.

Qualitative data are rich and powerful with the potential for revealing complexity. These data provide "thick descriptions" that are vivid, are nested in a real context, and have a ring of truth that has a strong impact on the reader. They are usually collected over a sustained period of time, making them powerful for studying process (including history). Rather than gaining a snapshot view (such as that gained using the survey method), the researcher gets an intensely detailed view at the meaning of lived experiences, as related to the everyday healthcare needs of an individual, group, or community.

Lived Experience

Because naturalistic data emphasize people's lived experience, they are well suited for identifying the meanings people place on the events, processes, and structures of their lives. As the data gathering and analysis proceed, participants' perceptions, assumptions, judgments, and suppositions become clear and can be placed in context in the social world around them.

Power of Qualitative Data

A final feature of qualitative research is its power of data: it is the best strategy for exploring a new area and developing hypotheses; it has a strong potential for testing hypotheses; and it is useful when one needs to supplement, validate, explain, illuminate, or reinterpret quantitative data gathered from the same setting (Creswell, 2007). The power of stories and narratives collected directly from participants or by embedding oneself in the daily lives of the individual, group, or community leads to rich and powerful insights, related to a healthcare issue or a change in public health policy that may come from people who advocated for themselves.

Recurring Features of Qualitative Research

Although qualitative research may be conducted in dozens of ways, there are some recurring features of the methodology. A slightly modified version of a list of such characteristics by Miles and Huberman (1994) follows:

■ Qualitative research is conducted through intense and prolonged contact with a "field" or life situation. These situations are typically "normal" ones, reflecting the everyday life of individuals, groups, societies, and organizations.

■ The researcher's role is to gain a holistic overview of the context under study: its logic, its arrangements, its explicit and implicit rules. The researcher adopts a learner role, learning from the participants and their surroundings.

■ The researcher attempts to capture the perceptions of local actors from a phenomenological viewpoint, through a process of deep attentiveness, empathetic understanding, and suspending preconceptions about the topics under discussion.

■ Reading through the data, the main task is to explain the ways people in particular settings come to understand, account for, act on, and otherwise manage their day-to-day situations.

■ Many interpretations of this material are possible, but some are more compelling for theoretical reasons and because they meet the goals of the particular study.

■ Questioning occurs simultaneously with collecting information and making sense of it. One process drives the other and results in the reformulation and refinement of the problem and the structuring of smaller questions, which are then pursued in the field.

■ Relatively little standardized instrumentation is used. The researcher is essentially the main "instrument" in the study.

■ Most analysis is done with words. The words can be assembled, clustered, and broken into segments. They can be organized to permit the researcher to contrast, compare, analyze, and search for patterns and themes.

Qualitative Strategies

As more health professionals have come to embrace naturalistic research, it is useful to see what can be learned from the strategies employed by other disciplines. Some of these strategies are more useful than others for health care professionals. They are listed here to show some of the creative methods that investigators have used to study particular topics.

Health professionals can gain some ideas for their own needs by studying how others have tackled challenging study topics.

- **Ethnography:** Ethnographies are studies that attempt to describe a culture or aspects of culture. The ethnographer's goal is to share in the meanings that the cultural participants take for granted and then to depict the new understanding for the reader (Creswell, 2007).
- **Ethnography of Communication:** This style of ethnography focuses on gaining an understanding of the culture by studying all forms of communication within the culture, including verbal, nonverbal, and symbolic. Communication between the cultural participants is seen as the key to understanding the culture.
- **Ethnomethodology:** This term, coined by Harold Garfinkel, refers to the subject matter researchers will investigate. That is, they will study how individuals create and understand their daily lives; how people see, explain, and describe the world in which they live. The subjects for ethnomethodologists are people in our own society rather than members of primitive tribes. Researchers in education have been heavily influenced by Garfinkel's approach.
- **Phenomenology:** Researchers in phenomenology are studying culture from the informant's own point of view, emphasizing the subjective aspects of their behavior. They attempt to understand the meaning of events and interactions to ordinary people in particular situations, trying to gain entry into the conceptual world of their subjects in order to understand how and what meaning they construct around events in their daily lives (Creswell, 2007).
- **Unobstrusive (Nonreactive) Research and Observer Studies:** In these types of studies, the investigator takes the role of an observer, making an effort to be unobtrusive. The goal is to gather most of the data for the study solely through observation, thus influencing the participants and environment as little as possible; in this way, the investigator gathers "uncontaminated" data.
- **Participant Observation:** This research strategy builds on the observer strategy, in that the investigator does take part in the participants' world to some degree in order to obtain more data.
- **Interview Strategies:** These strategies include investigative journalism, biography, and oral history; the researcher interviews participants in order to learn about their personal experience.
- **Archival Strategies:** Archival strategies include literary criticism, historical research, retrospective, content analysis, and philosophical research, in which documents and artifacts are used to gather data.

The following four major research designs are particularly useful for the type of topics often studied by healthcare professionals: ethnography, case methods, phenomenology, and narrative inquiry. The ways to conduct these particular styles of research will be described in greater detail later in this chapter. Meanwhile, the following is a brief description of some of the features of these four designs.

The Ethnographic Research Design

The attempt to describe culture or aspects of culture is called *ethnography*. Some anthropologists define culture as "the acquired knowledge people use to interpret experience and generate behavior." Thus, culture embraces what people do, what people know, and things that people make and use (Creswall, 2007, p. 10). Using this perspective, a researcher might think about events in the following way: "Ethnography should account for the behavior of people by describing what it is that they know that enables them to behave appropriately given the dictates of common sense in their community" (McDermott, 1976, p. 159). It has been said that ethnography succeeds if it teaches readers how to behave appropriately in the cultural setting, whether it is among patients in a rehabilitation hospital, residents in a community residence, workers in a sheltered workshop, elderly patients in a day program, or psychiatric patients in a day treatment facility (Box 8-5).

The writing of ethnography can be seen as writing thick, detailed descriptions, as described earlier. When culture is examined from the perspective of thick description, the ethnographer is faced with

---

BOX 8-5 ■ Ethnographical Research Design

This study by sports and exercise physiologists provided insight into how mountain climbers stay motivated and overcome the obstacles that are inherent in the activity when they perform on the mountain. This ethnographic study explored the multidimensional experience of feel and motivation of a small group of Mount Everest climbers (N = 4) as they scaled the mountain in order to shed light on factors that sustained their drive toward reaching their goals. The results indicated that the climbers' motivation was influenced by the way they felt climbing once on the mountain. Differences and similarities between the lived experiences of the climbers, and their ability to regulate how they felt through preparation and how they responded to obstacles in order to sustain their motivation, are discussed (Burke, Bush, & Doell, 2011).

---

a complicated interpretation of a slice of life and an understanding of the community under study based on common sense. The ethnographer's goals are to share in the meanings that the participants take for granted and then to depict their new recontextualized understanding for outsiders.

The Case Method Research Design

Case studies in the health sciences tend to draw from other disciplines for their theoretical base and format. Anthropology, sociology, psychology, history, and business have cultivated the qualitative case method in the health care professions. As in other qualitative research methods, case methods can be differentiated according to their purpose and end product. Some are descriptive, some interpretive, and still others evaluative.

Other disciplines have traditionally taken a broad view of the case method, readily viewing "the case" as a naturally occurring group of people rather than as an individual. Health professionals, on the other hand, have more commonly used a single patient as

the case, and have only recently begun treating groups of people as cases or units of study. This change in attitude brings health professionals more in line with the disciplines that developed ethnographic, phenomenological styles of research and allows health researchers to use these research approaches to the case method in the way they were intended (Box 8-6).

The case method, then, can be used to study individuals or groups of individuals as a case series, such as a group of patients in a nursing home, a support group for caregivers of people with Alzheimer's disease, or a group of people at an Alcoholics Anonymous meeting. Case studies can also use one depository of documents or one particular event as a data source.

The Historical Research Design

It is interesting to note that Bogdan and Biklen (1982) have listed historical organizational case studies as a distinct type of historical study. These studies focus on a particular organization over time and trace the organization's development. Therapists can use this type of design to study, for example, the American Physical Therapy Association or American Massage Therapy Association and the history of licensure, treatment intervention, and practice standards. The task may be to use the historical research methodology to trace how and for what reason the organization came into being, who was involved in starting the organization, what events and changes have happened

---

BOX 8-6 ■ Case Study Research Design

Henshaw, Polatajko, McEwen, Ryan, and Baum (2011) conducted two in-depth case studies related to the usefulness of the Cognitive Orientation to daily Occupational Performance in stroke rehabilitation. The case studies describe in detail the process and outcome of the CO-OP. In both case studies, preliminary measures were administered in three initial encounters, followed by 10 CO-OP sessions and immediate follow-up testing. Field notes and a posttest interview were conducted in an effort to capture the participants' perspectives.

---

over time, what it is like now, and how it came close to being what professionals wanted it to be (Box 8-7).

The Narrative Analysis Inquiry Research Design

Bochner (2001) notes, "Narrative analysis inquiry honors individuals' stories as data that can stand on their own as pure description of experience, worthy of narrative documentary of experience or analyzed for connections between the psychological, sociological, cultural, political, and dramatic dimensions of human experiences" (p. 116). Patton (2002) presents the following as foundational questions of narrative analysis: "1) What does this narrative or story reveal about the person and world from which it came? and 2) How can this narrative be interpreted so that it provides an understanding of and illuminates the life and culture that created it?" (p. 115). These foundational questions are in contrast to phenomenology where interviews may take the form of stories; however, according to Patton (2002), the foundational question is, "What is the meaning, structure, and essence of the lived experience of this phenomenon for this person or group of people?" (p. 104). From these foundational questions it was gleaned that in narrative analysis the focus is on the *texture* of the story and the *culture* that shaped it. In comparison, the foundational question in phenomenology is focused on the *meaning* of the lived experience (Box 8-8).

Preparing for a Qualitative Research Study

To prepare for a qualitative study, the researchers must identify the problem they wish to study and generate research questions concerning the problem. Review the literature to gain an understanding of the depth and parameters of your problem, as well as other people's views on the topic. (It should be noted that some qualitative researchers disagree with this, believing that it is better to read after data collection to minimize their preconceived ideas.) You will need

---

BOX 8-7 ■ Historical Research Design

DeLany (1999) utilized an oral history method to discern "the learning paths of a purposive sample of African American women who held positions of prominence within a predominantly female Caucasian allied health profession [occupational therapy]. Specifically, it sought to understand the processes by which these women learned and developed throughout their life span; the personal, family, and societal expectations and support systems they experienced as well as the opportunities and barriers they encountered during their life span; and the strategies they employed to succeed in their educational and career paths" (p. iii). The dissertation is available in full-text at http://search.proquest.com.ezaccess.libraries.psu.edu/docview/304540347.

BOX 8-8 ■ Narrative Analysis Research Design

This narrative analysis inquiry addressed how mothers with inflammatory arthritis experience mothering occupations in the presence of arthritis and how this experience affects participation and occupational identity. The data collection included two interviews, participant observation, and document review. Analysis focused on the stories of the mothers and then there was a comparison of the group's stories to develop an overarching storyline. Storylines were presented as narratives that describe the mothers' experiences of identifying with the role of mother, participation, fatigue, and the social context in which mothering occurs. "Just because I can't do, doesn't mean I'm not a mom" emerged as the main storyline. The main theme of the stories as a whole was that the mothers' doing and knowledge offset many of the negative effects of arthritis (Smith, Suto, Chalmers, & Backman, 2011).

to formulate background material and decide on a theoretical base within which to design the study. Finally, you will choose a research design encompassing data collection and analysis techniques. Even the format for the final write-up should be considered in the early stages of the project. The early chapters of this book, therefore, are just as relevant to qualitative research projects as to quantitative studies.

General Components of Qualitative Research

All qualitative researchers tend to use similar principles, techniques, and approaches. When using a qualitative approach, the investigator will interview relevant people, observe various interactions and events, examine written documents, make decisions about the resulting information, and write a narrative for professional colleagues. As stated earlier, before a naturalistic researcher begins to ask the first question in the field, a problem, a theory or model, a research design, specific data collection techniques, tools for analysis, and a specific writing style will have been formulated.

Although researchers begin with planned research designs, naturalistic work tends not to be orderly. The researcher must be ready to follow where the data and the informants lead, which means being open to serendipity, creativity, luck, and a lot of hard work. In contrast to quantitative research, data collection and data analysis in qualitative research begin and continue simultaneously. Data collection typically yields an enormous amount of data, and a preformulated data analysis technique is needed to make sense of data.

The Problem

Qualitative research begins with a problem or issue of interest that guides the entire project. It will dictate the style of the research design, the data collection techniques, and even the presentation of the findings.

Theory

Similarly, no study, naturalistic or otherwise, can be conducted without an underlying theory or model. It may be a formal anthropological or psychosocial theory or a personal model about how things work, but

theory is crucial in the definition of the problem and in deciding how to tackle it.

A typical model for naturalistic studies is based on phenomenology. Because qualitative researchers are interested in allowing the participant to take an in-depth personal approach to being involved in the study, the phenomenological model allows them to adopt the view that all things are relevant only from the participant's perspective (Box 8-9). Phenomenologically driven studies are usually inductive; their results are generated from the study data, and few explicit assumptions are made ahead of time about study informants or events. Creswell's (2007) grounded theory method of analysis is entirely based on such an approach.

Other theories used to guide naturalistic studies include cognitive theory, which assumes that we can describe what people think by listening to what they say (using linguistically driven techniques), and cultural or personality theory, which encompasses psychoanalytic theory. Some qualitative researchers adopt materialist theories and view the world according to observable behavior patterns related to class consciousness, class conflict, social organization, and economic

---

BOX 8-9 ■ **Theoretical Perspective: Phenomenological Perspective**

Peed's (2010) study investigated the **resilience** from the perspective of individuals who have experienced it and utilized Giorgi's descriptive phenomenological psychological method. Purposeful sampling was utilized to find individuals who had experienced a traumatic motor vehicle accident and had survived and thrived through resilience. The individuals represented different years of age and gender. Open-ended guided interview questions were used, and the interview was audio recorded and transcribed for gathering data. Findings from the data were consistent with prior research on components of resilience, specifically spirituality, a sense of coherence, positive adaptation and temperament, locus of control, and self-efficacy.

forces. Theories need not be elaborate sets of constructs, assumptions, propositions, or generalizations. Healthcare professionals engaging in qualitative research may choose similar theories to those chosen for quantitative studies, which are often psychologically, sociologically, or medically oriented (Table 8-1).

Research Questions

Although the qualitative researcher will have developed some research questions during the research design phase, many more questions will typically be generated during the initial survey phase of field work. Research questions are fluid in qualitative research and they guide the flow of the inquiry. Some questions may be dropped as irrelevant; some may be modified as additional data are gathered; and new questions may be added as the study proceeds. In qualitative research, the final report may be written in the form of hypotheses with supporting material. In this case, researchers frequently request that others test their proposed hypotheses further, under different conditions, or they may do so themselves in later studies.

Table 8-1 ■ Variety in Qualitative Inquiry: Theoretical Traditions

Perspective	Disciplinary Roots	Central Questions
Ethnography	Anthropology	What is the culture of this group of people?
Autoethnography	Literary Arts	How does my own experience of this culture connect with and offer insights about this culture, situation, event, or way of life?
Reality Testing: Positivist & Realist Approaches	Philosophy, social, sciences, and evaluation	What's really going on in the real world? What can we establish with some degree of certainty? What are plausible explanations for verifiable patterns? What's the truth insofar as we can get at it? How can we stay a phenomenon so that our findings correspond, as much as possible, to the real world?
Constructionism and Constructivism	Sociology	How have the people in this setting constructed reality? What are their reported perceptions, "truths," explanations, beliefs, and worldview? What are the consequences of their constructions for their behaviors and for those with whom they interact?
Phenomenology	Philosophy	What is the meaning, structure, and essence of the lived experience of this phenomenon for this person or group of people?
Heuristic Inquiry	Humanistic psychology	What is my experience of this phenomenon and the essential experience of others who also experience this phenomenon intensely?
Ethnomethodology	Sociology	How do people make sense of their everyday activities so as to behave in socially acceptable ways?
Symbolic Interaction	Social psychology	What common set of symbols and understandings has emerged to give meaning to people's interactions?

Continued

Table 8-1 ■ Variety in Qualitative Inquiry: Theoretical Traditions—cont'd

Perspective	Disciplinary Roots	Central Questions
Semiotics	Linguistics	How do signs (words, symbols) carry and convey meaning in particular contexts?
Hermeneutics	Linguistics, philosophy, literary criticism, theology	What are the conditions under which a human act took place or a product was produced that makes it possible to interpret its meanings?
Narratology and Narrative Analysis	Social sciences (interpretive): literary criticism, literary nonfiction	What does this narrative or story reveal about the person and world from which it came? How can this narrative be interpreted to understand and illuminate the life and culture that it created?
Ecological Psychology	Ecology, psychology	How do individuals attempt to accomplish their goals through specific behaviors in specific environments?
Systems Theory	Interdisciplinary	How and why does this system as a whole function as it does?
Chaos Theory: Nonlinear Dynamics	Theoretical physics, natural sciences	What is the underlying order, if any, of disorderly phenomenon?
Grounded Theory	Social sciences, methodology	What theory emerges from systematic comparative analysis and is grounded in fieldwork so as to explain what has been and is observed?
Orientational: Feminist Inquiry, Critical Theory, Queer Theory, among Others	Ideologies: Political, cultural, and economic	How is X perspective manifest in this phenomenon?

From Patton, M. Q. (2002). *Qualitative research & evaluation methods* (3rd ed.). Thousand Oaks: Sage.

Participant Selection

Qualitative research can be characterized as an inquiry in which the researcher observes and questions participants in their own setting, to learn their perspective on things—a naturalistic inquiry. Therefore, researchers will use purposeful sampling to choose participants who can offer the fullest and most relevant information about the topic under study. In purposeful sampling, you must establish the criteria or conditions necessary to be included in the study, then purposefully choose a case or cases that match these criteria. The participants who turn out to be the most reliable and informative become the key informants.

Others may have useful information to add and will be seen as secondary informants.

There are several types of purposeful sampling in qualitative research and they are chosen according to the researcher's needs for a particular study. Some of the most popular types are:

- **Typical:** A case is chosen because it is thought to be like the majority (i.e., typical). For example, a therapist might want to see how a typical person with hemiplegia proceeds through a particular rehabilitation program.
- **Extreme or Deviant:** After the norm for a typical case is established, the researcher might want to

explore extreme cases in order to make a comparison; for example, a person with hemiplegia who does not complete the rehabilitation program or a person who completes the program in an extremely short time.

■ **Comprehensive:** A situation in which all the cases in a sample can be examined; for example, all the people with hemiplegia completing rehabilitation programs with a particular treatment regimen.

■ **Unique-Case Selection:** Selection is based on unique or rare attributes; for example, a person with double lower extremity amputations who becomes an athlete.

■ **Reputational-Case Selection:** A case is chosen on the recommendation of experienced experts, based on its reputation; for example, a highly successful caregiver support program for persons caring for a spouse with Alzheimer's disease. The program is recommended by an expert in caregiver support programs because of its excellent reputation.

■ **Comparable-Case Selection:** Selecting cases on the same relevant characteristics over a period of time in order to compare results for replication; for example, selecting one person with hemiplegia who successfully completes a rehabilitation program for each month over a 6-month program.

■ **Critical Case Selection:** The one case that makes the point dramatically; for example, a program succeeding in a particularly difficult location, a successful program with especially low overhead costs, or a rehabilitation program showing an extremely high success rate with severely disabled clients.

Data Collection

Often, the only data collection "instruments" used during qualitative research are the investigators themselves. Although some quantitative methods rely heavily on physical instruments such as paper and pencil tests or goniometry, qualitative researchers generally collect data via observation, interviewing, and tape recording in the field. Because they are the ones observing the events and asking the questions, they are considered the data collection "instrument."

Some of the actual processes for collecting data include observation, interviewing, filming, photography, and record and artifact review.

Data Analysis

Qualitative data analysis is the process of systematically organizing the field notes, interview transcripts, and other accumulated materials until you understand them in such a way as to address the research questions and can present that understanding to others. Several techniques can be used to analyze qualitative data; the technique chosen depends on the goal of the study. For example, if you wish to generate new theories about devalued people living in group situations, the grounded theory approach and its attendant techniques is suitable; if you wish to understand what participants perceive to be the curative factors in a helping group (Creswell, 2007), you can appropriately use a priori or a posteriori coding. Naturalistic researchers may even select specific techniques from different approaches for the same study, using their experience to judge what will best serve the project's goals.

Report Writing

Naturalistic reports generally take the form of long narratives, sometimes interspersed with pictorial presentations. There are many formats to choose from. Again, what you plan to produce with the data will lead you to the appropriate choice. If you are writing a thesis or dissertation, certain format and style conventions will prevail. If you are producing an article or research report, there may be more flexibility. However, as Wolcott (2009) points out, you will still need a beginning, a middle, and an end.

The beginning portion of the report should include a general background to help readers understand the focus of your article's design. The introduction often concludes with a description of the design of the rest of the article. The description should include a discussion of the research methods and techniques used, the time and length of the study, the number of settings and subjects, the nature of the data, where and how the documents were located, researcher-subject relations, checks on data, and other information that might help the reader evaluate the soundness of your study.

The middle of the article makes up the bulk of the work. This is where you argue your thesis, present your theme, and illuminate your topic. Everything in the core of the article should relate to the focus specified in the introduction. The material comes from the data analysis and can be organized around the patterns, themes, and relationships that arose from coding and categorizing the data. Use the most salient quotations you can find judiciously to illustrate the main points of the thesis.

The end section should be written as a conclusion. Often the focus is decisively restated, the arguments reviewed, and the implications elaborated. For more pointers, read Harry F. Wolcott's excellent booklet *Writing Up Qualitative Research* (2009).

Qualitative Research Designs

It is difficult to differentiate types of qualitative research designs in the same clear-cut manner in which quantitative designs can be specified and described. Qualitative designs do not have strict boundaries; the same researcher may use one set of procedures in one study and a different set in another, depending on the study's purpose. However, some qualitative designs have distinguishing characteristics and can be discussed as discrete entities. For an ethnography or historical study, for example, researchers may begin with different mindsets but may use the same data collection and data analysis techniques.

The designs we will consider are:

1. The ethnography research design, studying the culture within a program, institution, or other group setting.
2. The case method research design, studying an individual person, program, or institution.
3. The historical research design, studying a past event, a person or group of persons in the past, or the development of a phenomenon such as a profession or an organization.
4. Narrative analysis inquiry as a research design in which a narrative or story is revealed about the person and world from which they came. The

story is then interpreted to understand and bring forth the life and culture that created it.

Research Design: Ethnography

Strict ethnography, as opposed to simply applying ethnographic techniques and approaches, is the art and science of describing a group and its culture. The description may be of the healthcare system in another country or of an inner-city clinic in urban America. Ethnography is characterized by the concept of culture as the organizational or conceptual principle for interpreting data.

The ethnographic research design originated in the field of anthropology and has occasionally been borrowed by health scientists to describe such settings as hospitals, special schools, sheltered workshops, and group homes. There has been a growing interest in healthcare research to find paradigms that relate to the holistic nature of the client, environment, and everyday living patterns.

Ethnographers, of course, have biases and preconceived ideas about the group under study, just as other researchers do. Controlled biases can focus and limit the study, whereas uncontrolled biases can undermine the quality of the research. The first task of ethnographers is to make specific biases explicit to themselves and, eventually, to the readers. Ethnographers try to achieve an open mind before going into the field because they are vitally interested in understanding and describing events and perspectives from the study participants' point of view, the emic perspective. This is crucial to ethnography.

The research design for ethnography will list each step of the study in sequence, guiding the investigation toward an effective solution to the identified problem. Each step will build knowledge and understanding about the nature of the people or organization under study. Fieldwork is the main element of any ethnographic research design. The researcher will go out to the scene to meet the informants in their own setting, to observe events in context, and to view the environment itself. All fieldwork is exploratory, aimed at finding out as much as possible about the site, as well as the participants and their lives.

Fieldwork

The early stages of fieldwork are concerned with learning the basics about the culture. Let's say the culture under study is a particular rehabilitation department where an innovative, complex treatment regimen has been introduced. The ethnographer is trying to determine the long-term effect on the staff, the patients, and the overall functioning of the department, including its relationships with the rest of the facility and with other similar facilities. In the initial fieldwork, the researcher focuses on learning about the basic structure and function of the culture (the department, facility, and similar facilities); how many people are involved and something about their demographics; the relationships between all the people involved in the program; the language used by patients, staff, and administrators; and some historical data about the department and previous treatments.

The first few sessions at a fieldwork site can be awkward and painful for a researcher. Bogdan and Biklen (1982) have some suggestions to make this an easier time:

■ Do not take what happens in the field personally. What you are going through is a typical part of the fieldwork process.
■ Set up your first visit so someone is there to introduce you. One of the people who gave you permission [would be a good person to] do it. . . .
■ Don't try to accomplish too much the first few days. Ease yourself into the field. Have your first day be a short visit (an hour or less); use it as a time to get a general introduction and overview. . . .
■ Remain relatively passive. Show interest and enthusiasm for what you are learning, but do not ask a lot of specific questions, especially in areas that may be controversial. . . .
■ Be friendly. The first days in the field, subjects will ask about why you are here. Repeat what you told the people who gave you permission. . . but try to use abbreviated explanations. Most suggestions on how to behave in the field parallel the norms governing nonoffensive behavior in general. . . (p. 127).

Once the ethnographer feels comfortable with baseline data on the culture, data collection and analysis begin in earnest. A distinct line is rarely drawn between baseline data gathering and "real" data collection; all of the information is usually used in the data analysis. How long baseline data collection takes varies enormously, depending on the investigator's previous knowledge of the culture, the complexity and size of the culture, and the complexity of the problem being studied.

Similarly, the amount of time spent in overall fieldwork varies significantly, depending on the same factors. The data for some very simple studies may be collected during 1 day per week for 6 weeks, for example, whereas a comprehensive study of a complex culture may take 2 or 3 years full-time in the field. The latter are typical anthropological studies of foreign cultures in distant lands, whereas the former are more typical of the recent ethnographic studies, sometimes called microethnographies, being undertaken by our colleagues in therapeutic environments. Most ethnographic studies probably fall on a time line somewhere between the two.

Ethnographers in the field do their best to be unobtrusive. They try to blend in with the routines and appearance of the "natives," be they members of a foreign culture or therapists in a rehabilitation facility. Although ethnographers attempt to minimize their effect on the setting, a stranger who is asking questions and watching activities will always have some impact. Investigators need to keep a careful record of their own behavior to assess its possible influence on informants and the ensuing data collection.

The first problem in fieldwork is to gain access to the population under study. If it is impossible to get permission to enter the field, some researchers conduct covert or undercover research, collecting data without the subjects' knowledge. This approach was used very successfully in a classic study of a mental hospital in which the researchers had themselves admitted as patients. This approach is not recommended for new ethnographers, however; you will be more successful reaping the advantages of being free from the constraints of a regular participant, gaining access to a variety of informants, and, perhaps most importantly, not having to deceive others and risk the embarrassment of being caught.

As to the degree to which you should participate in the activities of the setting, you may choose from a continuum ranging from one of a complete observer role to one of an active participant observer role. The complete observer does not participate in any activities and looks at the scene as though through a one-way mirror. At the other end of the continuum is the field-worker who is deeply involved in the site activities, with little discernible difference between the observer and the informants. Most field-workers settle on a role somewhere between these two extremes. If you are observing a classroom or a treatment setting, it is often inappropriate to take part in the teaching or treating. On the other hand, informants may ask you to act as an assistant; this may be perfectly suitable and not distract you from your task of observing. In the latter case, though, the students or patients will view you in a certain way—as other than solely an observer—and this must be accounted for in the data analysis.

Data-Gathering Techniques

There are several ways to gather information during ethnography fieldwork. The two most important techniques are observation, together with the resulting field notes, and interviews. Others include photography and examination of written documents and artifacts.

An important consideration is how to decide what and when to observe, whom to interview, how many and which documents and artifacts to examine, and what to photograph. In ethnography, this is the question of participant selection or internal sampling. If the focus of the study is narrow, you may be able to talk to all the subjects in the setting, review all the documents, or observe all the important events. If you are unable to do this, it is important to sample a range of people and materials, so that you have a diversity of perspectives on the setting.

Some informants are more willing to talk, have a greater experience in the setting, or are especially insightful about what goes on. These people become key informants and probably will be interviewed more frequently and for longer periods than other participants. Events and activities that are deemed important

because they offer insight into the culture will be selected for observation; they are called *key events*. Some examples might be dinnertime in a group home for mentally challenged adults or the weekly staff meeting in a physical therapy department. Similarly, some documents, such as treatment plans or minutes of staff meetings, may be extremely fruitful and deserve more time than other documents. Photographs can be used to take inventories of objects in a setting, and are also useful in reducing the need for descriptive field notes of those objects. They might include such things as a bulletin board, the writing on a blackboard, or the arrangement of furniture.

Often the timing of the ethnographer's visits affects the nature of the data collected. It is important during the initial fieldwork period to find out as much as possible about routines, when certain events happen, and who attends. Selecting when to observe and interview, or time sampling, will depend on the study's purpose. If the goal is to gain a perspective on the overall functioning of a rehabilitation department or of a group home, then the investigator should sample widely from different times of the day, week, and year. If, on the other hand, the goal is to gain insight into the morning meeting on a psychiatric ward, sampling should obviously occur during the morning meeting, perhaps 5 days per week over a several-week period.

Choices about sample selection are always made in the context of the study, with an eye toward achieving the goals for this particular study. The researcher often steps back during the study and asks, "If I go in now, if I talk to this person, what will I miss? What will I gain?" Ethnographers realize that choices are being made throughout the study that will affect the data collected and, therefore, the results of the analysis. They simply use their best judgment in making those choices.

Leaving the Field

During the first few days in the field, you will probably feel awkward. As time progresses, you will become more comfortable and can do your job more easily. Eventually you will have accomplished your goal and the time will come for you to leave the field. Leaving can be quite difficult, as you likely will become interested in the setting and fond of the participants. It is not uncommon to feel as if you are deserting people you have come to know well, especially if they are working under difficult conditions with a devalued population. You may also feel that you will miss something important to the study once you stop visiting the site.

In any event, you must eventually tear yourself away. As health care professionals, we can use our knowledge of the termination process to leave gracefully, giving the informants due warning and easing out of the setting gradually. Frequently, ethnographers are asked to return to the setting at a later date to report on the findings, and occasionally it is necessary to return to collect some missing data. Otherwise, researchers need to recognize when they have reached the point of data saturation (when any new data collected simply repeats data they already have) and to say their good-byes.

Research Design: The Case Study Method

In the healthcare setting, case studies are used when we want to learn from individual clients, understand certain issues and problems in our clinical practice, and form professional and managerial policy. A case is a unit of study. This unit is often an individual, but may also refer to a situation, a family, a hospital ward, a nursing home, or any group setting.

Novice researchers are often advised to choose a case study as their first research project because case studies tend to be more "doable" than some other types of qualitative research. Although case studies vary in complexity, it is possible to design one that is confined to one site or one person, that has a time limit, and that has a limit on the sources of data (such as the participant, records pertaining to the participant, and the participant's therapist). This keeps collected data to a manageable amount so that analysis can be accomplished in a relatively short time. Also, the smaller volume of resulting material permits the study to be written up more easily than would a study generating a large volume of data.

Perhaps most commonly, the single-client case method design uses an ethnographic approach. The goal is to gain an understanding of that particular client's issues and circumstances, frequently concerning the person's disability and how it was overcome, so that our colleagues can better treat other clients in similar circumstances. Data-gathering techniques for a case method study are the ones that have been previously described, such as observation, interviewing, videotaping treatment sessions or the client's achievements, and reviewing related artifacts such as assistive technology. Documentary evidence is likely to play an important part in a case study; it may consist of patients' charts, minutes of meetings, reports of case presentations, patients' assessments and progress reports, or even institution newsletters and administrative memoranda.

Denzin and Lincoln (2008) describe the design of a case study as best represented by a funnel, the beginning of the study being the wide end, represented by researchers scouting around for possible sites or people they might wish to study and finding a few possibilities. They make a wide search to increase their chances of finding just the right case. Once they have found several possible sites, they collect some initial data, perhaps documents or an initial interview and observation. The researcher then studies the data, focusing in on the more promising aspects of the site. The researcher makes decisions about the study's direction, which participants they might eventually interview, which documents to access, and which events to observe. The researchers may discard some initial ideas and formulate new ones as they go along, modifying the design and choosing procedures that will enable them to learn more about the topic. Eventually, they decide which individual or event will be studied; now they have developed a focus. The data collection narrows at this point to the particular topic under study—putting the researcher at the narrow end of the funnel.

When conducting an ethnographic case study, the investigator must consider the following tasks: (1) studying the case in its naturalistic setting; (2) being concerned with meaning from the participants' point of view; (3) viewing the case from a longitudinal perspective; (4) using multi–data-gathering techniques; (5) reviewing the data, both alone and with the participant(s), to explicate the ways by which these particular people understand, account for, take action, and manage their day-to-day lives; (6) decontextualizing the data according to the study's goals; and finally, (7) analyzing and recontextualizing the data that is ready for presentation to colleagues.

Data are analyzed using the usual qualitative research analysis techniques. However, in a strictly case study approach, analysis is more than an intensive, holistic description of a person's circumstances. Rather, concern will be shown for the client's cultural context. Wolcott (2009) has made a distinction between simply using ethnographic techniques to study a case and performing an ethnography.

Sometimes the major data-gathering technique in case studies is participant observation. If the focus of the study is an organization, the researcher must decide which aspect of the organization to study. For example, if the organization under study is a rehabilitation hospital, the researcher may decide on a particular place within the hospital (such as the ward for people with quadriplegia); a specific group of people within the organization (such as the people with quadriplegia on that ward); or a specific activity or event within the organization (such as the daily routine of the people with quadriplegia on that ward).

Research Design: Historical

The goal of the historical research design, or historiography, is the same as those for many other qualitative research designs (i.e., to present a holistic description and analysis of a specific phenomenon whether it be event, person, or organization). Current behaviors or attitudes can often be better understood if the past is reviewed and examined in the light of current events. Thus, historical research is undertaken to test hypotheses or to answer questions about past events that may shed light on present behaviors or practices.

Schwartz and Colman (1988) presented the debate about whether individuals other than historians can perform historical research in their own professions. They held that therapists can learn historiography and are thus in a good position to examine the development of their own professions. A number of excellent

historical studies have been recorded in occupational and physical therapy literature. Loomis (1983) and Litterst (1988) have described the historical development of two schools of occupational therapy. Oral histories exploring the occupational and leisure history of women leaders have been used to identify the qualities that contribute to women's emergence as leaders (AOTA, 1977–1980). Gutman (1978) has described the influence of the U.S. military and occupational therapy reconstruction aides in World War I on the development of occupational therapy. One therapist has proposed that the origins of graded activity in occupational therapy lay in tuberculosis sanatoria of the late 1800s (Creighton, 1993). Another researcher posited that 19th-century practices of moral treatment and phrenology contributed to a loss of caring attitudes and actions in the treatment of mental illness (Peloquin, 1993). In physical therapy, Moffat (1994) has proposed the idea that therapists look to the evolution of their profession to decide whether they can move on to achieve their professional dreams or whether their past will thwart those dreams.

Historical research uses prescribed techniques for the collection, organization, and analysis of historical data. These include critical investigation of past events, careful weighing of evidence regarding the validity of sources, and interpretation and documentation of the investigation (Kerlinger, 1979). The historical researcher asks open-ended questions of individuals (or examines documents or artifacts) about a past event; uses thorough prior knowledge of the event to interpret the answers; and recontextualizes and documents the event in an interwoven narrative, thus providing the reader with a new explanation from which current events can be understood.

Thus, a historical study involves much more than making a chronology of an event. To understand an event and apply one's knowledge to present practice means knowing the context of the event, the assumptions behind it, and perhaps the event's impact on an institution or participants, both then and now. A good historiography, like any good research design, relies on asking well-formulated questions, identifying reliable sources of information, verifying evidence, and accurately interpreting data.

At the basis of the historical study lies a clearly formulated, precisely worded research question clarifying what information the researcher is seeking. Historical research questions tend to have several components, dividing the topic under study into its various parts. As with other research designs, care should be taken not to have more questions than can comfortably be answered in one study and not to ask questions outside the scope of the particular study.

The data for a historiography come from primary sources and secondary sources. A **primary source** is an original account of an event, such as an eyewitness account, minutes of a meeting, a photograph, or a treatment plan and progress notes written by a client's therapist. A **secondary source** is a source of information at least one step removed from the original source, for instance, a newspaper account (if the reporter did not actually observe the event), a book by another historian, a clinical consult by a consultant who has not seen the client. A basic rule of historiography is that data sources should be predominantly primary sources, though an occasional secondary source may be used for back-up. Facts get biased and altered in the telling from one person to the next; the greater the distance from the original source, the more distorted the story. The historian lacks the accuracy and perspective of the eyewitness; even the veracity of the primary source should be checked, as far as that is possible.

At the core of historical research is *hermeneutics*, the study of historical texts, from the Greek *hermeneutikos*, meaning the clarification of what is unclear (Patton, 2002). Often, written documents are the only source of data available for historical research. If this is the case, it is particularly important that the investigator conduct an initial search to be sure there are sufficient primary sources to support a worthwhile study.

There are various ways of obtaining historical documents. Reviewing a town's newspapers or an institution's newsletters are easy ways to get started. However, you will probably get access to even more material by letting it be known, perhaps in your association newsletter, that you are interested in old letters, scrapbooks, minutes of meetings, and so on. Once you have found the first source, that person will lead you to others and you will soon find yourself with a network of informants. Libraries, archival collections, museums, government offices, and private papers are all good sources of primary data (Schwartz & Colman, 1988).

One of the first tasks of the historian is to determine which data in the primary sources are actually facts and which are opinions or distortions. Facts are seldom stated in their pure form; they are usually mingled with the opinions of the source. The historical researcher must also assess the veracity of the data, while selecting only data that are relevant to the research question.

Interpreting data is an exceedingly difficult process, but doing it well is critical to the study's success. The researcher needs a sound understanding of the data, based on well-formulated inferences and logic, in order to formulate a good analysis. Because historical researchers cannot go to firsthand informants for verification of their analyses, as other qualitative researchers can, the burden is on them to check their work for integrity and logic.

When documents are the only source of data, the researcher cannot confirm that one event in the past caused another to occur. In this case, the investigator must make assumptions or draw inferences that assign causality. The more information uncovered about an event, the more likely the possible cause of the event will become known. Investigators must be careful to restrict interpretations about causes to the evidence gathered. Of course, if the investigator is fortunate enough to have access to persons who were involved in the event being studied, then triangulation can be used—checking one source of data against another for accuracy. Causality is a controversial subject among historians; studies obviously cannot be conducted under the controlled conditions of experimental research, and all variables are ex post facto. Most historical researchers confine themselves to describing conditions surrounding events and exploring associations that suggest emerging patterns and themes (Schwartz & Colman, 1988). Two further tasks of historians are generalization and argumentation. What distinguishes a historian from a collector of historical facts is generalization—the ability to discern commonalities or patterns in the data and to infer a general principle from them. This is achieved through a similar process to that used by Glaser and Strauss (1967) in their description of formulating grounded theory. Like the grounded theoretician's approach, the historian must make logical generalizations that are based on sufficient data and do not go beyond the scope and nature of the data.

Historical researchers will make inferences from the data that will form the basis of an argument. Argumentation is their way of proceeding from an initial premise to an end argument (using inferences along the way) in an orderly and rational manner. The argument represents the researcher's understanding of the data. It is expected that the historian will approach the data with an open mind and let the facts shape the argument. The argumentation forms the major portion of the written report resulting from a historiography. Schwartz and Colman (1988) feel that a final report should include an introduction, a statement of the problem, an identification of the assumptions and limitations of the research, a literature review, and a discussion of the findings (the argumentation). The report should take the form of a narrative and should describe and analyze the answers to the research question.

Recently, the volume of historical research in healthcare professions, particularly in physical and occupational therapy, has increased. These professions' rich heritage offers many opportunities for historical explorations. The more we probe our background, our roots, the more we will understand and be able to put into context our present practice.

Research Design: Narrative Analysis

Bochner (2001) notes, "Narrative analysis honors individuals' stories as data that can stand on their own as pure description of experience, worthy of narrative documentary of experience or analyzed for connections between the psychological, sociological, cultural, political, and dramatic dimensions of human experiences" (p. 116). Researchers may ask themselves, "How do stories you gather in a narrative analysis inquiry differ from the stories you gather in a phenomenological or ethnography inquiry?" The

answer is that it is not the stories but rather the interpretation of the intact story offered by the participant which is at the heart of narrative analysis (Leiblich, Tuval-Mashiach & Zilber, 1998; Patton, 2002). It is about listening to and attempting to make sense of individuals' learned and lived experiences through their personal stories. It relates to coming to know that storytelling is at the core of an individual's being (Wilcock, 2002).

It is the goal of narrative analysis inquiries to collect data that describes daily life (Clandinin & Connelly, 2000). Denzin (1989) offers the following description of a narrative:

> A narrative is a story that tells a sequence of events that are significant for the narrator and his or her audience. A narrative as a story has a plot, a beginning, a middle and an end. It has an internal logic that makes sense to the narrator. A narrative relates events in a temporal, causal sequence. Every narrative describes a sequence of events that have happened. (p. 37)

Within this and every narrative inquiry, the systematic study of narratives (stories) informs the researcher about the participants and the world they live in (Patton, 2002). Wilcock (2002) and Bloom (2002) suggest it is within the rich description of narratives where the participants truly come to know about their being and experience their becoming. Narrative research allows participants to speak for themselves.

Narrative analysis is typically selected as the methodology for a study because it allows for a concentrated focus on and the telling of an individual's life within their cultural environment. Simply asking general questions and seeking general meaning can be problematic secondary to the complex and contextual nature of the texture of an individual's life.

As Bruner (1990) asserts, it is the forging of links between the exceptional and the ordinary where the uniqueness of narrative inquiry blossoms. He states, "When you encounter an exception to the ordinary, and ask somebody what is happening, the person you ask will virtually always tell a story that contains reasons" (p. 49). Riessman (1993) expands on the same notion by stating, "Respondents narrativize particular experiences in their lives, often where there has been a breach between the ideal and real, self and society" (p. 3). The motivation for conducting a narrative inquiry is to actively put into text the tensions, solutions, and creation of new ways for individuals to consider personal stories of occurring in their everyday living.

Chapter Summary

This chapter discussed the main principles in qualitative research and described some of the qualitative designs. If you are planning to engage in qualitative research, now is the time to decide which design and data collection and analysis techniques will best serve your purpose.

SKILL-BUILDING TIPS

■ When you are completing a large project, such as a research study, it is important to relax, pause, assess where you are, make a plan for where you are going, breathe, and move forward each day. Even if it is cleaning up your space or writing one page, don't allow procrastination to come into your life.

■ When you feel like you can't write one more page, try to construct a diagram, write a poem, find a saying, or complete a drawing that supports what you are trying to get across with your research. This stimulates more thoughts and eases the flow of thoughts to move forth in the research process.

■ Embrace the chaos instead of being fearful of what is yet to come. It is typical for there to be many books and many pages of written work piled up in your work space. Instead of being overcome by the flood of information, embrace the knowledge and skills that you are gaining. Breathe. Take the process one day at a time.

■ It is helpful to make up a daily task schedule to post at your work space. For example, if you want to have all of your participant interviews completed by April 30, transcripts reviewed by May 30, so you can schedule a focus group with all participants by mid-June, put that on a task schedule, print it on bright yellow paper, and post it on the bulletin board right in front of your desk.

■ If you get stuck in the actual research process or with writing up the outcomes, take a moment to write down the obstacles in your path. Don't sit with a "stopper" too long; instead, identify it so you can move forward as quickly as possible.

● LEARNING ACTIVITIES

1. What research methodology do you think best suits your qualitative study and why? List five points of your preferred research methodology that will assist you in designing and carrying out your study.

2. Can you identify at least three resources that will assist you in carrying out your study?

3. What environmental factors are influencing the route you are taking with your qualitative research endeavor?

4. As you know qualitative research begins with the researcher's interests and perspectives. What is bringing you or calling you to complete this specific qualitative study?

REFERENCES

AOTA. (1977-1980). *The visual history series*. Bethesda, MD: Archives of the American Occupational Therapy Association.

Anderson, D. (2011). *The perceived therapeutic attributes of the SMART program from persons in seasoned recovery. ProQuest Dissertations and Theses*, n/a. Retrieved from http://search.proquest.com/docview/366657178?accountid=13158

Bloom, L. R. (2002). Stories of one's own: Non-unitary subjectivity in narrative representation. In S. B. Merriam & Associates, *Qualitative research in practice: Examples for discussion and analysis*, (pp. 289–310). San Francisco: Jossey-Bass.

Bochner, A. P. (2001). Narrative's virtues. *Qualitative Inquiry 7*, 131–157.

Bogdan, R. C., & Biklen, S. K. (1982). *Qualitative research for education: An introduction to theory and methods*. Boston: Allyn & Bacon.

Bruner, J. (1990). *Acts of meaning*. Cambridge: Harvard University Press.

Burke, S. M., Bush, N. D., & Doell, K. (2011). Exploring feel and motivation with recreational and elite Mount Everest climbers: An ethnographic study. *International Journal of Sport and Exercise Psychology, 8*(4), 373.

Clandinin, D. J., & Connelly, F. M. (2000). *Narrative inquiry: Experience and story in qualitative research*. San Francisco: Jossey-Bass.

Crabtree, B. F., & Miller, W. L. (1992). *Doing qualitative research*. Thousand Oaks: Sage.

Creighton, C. (1993). Looking back: Graded activity: Legacy of the sanatorium. *American Journal of Occupational Therapy, 47*(8), 745–748.

Creswell, J. W. (2007). *Qualitative inquiry and research design: Choosing among five traditions* (2nd ed.). Thousand Oaks: Sage.

DeLany, J. V. (1999). *African-American women in a predominantly Caucasian female profession: Learning paths to positions of prominence.* The Pennsylvania State University. *ProQuest Dissertations and Theses, 1-259.* Retrieved from http://search.proquest.com/docview/30454034

Denzin, N. K. (1989). *Interpretive biography.* Newbury Park: Sage.

Denzin, N., & Lincoln, Y. (Eds.). (2008). *Handbook of qualitative research* (3rd ed.). Thousand Oaks: Sage.

Geertz, C. (1973). *Thick description: Toward an interpretative theory of culture.* New York: Basic Books.

Glaser, B. G., & Strauss, A. L. (1967). *The discovery of grounded theory: Strategies for qualitative research.* New York: Aldine De Gruyter.

Glesne, C., & Peshkin, A. (1992). But is it ethical? Learning to do it right. In *Becoming qualitative researchers: An introduction* (pp. 109–125). White Plains, NY: Longman.

Gutman, S. A. (1978). Looking back. Influence of the U.S. military and occupational therapy reconstruction aides in World War I on the development of occupational therapy. *American Journal of Occupational Therapy, 49*(3). 256–262.

Henshaw, E., Polatajko, H., McEwen, S., Ryan, J. D., & Baum, C. M. (2011). Cognitive approach to improving participation after stroke: Two case studies. *The American Journal of Occupational Therapy, 65*(1), 55.

Kerlinger, F. N. (1979). *Behavioral research.* New York: Holt, Rinehart & Winston.

Kliening, G., & Witt, H. (2000). The qualitative heuristic approach: A methodology for discovery in psychology and the social sciences. Rediscovering the method of introspection as an example. *Forum: Qualitative Social Research.* Retrieved from http://www.qualitative-research.net/fqs

Lieblich, A., Tuval-Mashiach, R., & Zilber, T. (1998). *Narrative research: Reading, analysis and interpretation.* Thousand Oaks: Sage.

Litterst, T. A. (1988). *Boston School of Occupational Therapy.* Unpublished paper.

Loomis, B. (1983, April). Professional occupational therapy education in Chicago, 1908–1920. Paper presented at the Written History Committee Symposium, *American Occupational Therapy Association Annual Conference,* Portland, OR.

McDermott, R. (1976). *Kids make sense: An ethnographic account of the interactional management of success and failure in one first grade classroom.* Unpublished doctoral dissertation, Stanford University.

Miles, M. B., & Huberman, A. M. (1994). *Qualitative data analysis: An expanded sourcebook* (2nd ed.). Thousand Oaks, CA: Sage.

Moffat, M. (1994). Will the legacy of our past provide us with a legacy for the future? *Physical Therapy, 73*(11), 1063–1066.

Patton, M. Q. (2002). *Qualitative research & evaluation methods* (3rd ed.). Thousand Oaks: Sage.

Peed, S. L. (2010). The lived experience of resilience for victims of traumatic vehicular accidents: A phenomenological study. ProQuest Dissertations and Theses, n/a. Retrieved from http://search.proquest.com/docview/219925648?accountid=13158

Peloquin, S. M. (1993). Looking back. Moral treatment: How caring practice lost its rationale. *American Journal of Occupational Therapy, 48*(2), 167–173.

Pitney, W. (2010). A qualitative examination of professional role commitment among athletic trainers working in the secondary school setting. *Journal of Athletic Training, 45*(2), 198–204.

Riessman, C. K. (1993). *Narrative analysis.* Newbury Park: Sage.

Rossman, G. B., & Rallis, S. F. (1998). *Learning in the field: An introduction to qualitative research.* Thousand Oaks: Sage.

Schwartz, K. B., & Colman, W. (1988). Looking back. Historical research methods in occupational therapy. *American Journal of Occupational Therapy, 42*(4), 239–244.

Self, M., Driver, S., Stevens, L., & Warren, A. M. (2013). Physical activity experiences of individuals living with a traumatic brain injury: A qualitative research exploration. *Adapted Physical Activity Quarterly, 30*(1), 20–39.

Smith, L. D. F., Suto, M., Chalmers, A., & Backman, C. L. (2011). Belief in doing and knowledge in being mothers with arthritis: Occupation, participation and health. *Occupational Therapy Journal of Research, 31*(1), 40.

Tanyi, R., McKenzie, M., & Chapek, C. (2009). How family practice physicians, nurse practitioners, and physician assistants incorporate spiritual care in practice. *Journal of the American Academy of Nurse Practitioners), 21*(12), 690–697.

Wilcock, A. (2002). *Occupation for health volume: A journey from prescription to self health.* London: College of Occupational Therapists.

Wolcott, H. (2009). *Writing up qualitative research* (2nd ed.). Thousand Oaks: Sage.

Yerxa, E. J. (2000). Occupational science: A renaissance of service to humankind through knowledge. *Occupational Therapy International, 7,* 87–95.

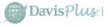 For additional materials, please visit **http://davisplus.fadavis.com, key word: Hissong.**

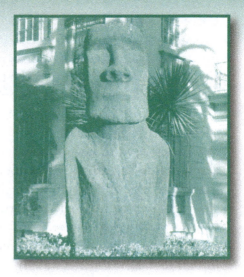

Chapter 9

Technical Aspects of Qualitative Research

Much to-do about the details, just try to be kind to yourself and remain focused.
—A. Hissong

LEARNING OBJECTIVES

The information provided in this chapter will assist the reader to:

- Understand the structure of a qualitative research study.
- Identify the need for assumptions, scope, limitations, subject criteria, and selection of participants for a qualitative study.
- List and explain data collection techniques in qualitative research.
- Understand the constructs of analyzing, reporting, and drawing conclusions related to qualitative research.

Establishing Boundaries for the Qualitative Research Study

A qualitative research study needs to be given boundaries and to be put into a suitable context for readers. Readers should be able to understand quickly where a study fits into the scheme of professional literature. They should also be made aware of any of the author's assumptions about the underlying principles of the study, glean the limitations of the study, and know if there are any overriding issues that are likely to influence the outcomes or interpretation of the outcomes. Finally, readers should be able to find the meanings of all terms used if they are not obvious. This information will enable readers to understand the qualitative researcher's general intentions and to follow the researcher's train of thought. The research report should include sections on the study's definition of terms, assumptions, limitations, subject criteria, and selection.

Assumptions and Limitations

The first step in establishing a study's boundaries is to think about your own assumptions regarding the study and the premises upon which it is formulated. Researchers customarily examine their assumptions carefully and state them to the reader near the beginning of the study. Readers need not agree with your assumptions but are able to follow the logic of your propositions and to understand why you approached the study as you did.

Assumptions are underlying principles that the researcher believes or accepts but that are difficult to

115

prove in any concrete way. In qualitative research, they are basic values or views about the world. They include such values as the notion that people are basically good or that people want to function independently in their day-to-day activities. These ideas are very difficult to prove with the population at large or even with a small research group. Two kinds of assumptions need to be examined: first, assumptions about the ideological principles upon which the study is based, and second, assumptions that are made concerning the processes used in the study. People adhere to certain ingrained principles that will affect the way they approach situations and, therefore, the way they design research studies. Making your assumptions known in the early stages of describing a study is important so the readers know where you stand on issues related to the research and where they should keep a critical eye on processes. Box 9-1 is an example of a researcher's assumptions for a narrative inquiry related to mothers living in a rural community and

their nurturance or care of self with the environmental variables.

Remember, only beliefs that are difficult to prove concretely, beliefs that are untested or untestable hypotheses, basic values, or views about the world should be included in the assumptions section.

Next, the research should identify the limitations of the study. Continuing with the example of the narrative inquiry conducted with mothers in a rural community, the researcher her identified the following limitations (Box 9-2).

Now that the researcher has identified the defining terms, assumptions, and limitations of the qualitative study, it is important to precisely define the parameters of participant criteria and selection of who will engage in the inquiry.

Participant Criteria and Selection

At this point, a word about the participants in your qualitative research project is in order. Although most

---

BOX 9-1 ■ Example of Assumptions of a Study

The following were the major assumptions that the researcher held as she entered into an inquiry from a feminist poststructuralist lens:

- For research to be valid and useful in the everyday lives of individuals, those individuals must actively participate and be actively represented in all aspects of the research process.
- The feminist poststructuralist perspective of constantly shifting identity (nonunitary self) is an empowering notion for women living in the 21st century.
- The process of motherhood has not been researched adequately in terms of the overall positive and negative effects it has on the health and well-being of women.
- The feminist poststructuralist theory is a powerful and meaningful lens to view the deconstruction of power and discourse within women's lives.

- Individual understanding of, and the engagement in, meaningful occupation is a positive aspect of personal health and well-being.
- The primary researcher is always present in the inquiry and the final product.
- Attending to my feminist poststructuralist sense of being, I am going into this research project thinking and feeling that the participants will want to speak for themselves in the data collection and data analysis section of this dissertation.
- The unique relationship that exists between researcher and coresearchers in a narrative inquiry presents a unique set of ethical considerations that reflect the unique relationship between researcher and coresearchers.
- An inquiry should challenge beliefs of *truth* that have held some women in bondage for generations—knowledge production outside of the box is empowering and emancipating.

qualitative studies, particularly those investigating the efficacy of treatment, use individuals to supply the evidence, some studies may also rely on documents, records, and verbal reports as evidence. Thus, data may be in the form of people's thoughts, beliefs, actions, or written materials. It is important that your readers know from which population the sample you studied came and how they were selected.

Let's examine purposeful sampling, which is a primary identifier of qualitative research. Patton (2002) states, "Qualitative inquiry typically focuses in depth on relatively small samples, even single cases (N = 1), selected purposefully" (p. 230). The participants for a qualitative study share a specific set of characteristics or criteria that have been established by the researcher. For example, for one study a researcher may recruit 24 physician assistants working in the United States who are from 40 to 60 years old working in a small private clinic to study the bias or philosophical thoughts about flu immunizations. For another study, a researcher may recruit 24 physician assistants from a regional area in Texas to specifically study the outcomes of work-related injuries and intervention within this specific part of Texas.

Primarily, the participant criteria of a qualitative study are determined from the researcher's guiding questions, which are informed by the literature review. Participant selection criteria are established gradually, as the assumptions and theoretical base of the study unfold. Additionally, in qualitative studies, the criteria are dictated by the theory behind why a researcher feels the intervention being studied will be helpful. For example, in a study that involves clients' compliance in the use of splints at their place of employment might include such information as the subjects' type of employment, how long they have been absent from their jobs, and any previous treatment they received for carpal tunnel syndrome.

Once the participant criteria are decided, the researchers use a qualitative study to actively and purposefully seek out individuals to engage in the research process with them. The researchers might, for example, set the criteria of the participants as adults in a specific rehabilitation system who have left hemiplegia, are between the ages of 45 to 65, who are dependent in dressing, and have lived alone for more than 5 years to be engaged in the research study. The goal is for the study to be useful in practice to as many similar individuals or groups as possible. The study is not intended to be replicated as is, but the parameters are clearly defined if someone else wants to conduct a similar study with a different set of participants, in a different geographical area, or under a different theoretical frame of reference or theory. Continuing with the study example in this chapter, in Box 9-3 you will see how the researcher defined parameters for participants.

Now that the assumptions, limitations, and participant selection criteria have been established for the study, the researchers begin to think about the data collection process.

Data Collection Procedures for Qualitative Research

In 2013, some skeptics still felt that qualitative research, by its very nature, cannot be reliable, that is, replicated to produce similar findings from study to study. Others find that validity, determining the extent to which conclusions effectively represent subjects' reality, is difficult to assess in a qualitative study.

BOX 9-3 ■ Example of the Participant Selection Criteria

Specifically, the selection of the participants in the rural mothers study was based on the following criteria:

1. Have at least two school-aged children;
2. Is over the age of 35;
3. Currently lives in, or has lived for 80% of her life in, a rural, religiously conservative, and patriarchal-driven community;
4. Work 20 or more hours outside of the home;
5. Identify self as the primary caretaker of children and household management;
6. Identify that motherhood has had an impact on learning about or the engagement in self-nurturance;
7. Identify that current or past religious affiliation has had an impact on learning about and engaging in self-nurturance;
8. Identify that living in a rural community has had an impact on learning about or engagement in self-nurturance;
9. Identify that issues of patriarchy in their family and community has had an impact on learning about or engagement in self-nurturance;
10. Identify that within the past year they have attempted a routine, course, or program related to self-nurturance for their mind, body, or spirit.

Most qualitative researchers ignore such criticisms, whereas others recognize that the credibility of their findings may be called into question and develop practices to address the criticism.

The information in this chapter will now move into the many reasons and ways qualitative research is a validated and valuable method of inquiry. Let's begin by addressing validity and reliability, and then conclude by providing the reader with a perspective on analyzing, reporting, and drawing conclusions from qualitative research data.

Validity

Many qualitative researchers feel that, contrary to the criticisms raised, validity is the strength of a qualitative study. This is especially true when one compares qualitative research to experimental studies, surveys, and other quantitative designs. Typically, the quantitative researcher gathers data in an "unreal" setting, asking subjects to perform in a contrived manner for a relatively short period of time. The qualitative researcher, in contrast, goes to the participants, observes them in their natural environment over a long period of time, and asks for their thoughts and opinions. Frequently, questions and observations are guided by what the participants feel is important and relevant, and data analysis is shared with individuals to see if it "feels right" before the researcher comes to any conclusions. Thus, as one can see, the qualitative study may be more likely to achieve validity than the quantitative study.

Steps can be taken to further the likelihood of a valid study. Qualitative researchers must decide, first, how much confidence to place in their own analysis, and second, how to present their analysis so that readers can validate and verify the findings for themselves. It is important to remember that, through a data analysis, one presents only a perspective on the data, and not the "truth." There are several ways to go about the task of validating and verifying that perspective. The six notions presented here are based on the work of Patton (2002) and Guba and Lincoln (2008).

Rival Explanations

Once the analyst has identified and described patterns, themes, and linkages from the data, it is important to look for rival or competing themes and linkages. This can occur inductively, by looking for other ways to organize the data that might lead to different findings; or it might be done logically, by thinking of other logical possibilities and seeing if these possibilities can be supported by the data. Failure to find strong supporting evidence for alternative themes or linkages helps increase the analyst's confidence in the original findings. There is unlikely to be clear-cut support for the alternative themes; rather, one must consider the weight of the evidence and look for the best fit between the data and analysis. Alternative themes that were considered should be noted in the write-up, as this will lend credibility to the final findings.

Negative Cases

Once patterns have been described, our understanding of those patterns can be increased by studying the instances and cases that do not fit within the patterns—the negative cases. For example, in a large rehabilitation program in which the majority of the participants complete the program and return to work, the most important analysis may be an examination of the program dropouts. Readers may then decide for themselves the plausibility of the reasons why dropouts do not fit the usual patterns.

Triangulation

Triangulation is the process of using different data-collection techniques to study the same program. Two kinds of triangulation contribute to validating and verifying qualitative data analysis: (1) checking for consistency of findings generated by different data collection methods, such as a survey and an interview; and (2) checking for consistency of different data sources using the same data collection method (e.g., obtaining verbal accounts of the same event from two people). Triangulation tests the quality of information gained and may be useful in putting findings in perspective.

Design Checks

The validity of findings in qualitative research may be compromised if there are flaws in the data-collection techniques. Nontypical events or occasions may be observed when the intent is to observe typical activities; problems may be caused by the people who were selected for observations or interviews; and problems may be caused by the time periods used for observations. It is important to acknowledge any such flaws in the write-up and to limit conclusions to those situations, people, and time periods sampled in the study.

Participant Reactions to the Analysis

Investigators can learn a great deal about the accuracy, fairness, and validity of their data analysis by having the people in the study react to what has been described. The analysis is credible only if it "feels right" to the participants. The participants' reactions can be included in the final write-up as an indication of the validity of the study findings.

Intellectual Rigor

The thread that runs through the previous suggestions for verifying and validating qualitative data analysis is the investigator's intellectual rigor. The effective investigator returns to the data over and over again to confirm categories, patterns, themes, and linkages, and to reexamine any interpretations to see if they really reflect the nature of the program or activity being studied. As Patton (2002) notes, "Creativity, intellectual rigor, perseverance, insight—these are the intangibles that go beyond the routine application of scientific procedures" (p. 339).

A great deal of rigor and detailed focus goes into qualitative research data collection. Furthermore, the data collected from a qualitative study is consistently guided by the theory and methodology that inform the study at its onset.

Reliability

Qualitative research reliability is more difficult to achieve than is validity. Generally speaking, reliability is concerned with replicability; it requires that a researcher using the same data collection and analysis techniques can obtain the same results as those of a previous study. **External reliability** addresses the issue of whether two different researchers would arrive at the same final themes and theories in the same study setting; **internal reliability** refers to the extent to which other researchers, given a set of previously generated codes and constructs, would match them with interview data and field notes in the same way the original researcher did.

Because qualitative research is concerned with naturalistic behavior (which is seldom repeated in the same way) in a unique setting and occasion (which will never be repeated because it is unique), replication for the purpose of establishing reliability is a tall order. Problems with uniqueness and idiosyncrasy may lead to the claim that qualitative studies can never be replicated; however, there are ways in which researchers can acknowledge and address issues of reliability. The following notions are based on the work of LeCompte and Goetz (1982).

External Reliability

Qualitative researchers can enhance external reliability by addressing five major problems: researcher status position, informant choices, social situations and conditions, analytic constructs and premises, and data collection and analysis techniques.

Researcher Status Position

No qualitative researcher completely replicates the findings of another because different researchers hold different social roles within the studied group and begin with different knowledge bases about the studied group. This problem can be eased by clearly identifying in the study report the researcher's role and status within the group investigated and the degree to which the researcher becomes involved with informants (i.e., where they fall on the spectrum between nonparticipant observers, with no personal relationships with informants, and participant observers who develop friendships that provide access to special knowledge).

Informant Choices

This concerns the problem of identifying the informants who provide the data. Different informants represent different interest groups within the study group. When researchers associate with one particular group, they may forfeit information from people in other groups, who may not be comfortable associating with the first group. Additionally, people who gravitate toward researchers or are sought out by researchers to be informants may be atypical of the rest of the group. For instance, they may be chosen because they are introspective and insightful about their own lives, a characteristic that might not be found in other members of the group. Threats to reliability posed by informant bias can be handled by careful description in the research report of those who provided the data. Such descriptions should include personal characteristics relevant to the research, as well as those that make the informants similar to or different from the rest of the group.

Social Situations and Conditions

The social context in which data are gathered may influence external reliability. Informants may not feel free to reveal certain information in some social environments. For instance, a patient interviewed may give one set of information while receiving treatment in the hospital but other information when interviewed at home after discharge. The informants may also be influenced by whether they are interviewed alone or in a group. Thus, it is important to state the social setting in which the data are gathered.

Analytic Constructs and Premises

Even if a subsequent researcher were to reconstruct the relationships and duplicate the informants and social contexts of a previous study, replication would be impossible if the constructs, definitions, or units of analysis of the former study were unclear. Analysts writing up their research must make clear the underlying assumptions, theoretical base, choice of terminology, and data collection and analysis techniques if a later researcher is to be able to replicate the study successfully.

Techniques for Data Collection and Analysis

Replicability is impossible without precise identification and thorough description of the strategies and techniques used to collect data. It is tempting to use shorthand descriptors because of the brevity that journals often require in manuscripts. Unfortunately, shorthand descriptors are not yet universally accepted by qualitative researchers; consequently, their use can lead to serious misunderstandings. More importantly, the strategies used for analyzing data are often poorly defined or not described at all. This is probably because the analytic process used with qualitative data is often vague, personal, intuitive, and idiosyncratic to the analyst. Researchers must specify their data collection techniques and their analytic strategies to ensure reliability within the study.

Internal Reliability

Internal reliability in a qualitative study concerns whether, within a single study, multiple observers agree. It is particularly important when several qualitative researchers plan to investigate the same problem at different sites, such as might be seen in an ethnographic inquiry. The important matter within internal reliability is that of **interrater or interobserver reliability**—the extent to which meanings held by multiple observers are sufficiently congruent that they describe phenomena in the same way and arrive at the same conclusions about them. Agreement is sought on the description or composition of events rather than on the frequency of events. The following five strategies are commonly used to reduce threats to internal reliability: low-inference descriptors, multiple researchers, participant researchers, peer examination, and mechanically recorded data.

Low-Inference Descriptions

Most guides to the construction of qualitative researcher field notes distinguish between two types of field notes. Low-inference descriptions, phrased in terms as concrete and precise as possible, include verbatim accounts of what people say as well as narratives of behavior and activity. The second category of notes may be any combination of high-inference interpretive comments and varies according to the analytic scheme chosen for the study.

Low-inference notes provide researchers with their basic observational data. Interpretive comments are then added, deleted, or modified, but the basic record of who did what under which circumstances remains unchanged. This basic material is analyzed and presented in excerpts to substantiate inferred categories of analysis. Studies rich in primary data, which provide the reader with multiple examples from the field notes, are generally considered most credible.

Multiple Researchers

The most effective guard against threats to internal reliability in qualitative research is the presence of multiple researchers. Ideally, investigations are conducted by a team whose members discuss the meaning of what has been observed until agreement is reached. The discussion period is regarded as training in interobserver agreement. However, most studies are conducted by a single researcher or pairs of researchers rather than larger teams or single researchers, because of funding constraints and because some qualitative research is often considered too time-consuming and labor-intensive for lone researchers. Two researchers who achieve interobserver reliability are considered preferable to a sole researcher for achieving internal reliability.

Participant Researchers

Some researchers enlist the help of informants to confirm that what the observer has seen and recorded is being viewed identically and consistently by both participants and the researcher. Sometimes participants serve as arbiters, reviewing the field notes to correct researcher misperceptions and misinterpretations. Other researchers work in partnership with participants, keeping two sets of accounts of observations and comments.

Quite commonly, researchers ask for reactions and feedback to their ongoing analyses from participants.

Peer Examination

Researchers may corroborate their findings with other researchers in three ways. First, they may integrate descriptions and conclusions from other researchers in their final report. Second, findings from studies conducted concurrently at multiple sites may be analyzed separately, and then compared. Similar findings across sites would support the reliability of observations. Third, the publication of study findings indicates that the material is offered for peer review and a debate of the findings is encouraged.

Mechanically Recorded Data

Qualitative researchers use a variety of mechanical devices to record data, such as audiotape and videotape recorders and cameras. The idea is to record and preserve as much of the data as possible, so that the veracity of the conclusions can be checked by other researchers.

Now that you have a better understanding about validity and reliability within a qualitative research study, the chapter will move into the tasks of analyzing, reporting, and drawing conclusions about the data.

Analyzing, Reporting, and Drawing Conclusions About Qualitative Data

Within the health-related fields, Law, Steinwender, and Leclaire (1998) offer the following criterion when researchers are considering qualitative research as the method for their study. First, the beliefs and worldviews of the researchers must be taken into consideration. Second, the researcher must ask themselves what is the nature of the end result desired. They suggest a qualitative study should be utilized when a researcher is seeking meaning and understanding about individual or group experiences. Third, they suggest that qualitative research requires a depth of understanding and description from participants. A moderate amount of emphasis is placed on the participants being able to tell the story of their lived experience.

Patton (2002) describes the first theme of qualitative research as involving the following design strategies—naturalistic inquiry; emergent design flexibility; and purposeful sampling. Within this study, naturalistic inquiry addressed the context simply as it existed, whereas the emergent design assisted in the flexibility and adaptability of the researcher. This allowed for the research to go outside of the boundaries of judgment.

The second theme involves data collection and fieldwork strategies—qualitative data; personal experience and engagement; empathy and mindfulness, and dynamic systems. Qualitative data is defined as observations, interviews, or documents that offer rich, detailed descriptions of the nature of an individual's perspectives of lived experience. Patton (2002) supports and encourages the researcher to become embedded in the environmental context of the study. In other words, the researcher's understanding of the lived experience is the starting point of the inquiry.

The third theme involves analysis of research strategies—unique case orientation; inductive analysis and creative synthesis; balanced perspective; context sensitivity; and voice, perspective, and reflexivity.

As Patton (2002) notes, without acknowledging or knowing about the context of the inquiry, a qualitative researcher has no eyes to see with or ears to hear the full meaning of a participant's personal story. The final and most discussed component in qualitative inquiry is that the researcher must own and reflect on his or her own voice and perspective, in relation to all aspects of the study. The researcher's ability to be reflexive addresses the credibility and authentic nature of qualitative research.

SKILL-BUILDING TIPS

■ If everything appears as if it is going smoothly or coming too easily, go back and check what you have done. Did you miss something? Is there more to the qualitative narrative?

■ Remember that your participants are living, breathing human beings. Sometimes they may have to reschedule an appointment or show up an hour late.

■ Buy yourself a special 5 x 7 notebook that you can keep with you at all times. Keep notes of everything you do during the research process. You may even find yourself waking up at 3 a.m. with a thought of how to

proceed with your study. Take pictures of the environment, record what kind of day it was when you were gathering data, and indicate how you are feeling about the research process. The time taken to document, document, and document will be invaluable.

LEARNING ACTIVITIES

1. Once again, find three to four related and well-written theses or dissertations. Now, spend time reading and reviewing your assumptions, limitations, theoretical constructs, and scope of study. Now spend some time fine-tuning your points.

2. Considerations of your study:
   ■ Do you have access to appropriate participants for your study?
   ■ List the criteria for participants who would be appropriate.
   ■ How many people will you be able to choose from?
   ■ How will you gain their permission to be participants?

3. List three points related to the scope and meaningfulness of this study. Also, consider how your study will be limited in scope.

4. List three reasons why this study will improve practice or the quality of daily living for your participants.

5. Identify potential audiences who may be interested in the outcomes of the study—other researchers, other practitioners, or policy makers.

REFERENCES

Guba, E. G., & Lincoln, Y. S. (2008). Paradigmatic controversies, contradictions and emerging confluences. In N. K. Denzin & Y. S. Lincoln (Eds.), *The landscape of qualitative research* (3rd ed., pp. 255–286). Thousand Oaks, CA: Sage.

Law, M., Steinwender, S., & Leclaire, L. (1998). Occupation, health & well-being. *Canadian Journal of Occupational Therapy, 65,* 81–91.

LeCompte, M., & Goetz, J. (1982). Problems of reliability and validity in ethnographic research. *Review of Educational Research, 52*(1), 31–60.

Patton, M. Q. (2002). *Qualitative research & evaluation methods* (3rd ed.). Thousand Oaks: Sage.

Evidence-Based Practice

Chapter 10

Understanding the Triad of Evidence-Based Practice: Evidence; Practitioner Skills and Knowledge; and Client Goals, Values, and Circumstances

As we work to create light for others, we naturally light our own way.
—Mary Anne Radmacher

LEARNING OUTCOMES

The information provided in this chapter will assist the reader to:

- Define evidence-based practice.
- Understand the three components of evidence-based practice—namely, evidence (research), practitioner skills and knowledge, and client goals, values, and circumstances.
- Differentiate evidence-based practice from ground-level research.
- Explore motives for evidence-based practice and consider challenges to engaging in it.
- Learn and apply five key steps for conducting an evidence-based practice project.
- Distinguish critically appraised papers (CAPs) from critically appraised topics (CATs).

- Classify research by its level of evidence.
- Critically appraise individual research studies.
- Synthesize multiple research studies to make recommendations for practice.
- Examine plausible clinical scenarios for application of evidence-based practice.
- Identify additional resources for evidence-based practice.

What Is Evidence-Based Practice?

The first step in becoming an effective evidence-based practitioner is gaining a clear understanding of the term. The most popular definition of evidence-based practice originated with the pioneer of evidence-based medicine, David Sackett. In his foundational article, evidence-based practice is described as "the conscientious, explicit, and judicious use of current best evidence in making decisions about the care of individual patients" (Sackett, Rosenberg, Gray, Haynes, & Richardson, 1996, p. 71). Although this definition emphasized the importance of using research in the clinical decision-making process, it failed to acknowledge the significance of the practitioner's knowledge and skills and the patient's goals, values, and circumstances. Thus, the definition was recently revised by Straus, Glasziou, Richardson, and Haynes (2011), who now identify evidence-based practice as "the integration of best research evidence with our clinical expertise and our patient's unique values and circumstances" (p. 1). Best evidence refers to the current applicable research available on the efficacy of treatments for particular diagnoses or conditions. This research could include quantitative, qualitative, or mixed methods designs. Although research purporting the value of a particular treatment technique is important, this information cannot be used in isolation. The knowledge, skills, and past experiences of the practitioner are critical to appropriately apply results of the research. In addition, consideration of each client's goals, values, strengths, weaknesses, and contexts is essential. A client's context can encompass his or her cultural background, personal demographics, virtual communication, stage of life, and physical and social environments (AOTA, 2008). The integration of these three components—best evidence; practitioner skills and knowledge; and client's goals, values, and circumstances—comprise evidence-based practice and is illustrated in Figure 10-1.

Evidence-based practice involves the practitioner searching and appraising available evidence on the treatment being considered or the condition a client presents with. For example, the practitioner might be considering the use of electrical stimulation to treat a client's low back pain, or he or she may be searching the literature to determine the best treatment(s) for low back pain because of a specific diagnosis, say lumbar stenosis. Once the available evidence has been garnered and evaluated, the practitioner needs to draw on past experiences, knowledge, and skills in treatment of this condition to determine the research's applicability to the current practice situation. At this point, the practitioner must consult with the client in order to make the most effective and appropriate

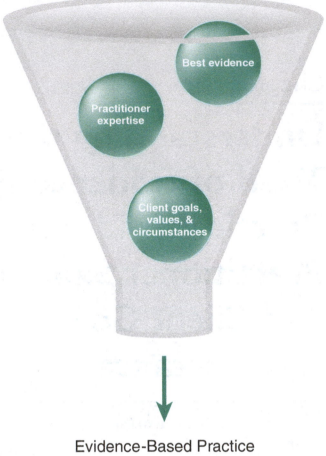

Evidence-Based Practice

Figure 10-1 Evidence-Based Practice

decision. Involving the client in the decision-making process emphasizes the collaborative relationship between practitioner and client (Gray, 1997).

Client-Centeredness

The term *client-centered* was first coined by Carl Rogers, in regard to the provision of psychotherapy, and is still gaining attention in all aspects of health care today. He used the label *client* to accentuate the even relationship between the therapist and the patient. The approach should be nonjudgmental and indirect with the goal "not so much to solve particular problems or relieve specific symptoms as to free clients of the sense that they are under the influence of malevolent forces beyond their control" (Miller, 2006, p. 1). Being client-centered allows the client to become an active member of the clinical team by voicing concerns, preferences, and expectations in regard to the proposed treatment. After consideration of the client's views, the practitioner may then need to use his or her clinical expertise to alter or adapt the interventions to best support the client.

Evidence-Based Practice Versus Research

As the concept of evidence-based practice has grown, students and practitioners alike have made the mistake of confusing it with ground-level research. In ground-level research, the aim is to generate new information on a particular condition, treatment, or phenomenon through testing some hypothesis. Researchers are attempting to describe lived experiences, assert connections among study concepts, or suggest cause-and-effect relationships. Evidence-based practice differs in that **already existing** literature is reviewed, appraised, and then applied to practice situations. Instead of generating new knowledge, the aim of evidence-based practice is to apply existing knowledge in a systematic way. One cannot assume that just because research is published or disseminated, it is of sound quality and appropriate for the current practice scenario. Therefore, critically appraising the evidence before integrating the findings with existing skills and knowledge and the client's goals and values is critical to the process.

Why Is Evidence-Based Practice Needed?

The interweaving of these three elements—best evidence, practitioner expertise, and client goals, values, and circumstances—culminates in effective evidence-based practice. When any one of these elements is omitted from the picture, the result might be an ineffective treatment, decreased quality of care, or an intervention devoid of client-centeredness. Evidence-based practice is needed for the following reasons:

- Clients deserve effective clinical interventions and high quality of care.
- Gaps often exist between evidence and practice. Evidence-based practice can help to bridge this gap.
- Ethical dilemmas exist when treatments are used that were shown to be ineffective.
- Many practitioners are faced with increased caseloads or productivity standards. Use of evidence-based practice can increase effectiveness and efficiency.
- Today, medical advances and changes in technology occur at a much faster rate than in the past.

New information is being produced daily, and treatments that were formerly accepted are now being questioned or dispelled.

- Practitioners have an ethical responsibility to ensure that they keep up-to-date on clinical practices. Past practice experiences, clinical judgment, or knowledge gained from initial schooling cannot solely drive practice decisions.
- Clients, families, policy makers, and third-party payors are demanding proof of efficacy for our treatments. Without evidence to support treatments, needed services may no longer be available in facilities, included in legislation, or reimbursed by payment plans.

Challenges to Evidence-Based Practice

Now that we have established the importance of evidence-based practice, we must acknowledge the challenges that need to be negotiated in order to effectively become an evidence-based practitioner. Barriers can be found at both the individual and organizational levels. At the individual level, perhaps the largest barrier to conducting evidence-based practice, as noted in multiple sources among the allied health professions, is the lack of time to retrieve, appraise, and apply best evidence to individual clients (Bennett et al., 2003; Dubouloz, Egan, Vallerand, & von Zweck, 1999; Ilott, 2003; Jette et al., 2003). Similarly, many practitioners lack the skills and confidence required to successfully search databases, to read and understand research articles, and to interpret and apply the results (Dubouloz et al., 1999; Fruth et al., 2010; Ilott, 2003; Schreiber, Stern, Marchetti, & Provident, 2008). Another concern is that not all research designs are readily applicable to real-life situations; perhaps a particular intervention was shown to be successful but only under strictly controlled conditions that cannot be replicated in the clinic or practice situation at hand (Jette et al., 2003; Salbach, Guilcher, Jaglal, & Davis, 2009).

Barriers at the organizational level include lack of support for research activities. Not all employers provide access to appropriate resources including memberships in professional organizations, libraries, and online journals, as well as reimbursement or time allotted for evidence-based continuing education (Houser, 2008;

McCluskey, 2003b). The work culture might also place greater emphasis on organizational goals, financial gains, and productivity standards, and practitioners may lack the authority to make decisions about some practice changes (Houser, 2008). Although these challenges pose threats to evidence-based initiatives, they are not insurmountable. Ilott (2003) proposes that success is likely when individual practitioners, employers, and policy makers collaborate. Investment of all parties in the process can lead to more competent practitioners, satisfied clients, and better clinical outcomes.

Employers can support practitioners by providing access to evidence-based resources, encouraging such activities in performance standards and appraisals (Salbach et al., 2009), and rewarding engagement in evidence-based practice via promotion or other means of recognition. Policy makers also need to balance their focus between cost-containment and quality of care. Creating local and national systems that support research and its real-life application can benefit practitioners and clients alike. In addition, a plethora of databases containing preappraised evidence, collections of evidence on specific topics, and systematic reviews have begun to emerge, all aimed at making the application of research less time-consuming and easier on the practitioner. Some examples are included in Table 10-1. Most professional organizations are also creating subsections, committees, and resource

Table 10-1 ■ Evidence-Based Practice Resources

Database	Website	Description
Cochrane Collaboration	www.cochrane.org	International network whose aim is to collect and disseminate systematic reviews
The Campbell Collaboration	www.campbellcollaboration.org	Nonprofit organization whose reviewers conduct and publish systematic reviews in social, behavioral, and educational arenas
National Guideline Clearinghouse	www.guideline.gov	U.S. Department of Health and Human Services public database of abstracts and evidence-based clinical practice guidelines
PEDro Physiotherapy Evidence Database	www.pedro.org	Free database of randomized trials, systematic reviews, and practice guidelines for physiotherapy
Clinical Evidence	www.clinicalevidence.com	Collection of systematic reviews on common clinical interventions
OT Seeker	www.otseeker.com	Database of abstracts of systematic reviews and randomized controlled trials relevant to occupational therapy
Evidence-Based Medicine	www.ebm.bmj.com	Journal that publishes, reviews, summarizes, and assesses applicability of international research
UpToDate	www.uptodate.com	Evidence-based clinical decision support system available on the Web and mobile devices
Bandolier	www.medicine.ox.ac.uk/bandolier/	Print and Internet journal focused on evidence-based care
Evidence-Based On-Call	www.eboncall.org/	Database of critically appraised topics

pages on their websites to assist their members in evidence-based practice efforts. Similarly to help bridge the divide between research and practice, researchers have been encouraged to express their findings in more user-friendly language to support practitioners in applying the results to real-life situations (Bennett et al., 2003; Jette et al., 2003).

Steps in Conducting an Evidence-Based Practice Project

Regardless of the scale and scope of the project, most evidence-based practice projects consist of five basic steps:

1. Identifying a need and an evidence-based practice question
2. Searching the evidence
3. Appraising and synthesizing the evidence
4. Applying the evidence
5. Evaluating the project

Identifying a Need and an Evidence-Based Practice Question

The evidence-based practice process begins by considering your practice setting and identifying an evidence-based practice question. What are your areas of interest? Do you see any unmet needs? Is there anything that could be done better? Consider who your clients are, what you are doing currently to serve them, and if you have proof of efficacy for these interventions. Your idea might stem from a clinical problem with a particular client or group of clients, or be driven by some larger need within your department, facility, or institution.

Needs Assessments

In clinical settings, practitioners conduct needs assessments before program development. A needs assessment is a systematic process used to clearly explain problems or existing voids and to lay out steps that will be followed for quality improvement. One of the most common types of needs assessments is a SWOT analysis. **SWOT** stands for strengths, weaknesses, opportunities, and threats. Each of these concepts is considered with regard to the facility, department, organization, or group of clients. You

will need to ponder each of these points in order to develop a meaningful evidence-based practice question.

Strengths and weaknesses are generally considered as internal aspects of the setting or situation. Reflecting on the strengths of your clients, clinic, and organization will be an important part of the process. Consider financial, physical, and emotional supports. Even if you have sound evidence to back up your plan, without the necessary supports in your setting, your project may fizzle. Considering the challenges (weaknesses) in your setting will help you to identify ways of circumventing these real issues. Envisioning problems ahead of time and devising a backup plan can greatly increase project success. Finally, the opportunities and threats present in the external environment have to be contemplated. In health care, this might include information about the current healthcare climate, the state of reimbursement for services, and the existing or proposed legislation. Each of these can present opportunities or threats, depending on the time and situation.

Rationale for the Project

Critically examining your practice situation and analyzing your clients' needs can provide a solid rationale for the project. Being able to justify your ideas will be important for getting buy in from other stakeholders, including clients, team members, and administration. Your rationale should be supported with references from multiple sources. Box 10-1 includes an excerpt from an evidence-based practice project aimed at training formal caregivers of clients with dementia. The practitioner has built the case for the project by including multiple statistics on the incidence and impact of dementia, thereby supporting the need to adequately train caregivers to handle these issues.

The Evidence-Based Practice Question

In this first phase of the project, you are essentially "setting the stage" for your idea. Supporting your points with observations, statistics, and a detailed description of your population and the problem are part of this foundational step. Defining key terms and the issues your project will address are precursors to identifying your evidence-based practice question. The evidence-based practice question (PICO question) will define the population (P), the intervention (I),

---

BOX 10-1 ■ **Example of Rationale for an EBP Project**

It is believed that by 2013, 34 million people in the world will have dementia (Gitlin & Corcoran, 2005). While there are unique features in different types of dementia such as Alzheimer's, for the purpose of this project the term dementia will be used to reflect the general course and progression of this group of diseases. Approximately 4.3 million people are believed to have dementia in the United States with this number growing daily (Gitlin & Corcoran, 2005). This is a staggering statistic alone but when combined with the reality that there is no known cure for dementia and that one in four people can expect to be a caregiver for a family member with dementia in their lifetime, the impact of this disease as a public health concern is significant. The Alzheimer's Association report for 2008 stated that 9.9 million US family members, friends and neighbors provided informal or unpaid care to people with dementia (Schaber & Lieberman, 2010). The value of the services these caregivers provide is estimated at close to $200 million per year with the total cost in productivity exceeding $11 billion annually (Gitlin & Corcoran, 2005). These statistics are just a glimpse into the devastating, unpredictable and grueling consequences of this rapidly growing disease (Bickmore, 2011, pp. 5–6).

---

the comparison intervention (C, if applicable), and the expected outcome (O). A well-constructed question will effectively guide the literature search and subsequent evidence-based project.

In theory, formulating just one question seems like a relatively simple task; however, it might take a few weeks to narrow your focus and adequately define each element in the question. Sufficiently narrowing your population and intervention of focus will allow you to locate literature that specifically relates to your situation at hand. Conversely, narrowing the topic too much could yield very limited results from your literature search. Conducting a preliminary search of the literature in your area of interest can help you to solidify your question, or to show you where you might need to refine it. Sharing your ideas with your peers, coworkers, mentors, or supervisors can help you determine if the question is specific enough, makes sense, and is applicable to the current practice situation. Your initial question may continue to evolve as you go through the evidence-based process. Also remember that at this point, you need not be concerned with what you will actually do in your project or intervention—you should only be concerned with formulating a workable question. Figure 10-2 includes several examples of evidence-based practice questions.

In developing a new program or conducting an evidence-based practice project, a formal report of

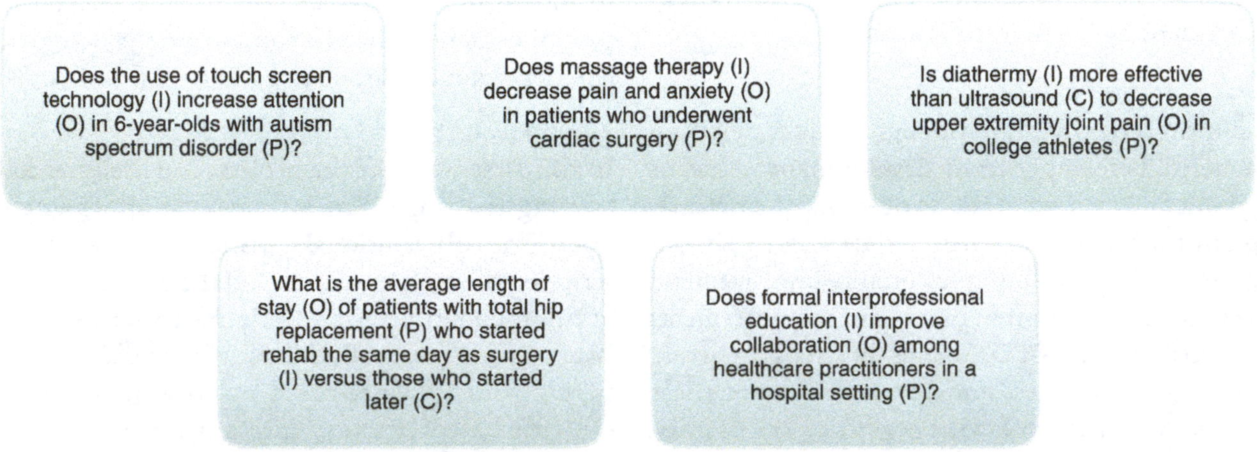

Does the use of touch screen technology (I) increase attention (O) in 6-year-olds with autism spectrum disorder (P)?

Does massage therapy (I) decrease pain and anxiety (O) in patients who underwent cardiac surgery (P)?

Is diathermy (I) more effective than ultrasound (C) to decrease upper extremity joint pain (O) in college athletes (P)?

What is the average length of stay (O) of patients with total hip replacement (P) who started rehab the same day as surgery (I) versus those who started later (C)?

Does formal interprofessional education (I) improve collaboration (O) among healthcare practitioners in a hospital setting (P)?

Figure 10-2 Examples of Evidence-Based Practice (PICO) Questions

the previous information is often prepared. The information is typically arranged into chapters; more details about writing the report will be provided in Chapter 12. See Box 10-2 for a suggested formalized chapter outline for an evidence-based practice project.

Searching the Evidence

After you have formulated an evidence-based practice question, it is time to begin the somewhat-daunting task of searching the literature. Initially it is effective to spend some time exploring the literature in your area of interest. Use broad search criteria and see what results you get. Then narrow the search terms to see how the results change. Do you find that some databases and sites have more information in your area of interest? It is a good idea to explore as many resources and databases as you can, just to get a feel for what is available. It will be time well spent, because locating the literature can be very time-consuming if you do not know how to approach it.

Once you are comfortable with your school's or institution's online library and the other databases

---

BOX 10-2 ■ **Evidence-Based Practice Project Outline**

Abstract

Chapter 1 **Introduction and Overview of the Topic of Interest**

Section 1.1 Description of Project Setting
Section 1.2 The Need and Rationale for the Project
Section 1.3 Identification of Supports and Barriers in the Setting
Section 1.4 The Evidence-Based Practice Question

Chapter 2 **Literature Review**

Section 2.1 Methodology of the Literature Search
Section 2.2 Synthesis of the CAT Portfolio *(See Appendix A: Individual CAP Outlines) Subsections will include:*
  - *Description of the Portfolio*
  - *Additional subsections will be individualized to your project and will be organized around common themes in the literature*

Chapter 3 **Methodology**

Section 3.1 Frameworks or Models of Practice Guiding the Project
Section 3.2 (Proposed) Activities of the Evidence-Based Project
Section 3.3 Assumptions
Section 3.4 Approach to Client-Centeredness

Chapter 4 **Implementation and Results**

Section 4.1 Description of the Participants
Section 4.2 Modifications to the Evidence-Based Plan
Section 4.3 Description of Implementation *Subsections will be individualized to your project. Subsections may be organized according to project phases, individual sessions, or individual participants, for example.*
Section 4.4 Quantitative Outcomes (if applicable)
Section 4.5 Qualitative Outcomes (if applicable)

Chapter 5 **Evaluation, Discussion, and Conclusions**

Section 5.1 Evaluation of the Project and Correlation with Literature
Section 5.2 Limitations
Section 5.3 Recommendations for Practice, Policy, and Education

References

Appendix A: **Individual CAP Outlines**
  - *You will likely have additional appendices that include items such as tools used in the project, lengthy tables and graphs, and so on.*

that you have at your disposal, the formal literature search can begin. In addition to the evidence-based resources already identified, some of the most popular databases for the allied health professions include Medline, OVID, PubMed, CINHAL, Academic Search Premier, ERIC, and SAGE Publications. Some of the databases include online tutorials to assist with the literature search. One example is PubMed (http://www.nlm.nih.gov/bsd/disted/pubmedtutorial/index.html); although it is designed to help you navigate their database specifically, it also provides information basic to a literature search anywhere.

To begin, consider the search terms you might use, which databases will be helpful, and the time period of the evidence you are seeking. If you are looking for evidence on treatment interventions, limiting your search to articles published within the last 5 to 10 years will likely yield the most appropriate results. However, you may want to go back further in time if you are looking for information on the origin of a particular treatment or for a more foundational intervention that has been shown to stand the test of time. Additional search terms could be reflective of the specific intervention that you are interested in, the client population, diagnosis or condition, or the outcome that you hope to achieve. Use of a combination of search terms is typical, and most databases allow you to limit results based upon a variety of criteria, including those discussed here.

Tracking Your Literature Search

During your literature search, it will be important to keep track of the databases that you searched, the search terms used, your rationale for your search criterion, and any additional search techniques employed. For example, one method commonly used is scanning the reference list of an article you identified as appropriate in your initial database search, to determine if any articles in the reference list should be pursued. This technique has been referred to as *snowballing* (Greenhalgh & Peacock, 2005, p. 1064) or *citation tracking* (Taylor, 2008, p. 150). An important part of evidence-based practice is being able to replicate the literature search. You may need to go back and revisit something you saw previously, and your search techniques should be included in your formal report. It will be much easier to organize this information from the beginning rather than trying to recall it later. Detailed information about the search methodology, key search terms used, and inclusion and exclusion criteria for the articles is usually included in the formalized report (see Box 10-2). Table 10-2 is an example of a research log which you can use to track your literature search; a full version of the form is available on the DavisPlus website (http://davisplus.fadavis.com, keyword: Hissong). The methodology of the literature search for a project on professional leadership might look similar to the example appearing in Box 10-3.

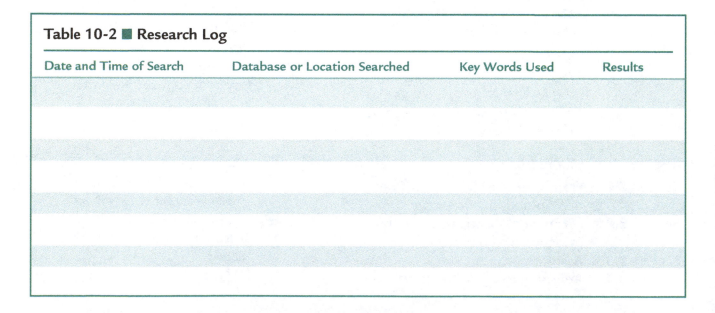

Table 10-2 ▪ Research Log

Date and Time of Search	Database or Location Searched	Key Words Used	Results

BOX 10-3 ■ **Methodology of the Literature Search**

Fifteen articles published between 2002 and 2012 were critically reviewed for this project. Search terms used included *leadership development, leadership confidence, mentoring, leadership recruitment, leadership skills,* and *commitment.* Databases searched included: MEDLINE, CINAHL, PubMed, ERIC, and GoogleScholar. Search terms were used individually and in combination, and the reference lists from previously located articles were hand-searched for any additional studies, in order to ensure an exhaustive search. The following inclusion criteria were also applied to the searches. First, research was primarily limited to the previous 10 years, so as to provide the most recent literature. Second, only research studies published in English were included.

How Many Articles Are Needed?

The number of articles you need to locate on your topic will largely depend on your goals and the quality of evidence found. A few articles may be enough if they are deemed of sound quality, include one or more systematic reviews, or will be applied to only a small client group. More studies might be indicated if the studies conducted were less rigorous, if you wish to develop a completely new program at your site, or if you want to apply the research across a larger population. Conducting a thorough search of the literature will ensure that you gain a clear picture of the intervention in question and the outcomes you can expect with its use. You will know that your literature search was exhaustive when your continued search attempts do not yield any new results when compared with what you located previously.

Appraising and Synthesizing the Evidence

Following the literature search, you will appraise and synthesize the articles that fit your criterion. Understanding scientific inquiry and research methods is important in determining the value and relevancy of the articles that you located. Understanding and applying research to practice is necessary to be on the cutting edge of today's practice. Ultimately, it is up to you to evaluate the rigor and applicability of each study.

CAPs and CATs

Critically Appraised Papers (CAPs) or **Critically Appraised Resources** (CARs) are short analyses of individual studies, whereas **Critically Appraised Topics** (CATs) are summaries of multiple studies on a single topic or practice concern. CATs are similar to systematic reviews in that they include synthesis of numerous studies, but they are generally less rigorous, more concise, and more limited in focus, with the emphasis on practical application of research. Systematic reviews are usually undertaken by researchers, whereas CATs are typically conducted by clinical practitioners. In practice, CAPs are completed on individual studies and compiled for the CAT portfolio. A variety of templates exist for completion of the individual CAPs; one example is shown in Table 10-3. After reading an individual study, you will highlight the purpose, the setting, the participants or sample used, the study design or methodology, the level of evidence, the main outcomes and findings, any limitations, and how and why the article was deemed applicable to the question at hand. An explanation of each area is included within the template in Table 10-3. It is a good idea to number each CAP, as this number can be used to quickly identify individual sources when you begin to make notes and synthesize the articles.

Levels of Evidence

During appraisal, it will be necessary for you to assign each article to the appropriate level of evidence. A number of scales exist for the purpose of classifying research studies (Greenhalgh, 1997; Howick, 2009; Law & MacDermid, 2008), and it matters not which scale you use as long as you identify it for the reader. One of the most common is the scale from the Centre for Evidence Based Medicine (Howick, 2009). For our purposes, a simplified version adapted from a number of scales is included in Figure 10-3.

On this scale, the levels correspond to the relative strength of the research study—with a level I study possessing the greatest strength or rigor and a level V

Table 10-3 ■ Critically Appraised Paper Template

CRITICALLY APPRAISED PAPER # _____

List PICO Question Here

Put APA Formatted Citation Here

Purpose of the Study	Briefly state the purpose of the study. How does the study apply to your discipline or your PICO question?
Setting	Examples: inpatient rehab unit, SNF, public school system, drug and alcohol clinic, health club, community senior housing complexes, and so on.
Participants or Sample	Include any information that is available regarding number of participants, diagnoses, how participants were recruited, if the sample was random, convenience, purposive, and any other pertinent demographics.
Study Design and Methodology	What type of research design was used? Examples: Systematic review, RCT, cohort, single case design, ethnography, grounded theory, and so on. Briefly describe the methodology (in other words, what did the researchers do?).
Level of Evidence	I, II, III, IV, V or Qualitative Study (see Figure 10-3 and the corresponding text for an explanation of levels of evidence).
Outcomes and Main Findings	Clearly state the results. Were the results statistically significant or clinically significant? Were the outcome measures valid and reliable?
Intervention Highlighted Through the Research	In a short phrase, what intervention was highlighted? (This does not mean the results have to be positive.) Examples: Use of a multisensory environment to decrease symptoms of pain, use of aromatherapy to increase appetite, use of therapeutic exercise to decrease contractures, and so on.
Limitations	List any limitations in the study that you need to consider in evaluating the results.
This Study Was Identified as the "Best" Evidence and Selected for the Portfolio for the Following Reasons:	■ Include bullet points here to identify why you included this study or article. ■ Write in your own words why it is important; what are the implications for your project or intervention? ■ Keep in mind that you can glean valuable information from ALL studies regardless of whether or not the results are positive. For example, say you are looking at fall prevention and you believe that use of appropriate footwear can decrease the risk of falls. Then you locate a study that reports this is not true. It would **still** be important to include this study—remember that "best" evidence combines the research with your skills and knowledge and the needs of your client or population. You also have to consider how applicable this study is to what you are proposing.

*The information in the column to the right in the table has been provided for explanation purposes. You should delete this information and use this template for each resource.

study possessing the least. Each study's level is dictated by the research design, including whether or not the study groups were randomized and if a control group was used. Keep in mind that certain topics lend themselves more easily to rigorous study, whereas others cannot be studied under such strict conditions. For example, if you are looking for research on a rare neurological disorder, you are likely to find case studies or accounts from experts who have treated clients with this condition. However, practitioners

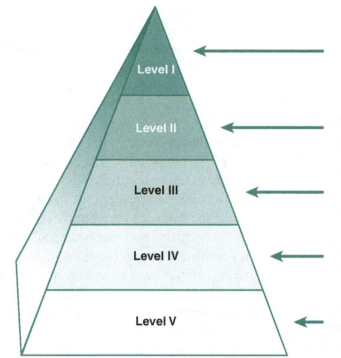

High quality RCTs or Systematic Reviews (SR) of these studies, meta-analysis

Small-scale RCTs, non-randomized studies *with* a control group such as cohort studies, case-control, pretest-posttest designs, or SRs of these studies

Non-randomized studies *without* a control group such as pretest-posttest designs, time series or longitudinal studies, and cross-sectional studies

Descriptive studies including single subject designs, case studies, normative studies, and survey studies

Expert opinion, literature reviews, laboratory research (research not performed on human subjects)

Figure 10-3 Levels of Evidence

interested in more commonly occurring diagnoses or treatments might expect to find larger scale studies in a multitude of settings. So, although a level I study boasts greater rigor and confidence of results, not all practice areas can be studied under these conditions.

Considering each study's design is vitally important in determining the validity and reliability of the findings. You must ask yourself if the researchers actually observed and measured the constructs they intended to. In other words, does the study have internal validity? The quality of the design and instruments used, the integrity of the procedures, and the inter-rater reliability can all impact validity. Similarly, you must contemplate the transferability, or external validity, of the study's findings. Was the study conducted in such a way that allows application to other groups, namely, those in your current practice setting? Finally, are the results statistically or clinically significant? What impact will this have on your practice?

Synthesizing Results From Multiple Studies

Once you have appraised each article individually, it is time to synthesize the findings from all of your articles and make recommendations for practice.

Synthesizing involves integrating the findings from all the individual studies you appraised to determine your course of action. This can be one of the most labor intensive parts of the process, but well worth the effort to gain a clear picture of the phenomenon in question. Did any common themes emerge among the studies? Did you find some studies that supported the treatment you are considering and others that did not? It will not be enough to just restate the evidence; you will need to comprehensively integrate the findings from all the studies in your portfolio.

Spend some time thinking about your literature review and start to conceptualize some of the sections or themes in your mind. **Themes** are central concepts or findings occurring in more than one study. If multiple studies have the same or similar findings, this adds strength to the conclusions and increases the likelihood that results can be generalized to similar situations and populations with the same outcome. Using a notebook with one page devoted to each theme is a good way to organize the process initially. As you identify each theme, record it on a separate page in the notebook; then, review each individual CAP and add notes, quotations, and statistics from it to the corresponding themes in your notebook. You may also perform this same procedure by creating separate electronic files for each theme, if you prefer.

Completing a CAT

The CAT can take several forms depending on the nature of the project and setting. In narrative form, the information from the literature review and corresponding synthesis and conclusions are typically included in Chapter 2 of the formalized report (see Box 10-2). A description of the CAT portfolio and a discussion of the common themes and findings should be included. The description of the portfolio is usually a straightforward review of the number of articles, study designs, time frame of the studies, where the studies took place, and the general themes. Box 10-4 contains an example of a portfolio description for the previously discussed professional leadership project. Following these paragraphs, one would expect a detailed description of the various themes, with multiple citations from the referenced articles to support each point, as well as a summary of the recommendations for practice. Remember that themes can only be

identified when more than one study yields the same or similar findings.

In other cases, a simpler, more-concise format can be utilized for the CAT. Several templates and tools exist online including CATmaker (CEMB, 2009), Clinical Appraisal Skills Programme (CASP UK, 2012), and CAT Template (McCluskey, 2003a). An additional template has been included in Table 10-4. An explanation of each area is included within the template in the online materials.

In any case, determining the "bottom line" or answering the evidence-based practice question based upon the available evidence is the goal. Although you can complete this process alone or with a group of your peers or colleagues, previously completed CAPs and CATs are often made available through a variety of organizations and websites. Checking the resources contained in Table 10-1, and some additional ones in Table 10-5, could save you valuable time if someone already reviewed the research in your area of interest.

In many cases, these recommendations are formally published as **clinical practice guidelines**. Conditions for publication typically include collaboration by multiple individuals to critically appraise the literature and set forth practice recommendations. Expert consensus may also be used when the involved parties have extensive experience or advanced training in the subject area. The popularity of clinical practice guidelines has grown as a result of their proven ability to enhance clinical practice, contain costs, and improve patient outcomes.

Applying the Evidence

Novak (2010), as adapted and cited by Glegg and Barrie (2012), proposed a framework for applying research to clinical practice. They use the metaphor of a traffic light to explain the process. Less rigorous levels of evidence or evidence proven to be ineffective or to cause harm is given a red light—meaning the recommendation is to abstain from using the treatment in question. Application with caution (yellow light) might be recommended for treatments with limited evidence, inconclusive evidence, or no evidence, or if the studied population differs from your clients. Clinical judgment is essential, so one must consider the clinical situation, practitioner's skills, and client's

---

> ### BOX 10-4 ■ Description of the CAT Portfolio
>
> The final portfolio contains 15 research articles from both national and international journals. Study designs include three randomized controlled trials, two longitudinal studies, eight experimental pre- and posttest designs, one case study, and one mixed methods design. All studies relate directly to components of the evidence-based practice question and will be used to draft new practice guidelines for mentoring new managers in health care.
>
> Five of the articles specifically describe characteristics of effective leaders with commonalities noted between articles. The other 10 articles address the process of mentoring new leaders. These themes will be discussed in detail.

Table 10-4 ■ Critically Appraised Topic Template

Evidence-Based Practice Question

Include the PICO question. Be as specific as possible with each element of the question in order to sufficiently narrow your search.

Clinical Scenario

Briefly describe the clinical situation or problem that motivated this investigation of the literature. What is your rationale for pursuing this topic?

Databases Searched

Include all databases or websites searched.

Search Methodology and Terms

PICO Question Categories	Search Terms Used
Population	Include applicable search terms for each category.
Intervention	
Comparison	
Outcomes	

Inclusion Criteria for Articles

Include any inclusion criteria. Examples might include particular study designs, full text articles, articles published only in English, studies conducted with specific diagnoses or ages, or those occurring in a particular setting.

Exclusion Criteria for Articles

Include any exclusion criteria. Examples might include studies occurring more than 10 years ago; less rigorous research designs, such as qualitative or Level V studies; or literature reviews.

Review Process

Discuss specifically how the process of the review was conducted. Include the following:

■ How was the question developed?

■ How were search criteria determined and databases selected?

■ How were the inclusion and exclusion criteria applied? For example, the abstracts of articles returned in the initial search might have been scanned to determine if each study met the basic criteria and should be explored further.

■ How were individual analyses completed on each study? In essence, how did you complete the individual CAPs?

■ What did you do to ensure quality control in the process? For example, did a mentor or expert in this content area review your analyses or did you use some other method of peer review?

Search Results by Level of Evidence

Level of Evidence	Study Design	Number of Articles Included
I	High-quality RCTs or Systematic Reviews (SR) of these studies, or Meta-analyses	Include number of articles in each category
II	Small-scale RCTs, non-randomized studies **with** a control group such as cohort studies, case-control, pretest-posttest designs, or SRs of these studies	

Continued

Table 10-4 ■ Critically Appraised Topic Template—cont'd

Level of Evidence	Study Design	Number of Articles Included
III	Nonrandomized studies **without** a control group such as pretest–posttest designs, time-series or longitudinal studies, and cross-sectional studies	
IV	Descriptive studies including single subject designs, case studies, normative studies, and survey studies	
V	Expert opinion, literature reviews, laboratory research (research not performed on human subjects)	
Qualitative Studies	Examples include phenomenology, ethnography, and grounded theory	
	TOTAL ARTICLES REVIEWED:	

Main Findings		
Level I	Use bullet points to list main findings for the studies under each level.	
Level II		
Level III		
Level IV		
Level V		
Qualitative studies		

Limitations		
Level I	Use bullet points to list limitations for the studies under each level.	
Level II		
Level III		
Level IV		
Level V		
Qualitative Studies		

BOTTOM LINE AND RECOMMENDATIONS:

Use this space to summarize your findings as they relate to clinical practice. Provide a clear and concise answer to your evidence-based practice question. Clearly state your recommendations.

Do you recommend:

1. Using the intervention (proven effectiveness)
2. Using the intervention with caution (conflicting evidence, no evidence, or insufficient evidence)
3. Not using the intervention (proven ineffective or the potential for harm) (Glegg & Barrie, 2012)

Table 10-4 ■ Critically Appraised Topic Template—cont'd

REFERENCES
- **Include appraised articles here in bold.**
- Include any other sources used to make your appraisal (not in bold).

Name of Appraiser(s):   Date Completed:

Table 10-5 ■ Sites Disseminating Completed CAPs and CATs

OT CATS: Occupational Therapy Critically Appraised Topics	http://www.otcats.com/intro.html
NSW Speech Pathology Evidence-Based Practice	http://www.ciap.health.nsw.gov.au/specialties/ebp_sp_path/caps.html
Journal of the American Academy of Physician Assistants	http://www.jaapa.com/critically-appraised-topic/section/699/
Evidence-Based Neurology CATS	http://www.cnsuwo.ca/ebn/cats/
Evidence in Motion	http://www.evidenceinmotion.com/
American Thoracic Society	http://www.thoracic.org/clinical/critical-care/evidence-based-critical-care/literature-reviews/index.php
Essential Evidence Plus	http://www.essentialevidenceplus.com/
Joanna Briggs Institute	http://www.joannabriggs.edu.au/Home

---

values in making these decisions. Finally, treatments substantiated with strong clinical evidence and studies conducted with similar populations and in similar situations to the current practice scenario would be given a green light—meaning the treatment is recommended.

After you have appraised the individual studies and synthesized all articles in the portfolio, considering the following questions will help you to move forward with your project:

1. Are the settings in which the studies were conducted similar to your current practice situation? Are the populations used in the studies similar to your client or client group? Context is extremely relevant. For example, a great level I study on the effect of sensory integration techniques with 3- to 5-year-olds is unlikely to be applicable to geriatric clients in a nursing facility.

2. What special skills, knowledge, and past experiences do you bring to the project?

3. How does the proposed project fit within your discipline's scope of practice?

4. What theoretical or conceptual frameworks will be used to guide the design of your project? Some models, such as a behavioral approach, a biomechanical model, or a model of change, can be applied across disciplines. In other cases, individual disciplines have developed unique models of practice to inform and guide their decision-making. Some examples of these include the

psychobiological adaptation model for physical therapists and the Model of Human Occupation for occupational therapists.

5. What are the values, goals, strengths, weaknesses, and circumstances of your clients?

Reflecting on your answers to these questions as well as the evidence leads to designing your evidence-based practice project. Unfortunately, there is no clear-cut way of integrating the evidence, your skills and knowledge, and the values and circumstances of your clients. This is where experience and sound clinical reasoning skills are important. In some cases, the evidence in favor of a particular treatment might be present and appropriate for your client, but you may lack the necessary certifications or skills to implement the treatment. Likewise, a proposed treatment, albeit substantiated by research and within your comfort zone to implement, might not mesh with your client's goals or circumstances.

Designing the Evidence-Based Project Plan

Most successful projects begin with a well-thought-out and detailed plan. In the early stages, creating a bulleted list of the proposed steps of your project can assist you to break it down into more manageable phases. Considering each phase individually allows you to adequately prepare and to navigate around expected and unexpected barriers. Sharing your list with your peers, coworkers, or mentors can also support you in identifying gaps in your plan. Some items warranting contemplation are:

▪ Do you need to secure permission from anyone to conduct the project?

▪ Do you need to recruit participants? How and when will you do that?

▪ Do you have to arrange for use of physical spaces or equipment?

▪ Do you need permission to use documents, assessments, or other tools?

▪ Do you need to purchase supplies, make copies, or organize schedules or other program content, such as lessons, presentation slides, or handouts?

In the preliminary phase, you will likely be concerned with setting up the logistics of your project. Your plan should be descriptive and include as many details as possible. Imagine someone other than yourself being responsible for carrying out the steps of your plan. Ensuring that your procedure is replicable will add credibility to your outcomes. In addition, be sure to include references to other sources that support the various steps of your plan. Including citations for activities within your intervention, or for certain forms or assessments used, allows others to easily see the connection between your project and the existing body of evidence.

Discussing any forms, assessments, or tools that you will use during the project is an essential step. Determining early on whether you choose to use a commercially available tool or one that you have designed yourself, such as a survey, will ensure that you can obtain appropriate information about your project after its completion. Being able to evaluate the success of your project is critical in making recommendations for future practice. Finally, consider who will be participating in your project. Are there specific inclusion and exclusion criteria or will everyone in your clinic or setting be invited to participate? Revisiting the goals for your project and the supporting evidence can assist you in making these decisions.

Other elements worthy of consideration include assumptions, limitations, and your approach to client-centeredness. In designing your project, assumptions are things that you assumed to be true or assimilated from a variety of sources, but which are difficult to prove. For example, you may have assumed that the clients in your clinic want to increase their independence or quality of life. Although you may not have definitive proof of this, you may have presumed this in designing your project.

Limitations are weaknesses in your project plan. Because you are not conducting ground-level research, there is no need to be overly concerned if you have a small number of participants or the presence of some bias. Some limitations that you might discuss include the lack of appropriate assessments to evaluate the phenomenon in question; limited timing of the intervention possibly related to the logistics of your setting, or assessment of more qualitative characteristics that can be subjective or difficult to isolate.

Lastly, you should consider how your intervention will be client-centered. Because this is a key element in evidence-based practice, reflect on who your clients are; how you will establish relationships with them; and how you will adapt, alter, or modify your program to support each client to the best of your abilities. Some interventions are inherently client-centered, whereas others might have to be tweaked to ensure this criterion is met. In today's healthcare climate, a cookie cutter approach, where each client receives the same treatments under the same conditions, is no longer acceptable. Your ability to tailor your program to fit each client's goals, values, and circumstances will impact success and client satisfaction. In a formalized report, the project plan as well as discussions of guiding frameworks or conceptual models, assumptions, limitations, and the approach to client-centeredness are included in Chapter 3 (see Box 10-2).

Project Implementation

In the implementation phase, you should follow your established procedures and document any deviations in the plan. Keeping accurate and detailed records is imperative in all aspects of health care today, and your evidence-based practice project is no exception. Administering assessments per standardized procedures and objectively evaluating client performance allows you to draw accurate conclusions. Just like research, evidence-based practice projects can yield quantitative data, qualitative data, or both, depending on the nature of the project and the treatment being implemented. Data collection may include use of standard documentation in your setting and the use of new tools identified or designed following your literature search. Observations of clients, surveys, and focus groups are also appropriate ways to gather data for an evidence-based practice project.

In most cases, healthcare practitioners are implementing evidence-based practice plans within their current practice settings and under their discipline's current scope of practice. It is important to remember that research is not being conducted, but rather existing research is being appraised and applied to the current practice situation with the goal of improving client outcomes. Clearly articulating your goals for the project and the evidence that supports it will assist you in gaining support from coworkers, administrators, and third-party payors (if the services are reimbursable). The description of the participants, a discussion of deviations from the original project plan, and a formal report of the outcomes of the evidence-based practice project are customarily included in Chapter 4 (see Box 10-2).

Evaluating the Project

As healthcare students and practitioners, the process of reassessment or evaluation throughout the client encounter is common practice. This allows us to see if our interventions have been successful, determine if there have been changes in the client's status, and make decisions about the course of treatment moving forward. The evaluation of your evidence-based practice project works in much the same way. Closely examining the outcomes of your project allows you to draw conclusions about the treatment in question and to decide if you will continue to use it with this population.

In evaluating your project, you will need to consider your results within the context of the existing evidence. Do your findings agree or disagree with what was reported in the literature? Why or why not? One caveat about evidence-based practice is that even though something happened in your project that is dissimilar to the literature, it does not mean something is wrong. Perhaps your client's values and circumstances differ slightly from those in the articles you appraised. Maybe you used different tools to measure your outcomes, or you adapted the intervention based upon your past experiences. Discussing these differences facilitates the comparison between what occurred in your setting and the existing literature. Referring to sources from your CAT Portfolio further strengthens the connection between research and practice.

Visual displays of outcomes may also be useful in explaining and evaluating your project. Similar to the research examples given in Chapter 12, tables of data or figures, including pie charts, bar graphs, line graphs, flowcharts, or other drawings, can be used to compare before and after data and to draw conclusions. If you used an assessment tool employed in existing studies, a visual aide could be used to plot your results next to the results of the prior studies. Taking the time to adequately evaluate the outcomes of your project leads to recommendations for future practice, policy, and education.

Making Recommendations for Practice, Policy, and Education

A worthwhile evidence-based practice project culminates with recommendations for the future. The recommendations could be for clinical practice in your setting or across settings; for policy impacting access and payment for services; or for continuing education for existing practitioners, entry-level education for new practitioners, or education of other parties. If your project was successful, how will you expand upon it or get the word out so others in similar situations can benefit from this information? Consider presenting your project within your facility or at a state or national conference; you may also seek publication in a discipline-specific magazine or journal or with one of the groups that disseminate evidence-based practice guidelines. See Tables 10-1 and 10-5 for some ideas to get you started. If you plan to continue the project, reflect on the outcomes to determine if it is necessary to alter or tweak the methodology for future success. Finally, if the project was ineffective, contemplate how this information can be put to good use. Even if the outcomes were not what you had hoped for, cautioning others who might be considering this approach, or discussing the issues at hand and how to circumvent them the next time, will be valuable. Evaluation of the project and recommendations for the future should be incorporated into Chapter 5 of the formal report (see Box 10-2).

Stories of Evidence-Based Practice

Now that you know the steps in conducting evidence-based practice, we will discuss some examples of how evidence-based practice can be integrated into clinical scenarios in real life. Ideally, evidence-based practice should be at the foundation of the clinical decision-making process regardless of the setting. Educators, practitioners, and students alike can use evidence-based practice for program development; guiding

decisions with unique or complex case scenarios; justifying the need for staff, equipment, or services; and mentoring, fostering teamwork, and motivating patients and clinicians.

Program and Protocol Development

One of the most common uses of evidence-based practice is to develop new programs or protocols. The following example will help to illustrate this point.

A group of physical and occupational therapists work together in a 120-bed skilled nursing facility in a rural community. The average age of their patients is 70 years old, and they frequently treat clients with primary or secondary cardiac diagnoses. The facility has recently implemented a specialized cardiac program aimed at more effectively managing all chronic cardiac conditions, specifically congestive heart failure, and decreasing the incidence of readmission to the hospital for this condition. The facility protocol is primarily limited to actions taken by nurses and the physicians; these include things like dietary restrictions, daily weights, and changes in medications for residents on the program. The facility is looking to increase marketing efforts for this patient group and the administrator has asked the rehab director if the rehabilitation department might be involved.

Before this time, clients with cardiac diagnoses have been evaluated for rehab services using standard evaluations and procedures. Cardiac precautions, including limited use of weights and reaching over the head during therapeutic activities, as well as education on energy conservation techniques have been instituted. Historically, therapists have also monitored blood pressures and oxygen saturation as necessary during treatment of these clients; however, no standard rehabilitation procedures exist for this client group.

In response to the administrator's request, the rehab director conducts a preliminary search of the literature through the American Physical Therapy Association's website (because she is a member) and through Google Scholar using a combination of the following search terms: "cardiac rehabilitation," "cardiac protocols," "congestive heart failure," and "rehab protocols." This quick search uncovers a plethora of information on patient education, evaluation and treatment protocols, assessments, and exercise and ambulation programs. At this point, the manager realizes that the team could be doing much more for this patient group and solicits the help of three other staff members to assist in this endeavor. Each staff member has goals on his or her performance review for program development so this task fits nicely into the plan.

Each member of the task group then volunteers to conduct a detailed search on a specific area. Breaking the information down into subcategories not only makes the task more manageable, but allows each clinician to select an area of interest. The rehab director takes on the task of searching the literature for evaluation and assessment procedures, whereas the other three staff members volunteer to delve deep into patient education, exercise and ambulation programs, and patient activities, respectively. They agree to look at literature limited to the last 5 years since the goal is to create a rehabilitation protocol for patients with congestive heart failure based upon the most current evidence.

The group is given 3 weeks to search the literature before they meet again. At that time, the group is charged with appraising the literature to determine if the information located is of sound quality and relevance to the clients at hand. The group uses a concise template similar to the one in Table 10-3 to assess the quality and applicability of the studies located. Those articles that pass the test are set aside for the next meeting, at which time the group analyzes them for common themes. Locating multiple articles that support a particular assessment, or exercise protocol, for example, will add strength to the findings and to the subsequent program.

Next, the group uses the identified themes, as well as their personal skills and experiences, and the perceived values and circumstances of clients typically encountered in their setting to create a rehabilitation protocol for clients with chronic congestive heart failure. The information is organized into a resource binder with tabs for procedures for the therapists, patient handouts, and exercise and ambulation protocols. Information for therapists includes how and when to monitor blood pressure, oxygen saturation, and perceived client exertion during evaluation and treatment. Protocols for exercise and ambulation are also included to help guide therapists during the rehab process. Patient education includes information on the use of adaptive equipment, energy conservation and work simplification techniques, stress management, and precautions, to name a few. The administrator and medical director approve use of the new program, and all rehab staff are provided with education before its formal implementation.

This new program serves two purposes. First, it provides the staff with an evidence-based program that can be easily implemented. The instructions are detailed and clear; references are included to support the procedures and activities. Second, it demonstrates the facility's and the rehab team's commitment to providing quality patient care for this population, which may aid in marketing efforts as well as obtaining continued coverage from third-party payors for this service.

The need for a new program may arise out of a quality improvement initiative, as in this example, or it may be necessitated by regulatory changes or citations on an agency, state, or national survey. Regardless of the motivation, evidence-based practice undertaken for this purpose is likely to require some extra time, effort, and research skills. Collaborating with others, as illustrated here, can disperse the workload, reinforce the need for teamwork among facilities and departments, and increase team morale by allowing everyone to have a voice in changes that will impact their practice.

Guidance for Unique Clinical Scenarios

Although evidence-based practice can be used on a large scale to impact whole programs affecting large groups of clients, it is also an effective tool for making clinical decisions about very unique or complex individual cases. The following example is used to clarify this point.

A 33-year-old female, diagnosed with Isaac's syndrome by her physician, independently seeks out a massage therapist for possible pain management for her condition. At the initial consultation, the massage therapist is hesitant to initiate any type of massage as he is unfamiliar with this diagnosis and the accompanying symptoms, contraindications, and treatments. He gathers some baseline data, performs a basic assessment with the client, and tentatively schedules her to return in a few days. Because evidence-based practice should actively involve the client in the decision-making process, he shares his concerns with her and explains that he would like to look specifically at the research on this diagnosis to determine what techniques might be most effective for her.

Later that day, the therapist conducts an initial Internet search on Isaac's syndrome. During this search, he finds that Isaac's syndrome is a rare neuromuscular disorder characterized by continual muscle contractions resulting in severe muscle cramps, joint stiffness, and pain (NINDS, 2011). His search leads him to the U.S. Department of Health and Human Services website on genetic and rare diseases, which includes information on clinical trials conducted with individuals diagnosed with this condition (U.S. Department of Health and Human Services, n.d.). Current research includes studies of the etiology of this condition as well as effective treatment options.

Because the condition is rare, he is unable to locate any studies that specifically examine the use of massage for pain management with Isaac's syndrome; however, preliminary findings suggest that range of motion and isometric exercise can be effective in managing the symptoms. He also finds several single case examples of individuals with Isaac's syndrome attesting to the benefits of deep tissue massage to decrease pain. This information coincides with his prior knowledge of other conditions involving muscle spasticity.

Although research has not yet been conducted to specifically examine the use of massage with Isaac's syndrome, this search has allowed the therapist to gain a full understanding of the condition and the current research. Armed with this information, he is now prepared for the collaborative discussion with his client when she returns. Using his skills and knowledge, as well as the recently discovered evidence on this rare condition, the massage therapist collaborates with the client at the next visit to determine the best course of action.

With advances in technology and medical science, new conditions or complex cases are identified more frequently than in the past. As the previous example illustrates, several organizations have been established specifically to research and disseminate information on them. Knowing that you could be faced with a unique scenario in clinical practice can be intimidating, but knowing how to use evidence-based practice to guide your decision-making can foster confidence and lifelong learning. Also be aware that in researching rare conditions, or very specific medical complexities, you may be unlikely to find large numbers of or very rigorous studies. Case studies, qualitative studies, or mixed methods designs with small sample sizes will be more common. In these cases, you have to examine the research that is available and integrate it with your skills and knowledge, as well as the client's goals and circumstances, to determine your course of action. Moreover, use of evidence-based practice can help to incorporate client preferences. In the prior example, remember that the client independently consulted the massage therapist for services, and therefore had a vested interest in collaborating to determine the best treatment.

Justifying the Need for Staff, Equipment, or Services

Evidence-based practice can be an invaluable means of justifying the need for additional staff, equipment, or services. Additional staff and equipment might be needed to meet the changing needs of your clinic or practice, or you might be asked to justify the treatments that you provide to administrators, supervisors, or third-party payors. Without adequate support, clients may be denied beneficial services, or you may lack adequate staff and equipment to complete your job. The following example reveals how evidence-based practice can be used in this endeavor.

A local high school places an advertisement for an athletic trainer to replace the current one who is retiring after 40 years of service to the district. Although the former athletic trainer seemed to meet the needs of the student athletes, the school board is looking to hire a recent graduate who has more cutting-edge knowledge in the field. After several rounds of interviews, a new trainer is hired and begins employment. Although the school board is excited about the innovative skills the new hire will bring to the table, they have not planned nor budgeted for new equipment.

After accepting the position, it does not take the new trainer long to realize that the equipment in the training center is far outdated, posing potential safety risks. She knows the board may not respond favorably to her requests so soon after beginning employment. To combat the problem, she solicits some help from the National Athletic Trainers' Association to locate research on the most cost-effective and clinically beneficial equipment (NATA, 2012). Her search reveals that a variety of budget-friendly equipment, including therapy balls, medicine balls, and resistive bands, have been shown to be just as effective as more costly weight-lifting machines. In addition, much of the literature substantiates her prior belief that the current free weights and outdated equipment pose serious risks to the athletes with continued use.

As a result, she selects the most rigorous and current studies on appropriate equipment for athletic training, assessing each for sound quality and procedures. She makes copies for the athletic director and prepares a concise two-page report pointing out the main findings from the studies as well as a list of potential risks if new equipment cannot be obtained. She schedules a meeting with the athletic director and presents her findings. In cases like this, the evidence often speaks louder than any words. Although the district needs to be mindful of its spending, the board found it difficult to deny the request when the students' safety was clearly on the line.

In this scenario, the trainer used evidence-based practice by integrating her knowledge of anatomy and physiology, injury prevention, and conditioning, as well as the goals of her students with current research to justify the need for some updated equipment. Similarly, this same procedure can be used to justify additional staff in a hospital rehab clinic, a clinical laboratory, or an academic setting. Although you may know firsthand the additional needs, looking to the literature can provide more objective support.

Evidence-based practice can also be used to validate use of specific assessment and treatment techniques in clinical practice. In some cases, third-party payors are denying coverage for various procedures deemed medically unnecessary or unlikely to result in significant changes in condition or function. You may have greater success in appealing each case if you can provide research that shows the success of the modalities or procedures you are requesting. In addition, providing support for what you do is not limited to insurance providers. Clients, families, and policy makers may also demand proof of efficacy for your treatments. Although using evidence-based practice can ensure best practice for your clients, it can also promote modification of current practice to increase efficiency and cost-effectiveness.

Mentoring, Teamwork, and Motivation

Whether you are a nurse, therapist, laboratory technician, or athletic trainer, you have a professional and ethical responsibility to provide your clients with the best treatment possible. In many settings, teamwork lies at the foundation of the process. Research supports a multidisciplinary approach to care, where individual team members approach the client from their area of clinical expertise, but also meet and coordinate the care with other professionals for maximum client satisfaction and benefit (DiGioia, Greenhouse, & Levison, 2007; Gabel, Hilton, & Nathanson, 1997; Murray et al., 2009; Tomita et al., 2009). Evidence can provide support for your clinical decisions and assist other team members to understand your approach. Likewise, when other professionals can justify their actions with sound evidence, you will gain a clearer understanding of their perspective. Often what you do will be impacted by the care provided by other professionals; ultimately, evidence can be used to collaborate with clients and families when the need arises to make tough clinical decisions.

Similarly, evidence-based practice can be used in mentoring relationships. Although you may clearly be the team's expert for one aspect of the client's care, using evidence to support and teach others about your practice will add to your credibility. Whether you are mentoring a student, a new staff, or a team member from another clinical discipline, evidence-based practice can strengthen the collaborative relationship and ensure that you are doing what is truly best for your client. Practitioners can often fall into the trap of "doing what they have always done." Integrating evidence with your clinical skills and knowledge as well as the goals and values of your clients can ensure best practice.

When evidence-based practice is used in teaching and mentoring relationships, the therapeutic relationship between client and practitioner is strengthened, and the cohesion among practitioners is increased. This sense of teamwork serves to improve client outcomes and team morale. Subsequently, enhanced satisfaction and motivation leads to continued use of evidence-based practice in the decision-making process. This cyclic relationship is illustrated in Figure 10-4.

Chapter Summary

Clearly the benefits to evidence-based practice outweigh the time and effort that it takes. Although the examples provided here are very distinct, you may find overlap of the reasons for using evidence-based practice. For example, you may be charged with developing a new program in your setting. During the process, you might mentor a student and a fellow staff member with limited knowledge of appraising research. This effort could serve as a quality improvement initiative for your facility, as well as a way to foster teamwork and motivation among staff and clients.

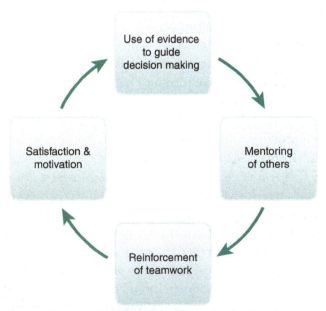

Figure 10-4 Use of Evidence-Based Practice for Mentoring, Teamwork, and Motivation

Furthermore, you may need new supplies and space to get your program started and using the evidence can provide justification to administration. Irrevocably, using evidence-based practice can ignite your passion for your profession and impact the clients that you serve.

SKILL-BUILDING TIPS

■ Use a small journal or an application on your phone or other mobile device to organize your thoughts and jot down ideas for your evidence-based practice project. You will find that you will spend a lot of time thinking about the evidence-based practice project in the preliminary stages and never know when a great idea will hit!

■ Change is often difficult to accept. Despite your drive to make positive changes through use of evidence-based practice, know that not everyone will be on board. Recognizing and learning how to work around the barriers is an important part of the process.

■ If you have difficulty locating literature on your subject, broaden your search terms. Likewise, if your search is returning too many articles, consider narrowing your search terms by focusing on a more specific treatment, population, or setting. Also, do not forget to search the literature in other countries and disciplines.

■ As you search the literature, do not be afraid to reach out to the authors of individual studies if you have questions. Most times, the authors contact information or e-mail is included in the article, and many are more than willing to assist others interested in their area of study.

■ In appraising the articles, do not let the statistics intimidate you. Consulting a basic statistical text such as Salkind's (2011) *Statistics for People Who (Think They) Hate Statistics* or seeking assistance from your supervisor or faculty mentor can help you make sense of the numbers.

■ Remember that all research is flawed. With evidence-based practice, your goal is to tease out the strengths and weaknesses of each study to determine if the findings can be applied to your current practice situation. Drawing on your skills and knowledge as well as the values and circumstances of your clients can help in the decision-making process.

■ Break the process down into smaller, more manageable steps. Set a reasonable time line for completion of each of the five steps of the evidence-based practice process discussed earlier. Be realistic and consider your other obligations and responsibilities.

■ Pursue evidence-based practice initiatives with others whenever possible. Support from others will increase your chances of success, and there is comfort in knowing that others are on the journey with you. Share your questions and concerns; problem-solve together, and most of all believe in yourself!

☁ LEARNING ACTIVITIES

1. What supports and barriers to evidence-based practice exist in your setting? Make a list of each and then contemplate how you might focus on the strengths to circumvent each barrier.

2. Can you identify a need in your setting that you could address through evidence-based practice? Furthermore, what facts, statistics, observations, or other information provide the rationale for the project?

3. What search criteria will you employ for your literature search? Consider what databases you will search as well as key terms, dates of publication, and disciplines or countries of publication that are most appropriate for your goals.

4. Ponder your own evidence-based practice story. How do you envision it playing out? Create a bulleted list of desired outcomes. As you design your plan, review this list to see if the plan aligns with your expectations.

REFERENCES

American Occupational Therapy Association [AOTA]. (2008). Occupational therapy practice framework: Domain and process (2nd ed.). *American Journal of Occupational Therapy, 62*(6), 625–668.

Bickmore, T. (2011). *The power of occupation: Living life with dementia—A training program for formal caregivers.* Unpublished manuscript, Department of Occupational Therapy, Chatham University, Pittsburgh, PA.

Bennett, S., Tooth, L., McKenna, K., Rodger, S., Strong, J., Ziviani, J., . . . Gibson, L. (2003). Perceptions of evidence-based practice: A survey of Australian occupational therapists. *Australian Occupational Therapy Journal, 50*(1), 13–22.

CASP UK. (2012). *Clinical appraisal skills programme: Making sense of evidence.* Retrieved from http://www.casp-uk.net/

Centre for Evidence Based Medicine [CEBM]. (2009). *CATmaker.* University of Oxford, UK.

DiGioia, A. M., Greenhouse, P. K., & Levison, T. J. (2007). Patient and family-centered collaborative care: An orthopaedic model. *Clinical Orthopaedics & Related Research, 463,* 13–19. doi:10.1097/BLO.0b013e31814d4d76

Dubouloz, C. J., Egan, M., Vallerand, J., & von Zweck, C. (1999). Occupational therapists' perceptions of evidence-based practice. *American Occupational Therapy Journal, 53,* 445–453.

Fruth, S. J., Van Veld, R. D., Despos, C. A., Martin, R. D., Hecker, A., & Sincroft, E. E. (2010). The influence of a topic-specific, research-based presentation on physical therapists' beliefs and practices regarding evidence-based practice. *Physiotherapy Theory and Practice, 26*(8), 537–557.

Gabel, M., Hilton, N. E., & Nathanson, S. D. (1997). Multidisciplinary breast cancer clinics. Do they work? *Cancer, 79*(12), 2380–2384.

Glegg, S., & Barrie, A. (2012). *Traffic lighting overview: Identifying the evidence on intervention effectiveness.* Vancouver, BC: Sunny Hill Health Centre for Children.

Gray, J. A. M. (1997). *Evidence based healthcare: How to make health policy and management decisions.* New York: Churchill Livingstone.

Greenhalgh, T. (1997). How to read a paper: Getting your bearings (deciding what the paper is about). *BMJ, 315*(7102), 243–246. doi:10.1136/bmj.315.7102.243

Greenhalgh, T., & Peacock, R. (2005). Effectiveness and efficiency of search methods in systematic reviews of complex evidence: Audit of primary sources. *BMJ, 331,* 1064–1065.

Houser, J. (2008). *Nursing research: Reading, using, and creating evidence.* Sudbury, MA: Jones & Bartlett.

Howick, J. (2009, March). *Centre for evidence based medicine: Levels of evidence.* Retrieved from http://www.google.com/url?sa=t&rct=j&q=&esrc=s&source=web&cd=3&ved=0CDcQFjAC&url=http%3A%2F%2Fwww.cebm.net%2Findex.aspx%3Fo%3D4590&ei=cFALU5eECuHXygH4t4HIBQ&usg=AFQjCNE_HiJhZsc5Evz1_BwdvVFgY0nnSQ&sig2=V-TK5vHLklRxTALL8V3ilA&bvm=bv.61725948,d.aWc

Ilott, I. (2003). Challenging the rhetoric and reality: Only an individual and systemic approach will work for evidence-based occupational therapy. *American Journal of Occupational Therapy, 57*(3), 351–354.

Jette, D. U., Bacon, K., Batty, C., Carlson, M., Ferland, A., Hemingway, R. D., . . . Volk, D. (2003). Evidence-based practice: Beliefs, attitudes, knowledge, and behaviors of physical therapists. *Physical Therapy, 83*(9), 786–805.

Law, M., & MacDermid, J. (Eds.). (2008). *Evidence-based rehabilitation: A guide to practice* (2nd ed.). Thorofare, NJ: SLACK Incorporated.

McCluskey, A. (2003a). *CAT template.* Retrieved from http://www.otcats.com/template/index.html

McCluskey, A. (2003b). Occupational therapists report a low level of knowledge, skill, and involvement in evidence-based practice. *Australian Occupational Therapy Journal, 50,* 3–12.

Miller, M. (2006, January). Client-centered therapy. *Harvard Mental Health Letter, 22*(7), 1–3.

Murray, M. M., Osaki, S., Edwards, N. M., Johnson, M. R., Bobadilla, J. L., Gordon, E. A., . . . Kohmoto, T. (2009). Multidisciplinary approach decreases length of stay and reduces cost for ventricular assist device therapy. *Interactive Cardiovascular and Thoracic Surgery, 8,* 84–88. doi:10.1510/icvts.2008.187377

National Athletic Trainers' Association [NATA]. (2012). *Public resources.* Dallas, TX: Author.

National Institute of Neurological Disorders and Stroke [NINDS]. (2011). *NINDS Isaac's syndrome information page.* Bethesda, MD: Author.

Novak, I. (2010, September 29). Closing the research-practice gap: Responsibilities and solutions. *Evidence Based Practice Workship.* Lecture conducted from Sunny Hill Health Centre, Vancouver.

Sackett, D. L., Rosenberg, W. M. C., Gray, J. A. M., Haynes, R. B., & Richardson, W. S. (1996). Evidence based medicine: What it is and what it isn't. *British Medical Journal, 312,* 71–72.

Salbach, N. M., Guilcher, S. J. T., Jaglal, S. B., & Davis, D. A. (2009). Factors influencing information seeking by physical therapists providing stroke management. *Physical Therapy, 89*(10), 1039–1050.

Salkind, N. J. (2011). *Statistics for people who (think they) hate statistics* (4th ed.). Thousand Oaks, CA: SAGE Publications, Inc.

Schreiber, J., Stern, P., Marchetti, G., & Provident, I. (2008). School-based pediatric physical therapists' perspectives on evidence-based practice. *Pediatric Physical Therapy, 20,* 292–302.

Straus, S. E., Glasziou, P., Richardson, W. S., & Haynes, R. B. (2011). *Evidence-based medicine: How to practice and teach it* (4th ed.). Maryland Heights, MO: Elsevier Churchill Livingstone.

Taylor, M. C. (2008). *Evidence-based practice for occupational therapists* (2nd ed.). Malden, MA: Blackwell Publishing.

Tomita, M. R., Tsai, B. M., Fisher, N. M., Kumar, N. A., Wilding, G., Stanton, K., & Naughton, B. J. (2009). Effects of multidisciplinary Internet-based program on management of heart failure. *Journal of Multidisciplinary Healthcare, 2,* 13–21. doi:10.2147/JMDH.S4355

U.S. Department of Health and Human Services, National Institutes of Health, Office of Rare Diseases Research. (n.d.). *Genetic and rare diseases information center (GARD): Isaac's syndrome.* Retrieved from http://rarediseases.info.nih.gov/GARD/Condition/6793/Isaacs_syndrome.aspx/Showall#Resources

DavisPlus| For additional materials, please visit **http://davisplus.fadavis.com, key word: Hissong.**

Common Tasks Along the Journey

Chapter 11

Before Implementing Your Plan: Important Steps and Considerations

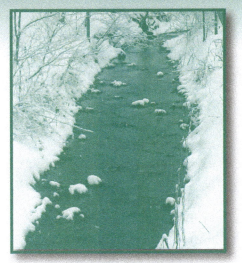

From a certain point onward there is no longer any turning back. That is the point that must be reached.
—*Franz Kafka*

LEARNING OUTCOMES

The information provided in this chapter will assist the reader to:

- Understand the Institutional Review Board (IRB) process.
- Acknowledge the many facets of healthcare ethics and professional behavior.
- Identify if inquiry should include a pilot study or survey.

Important Preparations

You are now almost ready to engage in the inquiry and evidence-based practice process. Just two more items need to be dealt with before you begin. First, you must gain permission from the relevant human participants committee(s). Second, you must double-check to make sure that you have everything needed to complete the inquiry process. For example, make sure that all components (i.e., required equipment, access to meeting rooms, or permission to utilize an evaluation tool) are granted before you begin your project. Before going further, it is important to note that the level or type of evidence-based practice process you are engaging in will determine whether or not you need to complete the human participants or Institutional Review Board (IRB) process. This chapter will also inform the researcher about the process, benefits, and limitations of conducting a pilot study. *From this point on, the chapter will refer to research, but the same policies and procedures may need to be followed for an evidence-based practice inquiry.*

Human Participants Committee Procedures

Before you implement your research study, you must submit a proposal describing your study to the human participants committee, the group responsible for safeguarding the rights of the individuals or groups you will be studying. (These committees may be known by other names, such as *Institutional Review Board* or *research protocol review committee*.) If you are a student, you will address the committee within your university; if you are a healthcare practitioner, you will approach the committee within or connected to your facility. Students planning to conduct research with patients frequently need consent from the human participants committees of both the university and the treating facility.

The purpose of the human participants committee is to ensure that individuals who are participating in a research study are protected and that ethical research standards are employed. This concern for the welfare of human participants in medical research studies was organized into a worldwide system in 1964, at the 18th World Medical Assembly in Helsinki, Finland. At that meeting, the *Declaration of Helsinki* was adopted by the assembly and has since provided the guiding principles for human subject research.

Before conducting research, you must present a proposal to the appropriate human participants committee(s) outlining the purpose, hypotheses, background, definitions of terms, and methodology of the study. The proposal should also describe procedures you will use to ensure the safety, confidentiality, rights, and so on, of the participants. When committee members are satisfied that their requirements have been met, they will give you permission to proceed with the research study. The committee will review the proposal to see if it meets the following criteria:

- The scientific logic on which the study is constructed is sound.
- The study is worthwhile.
- The proposed methodology is sound.
- Procedures are safe.
- The researcher has the skills to perform the study.
- There is provision for informed consent or agreement by participants.
- The benefits of participating in the study outweigh the risks.
- Participants may withdraw their consent to participate at any time.
- Participants' confidentiality will be protected.
- Necessary treatment will not be withheld.

The researcher should always check the IRB's requirements; however, the previous list displays the most common components of any IRB application. At this time, let's review the listed points in more detail:

Sound Scientific Logic: This issue will be addressed by the material you present to the committee on the background, literature review, and scope of the study. These sections of the proposal have already been prepared from the work you did in Chapters 3, 4, and 5, and a summary of these sections will explain the scientific logic of the study to the committee.

Study Is Worthwhile: This issue can be addressed by a summary of the sections you prepared on the purpose and significance of the study, following Chapter 4.

Sound Methodology and Safe Procedures: These items are addressed by the material in Chapters 5 to 9 containing the research design and the techniques for collecting and analyzing data. The committee will decide whether the method is appropriate to the study and whether it will achieve the purpose of the study.

Research Skill: Your qualifications for conducting the research may be substantiated by submission of a resume or by your presence before the committee to present your credentials.

Informed Consent: Participants must understand the nature of the project, what procedures will be used, and how the outcomes will be utilized (Box 11-1). Therefore, you must explain the study in lay terms. In survey research, participants give their tacit consent to participate if they return the survey. In experimental, quasi-experimental, and qualitative studies, participants give their consent in writing and must be offered a copy of the signed informed consent form. Samples of informed consent forms are given in Appendices F and G. If you feel that a subject is unable to give informed consent by virtue of cognitive or physical incapacity or age, you must obtain the legal guardian's consent. If the participants are children, you must obtain the consent of the parents or guardians. If the nature of the research dictates that you cannot tell participants the purpose of the study, because the knowledge may affect their participation in the study, that failure to disclose needs to be clearly explained in the informed consent.

Benefits Outweigh Risks: In the informed consent form, any risks or benefits that may result from participating in the study must be explained to participants (see Appendices F and G, and Box 11-1). The committee will expect that the benefits will outweigh the risks. You should point out possible

BOX 11-1 ■ Outline of an Informed Consent

Title:
Principal Researcher:
Advisor:

1. Purpose:
2. Procedures:
3. Discomforts and Risks:
4. Benefits:
5. Duration or Time commitment:
6. Statement of Confidentiality:
7. Right to Ask Questions:
8. Compensation:
9. Voluntary Participation:

You must be 18 years of age or older to consent to participate in this study. If you consent to participate in this study and to the terms above, please sign your name and indicate the date below. You will be given a copy of this form to keep for your records.

_____   _____
Participant Signature   Date
I, the undersigned, verify that the above informed consent procedure has been followed.

_____   _____
Researcher Signature   Date

side effects of the study and discuss precautions you will take to prevent harm to participants. You should also explain the place and length of time for the study sessions.

Withdrawal of Consent: The informed consent form should include a statement indicating that there will be no reprisal, regardless of the subject's willingness to participate (see Box 11-1). Occasionally, clients may fear that their treatment may be compromised in some way if they refuse to participate in a study; they may feel they will not receive the same quality of care as the study participants. This problem especially arises if the therapist implementing the study is also the clients' treating therapist. It must also be made clear in the written informed consent form that

participants can terminate participation in the study at any point without fear of reprisal (see Appendix F and G).

Confidentiality: If there will be any audiotape or videotape recording of participants' behavior or interviews, such as samples of participants' writing or art work, the document must state how the information from these recordings and actual tapes will be used and what will happen to them at the conclusion of the study (see Box 11-1). It is typical to offer participants, or their guardians an opportunity to view the materials if they wish. Participants must be assured that materials will be kept in a secure place during the study and told who will have access to them. If the results of the study are to be published, participants need to know that their anonymity is guaranteed. Separate written permission must be gained if photographs are to be used in the published material. Survey respondents also need to be assured that their anonymity will be guarded. This is usually accomplished by having them return the surveys anonymously. Survey respondents are not asked to sign a consent form, because responding to the survey is considered as consent to participate. If participants are to be paid for their participation in the study, payment should be based on work and time considerations rather than as compensation for any risk involved or as inducement to poor participants to participate.

Acknowledgement That Treatment Will Not Be Withheld: If experimental and control groups will be included in the study, participants might not be told to which group they are assigned. If the study is conducted to test a new procedure with the experimental group, the control groups may receive either the standard treatment or no treatment. Some facilities don't allow participants to be in control groups that do not receive treatment, which is understandable, as these individuals are usually in the facility for the express purpose of being treated. This expectation will dictate the activity of the control group, and researchers must abide by the facility's regulations.

Healthcare Research Ethics

Healthcare researchers are expected to behave ethically in all areas of their practice. It is the researcher's responsibility to know the rules of conduct. Professional associations have a code of ethics: a public statement of the values and principles expected of practitioners in that profession. Some of these ethical principles pertain to healthcare practitioner research behavior, as reviewed in Box 11-2 for occupational therapy practitioners. Each healthcare profession has published ethical standards that can be obtained readily through the national association or registry. Researchers must show integrity and be guided by ethical principles that include respecting the rights of participants, abiding by the research design, and reporting results accurately and truthfully.

It is particularly important to guard zealously the rights of participants who are in institutional environments, such as persons with developmental disabilities, persons with behavioral health issues, and persons who are imprisoned. Individuals in these settings are particularly vulnerable and are not usually in a position to serve as their own advocates; therefore, researchers

---

BOX 11-2 ■ **Example of Ethics in Research**

The following excerpt from the 2010 Occupational Therapy Code of Ethics pertains to research behavior (AOTA, 2010).

NONMALEFICENCE

Principle 2. Occupational therapy personnel shall intentionally refrain from actions that cause harm.

Nonmaleficence imparts an obligation to refrain from harming others (Beauchamp & Childress, 2009, as cited in AOTA, 2010). The principle of nonmaleficence is grounded in the practitioner's responsibility to refrain from causing harm, inflicting injury, or wronging others. Although beneficence requires action to incur benefit, nonmaleficence requires nonaction to avoid harm (Beauchamp & Childress, 2009). Nonmaleficence also includes an obligation to not impose risks of harm even if the potential risk is without malicious or harmful intent. This principle often is examined under the context of *due care*. If the standard of due care outweighs the benefit of treatment, then refraining from treatment provision would be ethically indicated. (Beauchamp & Childress, 2009)

Occupational Therapy Personnel Shall

A. Avoid inflicting harm or injury to recipients of occupational therapy services, students, research participants, or employees.

B. Make every effort to ensure continuity of services or options for transition to appropriate services to avoid abandoning the service recipient if the current provider is unavailable because of medical or other absence or loss of employment.

C. Avoid relationships that exploit the recipient of services, students, research participants, or employees physically, emotionally, psychologically, financially, socially, or in any other manner that conflicts or interferes with professional judgment and objectivity.

D. Avoid engaging in any sexual relationship or activity; whether consensual or nonconsensual, with any recipient of service, including family or significant other, student, research participant, or employee, whereas a relationship exists as an occupational therapy practitioner, educator, researcher, supervisor, or employer.

E. Recognize and take appropriate action to remedy personal problems and limitations that might cause harm to recipients of service, colleagues, students, research participants, or others.

F. Avoid any undue influences, such as alcohol or drugs that may compromise the provision of occupational therapy services, education, or research.

BOX 11-2 ■ Example of Ethics in Research—cont'd

G. Avoid situations in which a practitioner, educator, researcher, or employer is unable to maintain clear professional boundaries or objectivity to ensure the safety and well-being of recipients of service, students, research participants, and employees.

H. Maintain awareness of and adherence to the Code and Ethics Standards when participating in volunteer roles.

I. Avoid compromising client rights or well-being based on arbitrary administrative directives by exercising professional judgment and critical analysis.

J. Avoid exploiting any relationship established as an occupational therapist or occupational therapy assistant to further one's own physical, emotional, financial, political, or business interests at the expense of the best interests of recipients of services, students, research participants, employees, or colleagues.

K. Avoid participating in bartering for services because of the potential for exploitation and conflict of interest unless there are clearly no contraindications or bartering is a culturally appropriate custom.

L. Determine the proportion of risk to benefit for participants in research before implementing a study.

---

must be especially careful not to take advantage of them and know the boundaries of the research agenda. There is often an ombudsman or client advocate in these types of facilities, and researchers would do well to include such persons in the consent process.

Another ethical consideration is that researchers must abide by the research design as it was presented and approved by the human participants committee. Unexpected issues may arise that cause researchers to redesign their study. If this is the case, the revised design must be submitted to the committee to ensure that it still meets requirements. If any of the changes affects the informed consent form signed by the participants, they must also be informed and a new informed consent form signed.

Finally, there are definite ethical standards involving the reporting of research results. Sometimes, some findings support the hypotheses or research questions, whereas others do not. All findings must be reported. In a quantitative study, if findings are not at the identified level for statistical significance, they must be presented as found. In a qualitative study, it is important to report exactly what the participant said or identify themes that accurately relay what the participants meant when answering a question or making a point. It can't be stressed enough that the

highest integrity must be maintained in reporting on all phases of the study, exactly as they occurred in the moment of the inquiry.

Just a few more words are needed about ethical conduct in qualitative research. Qualitative researchers must remember the ethical issues raised when they first became closely involved in the events or situations under study, confidentiality of data that may be extremely personal, anonymity of participants who may provide idiosyncratic and identifiable data, readers' ability to distinguish between data and the researchers' interpretations, possible long-term effects of in-depth interviewing about personal issues, and knowledge gained from participants' unself-conscious acts during participant observation.

The Pilot Study: A Helpful Measure of a Researcher's Readiness

The pilot study is a preliminary trial of the study, or a mini-study, that may be performed before the final study. The pilot study has been suggested as a way to check on the feasibility of various components of the project, including the researcher's readiness to carry out the inquiry. The following paragraphs will examine what a pilot study should include, how it is done, and what can be learned from it.

Most of the steps in the final study should be included in the pilot study, but on a smaller scale. The number of participants will be considerably smaller than in the final study, but they should be selected from the target population, so that results are likely to be representative of those of the final study. The process will be the same as the one proposed for the final study, including the analysis of the data generated from the pilot group. As a result, the pilot study provides an evaluation of the proposed process and may be used to remove flaws.

A pilot study may reveal fundamental problems in the logic that leads to the study's conclusions, in which case a major revision of the research questions may be in order. Lesser flaws may require only simple changes in the measuring instrument or subject selection criteria to make the project satisfactory. Some modifications of the original proposal are almost always necessary, so pilot studies invariably improve the design and data of the final project. Therefore, it is worthwhile to take the time and effort to perform a pilot study.

The items that may be tested in a pilot study include methods and scientific logic. Those concerning scientific logic might include:

- Has the problem under study been too broadly or too narrowly defined?
- Are the variables suitable?
  - Will the resulting data address the purpose of the study?

Those concerning methodological issues might include:

- Are the survey questions clearly stated?
- Will the investigative methods generate information suitable for answering the research question?
- Are appropriate participants available?
- Are the variables discrete and can they be measured meaningfully?
- Is the measuring instrument accurate and practical?

Typically, certain items in each type of research design can be best evaluated by a pilot study. For example, in survey research, the way in which questions are composed is very important. A pilot study will tell the researcher if respondents understand the questions, if the questions elicit the information desired, and whether the survey is too long or too short. Respondents should know that they are answering a pilot study instrument and that they will be asked if they have any suggestions for improvements in the questions and the cover letter and how long it took them to complete the survey.

Performing a pilot study can be difficult in experimental research because the researcher may have access to only a few participants who meet the selection criteria. Consequently, if participants are engaged in a pilot study; there may not be a sufficient number of participants for the final study. In behavioral research, participants often cannot participate twice (once in the pilot study and again in the final study) because the effects intervention provided in the pilot study might influence the results of the final study. Sometimes this can be overcome by using a pilot sample of suitable participants from another facility or by using a slightly different population. This solution is often preferable to eliminating the pilot study altogether.

Sometimes experimental and quasi-experimental research studies are performed on very small samples with no pilot studies, simply because of constraints on time, money, or access to participants. The downside to not conducting a pilot study is that the results of such inquiries are often published with a list of limitations and disclaimers. In this situation it is preferable to regard the project as a pilot study, and then pursue a second study, amending philosophy and procedures to address the limitations of the pilot study. The results of the second study would then be more valid and meaningful (Boxes 11-3 and 11-4).

In methodological research, the pilot study is built into the research process at the stage when the newly developed measure is tested on a sample, changes are made, and the revised measure is tested again. The process may occur several times before the researcher feels satisfied with the results. This test and retest procedure serves the same purpose as a pilot study and may be considered as such.

In the summative component of evaluation research, the survey instruments used to garner data about the

BOX 11-3 ■ Example 1 of Pilot Study

Case study research is often conducted as a pilot study, in the sense that the individual case is used to generate hypotheses that will later be tested experimentally on a large sample of similar participants. However, if the researcher does not intend the case study to be a pilot for a larger study, portions of the case may be piloted ahead of time. Portions that may be pretested include the use of the equipment, the validity of the measuring instrument, or the usefulness of the data-gathering technique.

BOX 11-4 ■ Example 2 of Pilot Study

In discussing the design of qualitative research, Marshall and Rossman (2011) state that: . . . use of a pilot study can lend credence to the researcher's claim that he can conduct such a study. He can illustrate his ability to manage qualitative research by describing initial observations or interviews. . . . A description of initial observations demonstrates not only the ability to manage this research, but also the strength of the approach for revealing enticing research questions. Inclusion of a description of a pilot study or initial observations can strengthen the proposal.

program under study may appropriately be subjected to a pilot study. This ensures that the questions will elicit needed data and be understood by respondents.

In regard to qualitative research, an historical study does not lend itself to the use of a pilot study because it involves only one event or chain of events being studied. If the method of data collection proves unsatisfactory, no harm has been done to the historical event and other methods may be explored. Generally, it is considered part of the study method to try different forms of data collection and data analysis until satisfactory methods are found.

Similarly, ethnographic research is similar to historical research in this respect. One culture or program is under study, and data can be collected and analyzed in many ways until the process is considered satisfactory. Sometimes an event within the culture or program will occur only once (such as an unusual ceremony or a patient trying a rare treatment); in that case, the researcher must be ready with the best method to capture that event exactly when it occurs. This may require preparation by testing certain techniques ahead of time; in other words, running a pilot study, perhaps in a simulated situation. It is almost always methodology, rather than scientific logic or philosophical issues, that needs testing in this type of once-only research. In fact, in ethnographic research, proposing and rejecting philosophical issues in the data analysis is one of the main ways of interpreting data.

Finally, another important purpose of performing a pilot study is that it gives the researcher a chance to practice conducting research. Like most things, research becomes easier and improves in quality with practice. A pilot study gives the novice researcher a good opportunity to gain skill while achieving the all-important goal of improving the research design.

Implementing the Project

Practical issues must now be arranged. Depending on the type of research, these may be as varied as scheduling times and places to meet with participants, arranging access to rooms and equipment, training raters or data gatherers, copying and mailing surveys, locating suitable client records for review, or arranging to videotape a group procedure.

You are finally ready to carry out your research project. As you can see, it takes an enormous amount of work to prepare for the treatment or action component of a research study. Yet often this is the only component that people equate with the term *research*.

Chapter Summary

First, this chapter provides the reader with insights to the Institutional Review Board (IRB) process, which takes a considerable amount of planning and time to complete in addition to the inquiry or project. The reader is then reminded of the exacting policies, procedures, and professional behaviors that must be employed and followed when engaging in an inquiry. Lastly, readers are provided with insights to determine whether their particular inquiry should engage in a pilot study or a survey.

SKILL-BUILDING TIPS

■ Researchers often underestimate the length of time needed to gain permission from a human participants committee. This process can take anywhere from 1 to 6 months, depending on the frequency of committee meetings and whether all materials have been submitted correctly and completely. If the protocol needs to be revised, it may take even longer. You should probably submit the proposal to the committee just after the research protocol is written. This will allow sufficient time for notification by the committee before the start of data collection.

■ It is important to determine the exact requirements of the committee to which you are applying. All of the committees have detailed written instructions and most will have an electronic packet of instructions.

■ When describing a study to potential participants in order to obtain informed consent, it is sometimes difficult to know if the explanation has been fully understood. If there is any doubt about the participant's comprehension, it is a good idea for the person who knows the individual best to be present to assess how much is understood and perhaps to reword the explanation so that it is meaningful to the client. Some human participants committees require that a member of the committee be present on such an occasion, whereas others have a human rights officer, an ombudsman, or an advocate who will serve this purpose.

LEARNING ACTIVITIES

1. Find out which human participants committee is responsible for the participants you intend to study. Request a copy of that committee's requirements to review sooner than later.

2. Practice writing up an informed consent statement for your participants. (To assist with this review, see the examples of informed consent forms in Appendices F and G). Remember to:
   ■ Include the purpose of the study
   ■ Include the place and the amount of time the study will require of participants
   ■ Include a description of the procedure to be used
   ■ State that participation is voluntary
   ■ State that participation can be withdrawn at any time without fear of reprisal
   ■ List the risks and benefits of the study
   ■ Cite any costs that may be involved
   ■ Describe how confidentiality will be protected
   ■ Give the name of someone who will be available to answer questions about the research
   ■ State that a copy of this statement will be offered to participants
   ■ Provide a space for the subject's signature, a witness's signature, and, if needed, a parent or guardian signature
   ■ Provide a space for the date of the signatures

3. The committee will want to know details about the researchers involved in the study. List your qualifications as head of the research team, and state why you are qualified to carry out the proposed research project. If you have an advisor or mentors assisting you with the study, you will also need to list their credentials.

4. Decide whether your study lends itself to a pilot study. Will methodological issues, scientific logic issues, or both need to be piloted? List the parts you think could be improved by a pilot study and say why.

Methodological issues:

Scientific logic issues:

Is it feasible and wise to utilize participants for the pilot study sample?

If so, how will you select them?

If not, where can you find pilot study participants?

5. Write a protocol for a pilot study. It will resemble the protocol you wrote earlier and should contain the following:

- Subject criteria
- Subject selection method
- Research questions or hypotheses

- Variables
- Procedures for treatment (if quantitative research)
- Data collection techniques (if quantitative research)
- Data analysis methods (if quantitative research)
- Procedures for data collection and analysis (if qualitative research)

REFERENCES

Commission on Standards and Ethics, AOTA. (2010). Occupational therapy code of ethics. *American Journal of Occupational Therapy*, *64*, S4–S16.

Marshall, C., & Rossman, G. B. (2011). *Designing qualitative research*. Newbury Park, CA: Sage Publications.

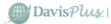 **DavisPlus** | For additional materials, please visit **http://davisplus.fadavis.com, key word: Hissong.**

Chapter 12

The Art of Writing Up the Research Study or Evidence-Based Practice Project

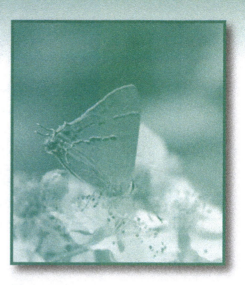

The difference between something good and something great is attention to detail.
—*Charles R. Swindoll*

LEARNING OUTCOMES

The information provided in this chapter will assist the reader to:

- Understand the sections that are typically included in a formalized report of a research study or evidence-based practice project.
- Determine the best way to present data and outcomes visually.
- Synthesize data with existing literature to effectively report study findings and draw conclusions.
- Explore styles of scientific writing and discover tips for becoming a better writer.
- Construct a formal report on a research study or evidence-based practice project.

In conducting a research study or an evidence-based practice project, a formal report of the background, methodology, outcomes, and analysis is often prepared. This information is typically arranged into chapters. A suggested formal chapter outline for a research study is included in Box 12-1; the suggested chapter outline for an evidence-based practice project can be found in Box 10-2 (Chapter 10 of this text). There are many similarities between the two reports, but some variations do exist related to the differing goals of research and evidence-based practice. Whereas the purpose of the research report is to convey information gained from scientific inquiry and procedures, the function of the evidence-based practice report is to illustrate application of existing research and evaluate the outcomes to inform practice and future program development. Each chapter of the reports and the suggested content will be reviewed.

Chapter 1: Introduction and Overview of the Topic of Interest

In both reports, Chapter 1 helps to "set the stage" for the study or project. In the research report, Chapter 1 serves to orient the reader to the topic investigated, to outline the scope of the study, and to explicitly review the research hypothesis or research question. For the evidence-based practice report, Chapter 1 commonly includes a detailed description of the

---

BOX 12-1 ■ **Research Study Outline**

Abstract			**Chapter 4**	**Implementation and Results**

Abstract

Chapter 1   Introduction and Overview of the Topic of Interest

Section 1.1   Background of the Topic
Section 1.2   Scope of the Study
Section 1.3   Hypothesis and Research Question

Chapter 2   Literature Review

Section 2.1   Methodology of the Literature Search
Section 2.2   Synthesis of the CAT Portfolio *(See Appendix A: Individual CAP Outlines)* *Subsections will include:*

- *Description of the Portfolio*
- *Additional subsections will be individualized to your project and will be organized around common themes in the literature*

Chapter 3   Methodology

Section 3.1   Frameworks or Models of Practice Guiding the Research
Section 3.2   Subject Selection and Recruitment
Section 3.3   Research Design and Procedures
Section 3.4   Assumptions

Chapter 4   Implementation and Results

Section 4.1   Description of the Subjects
Section 4.2   Results (quantitative, qualitative, or both, if applicable) *May include:*

- *Tables and figures to display data, outcomes, and statistical results*

Chapter 5   Evaluation, Discussion, and Conclusions

Section 5.1   Implications of Findings and Correlation of Results With Existing Literature
Section 5.2   Limitations
Section 5.3   Recommendations for Practice or Future Research

References

Appendix A: Individual CAP Outlines

- *You will likely have additional appendices that include items such as tools used in the project, lengthy tables and graphs, and so on.*

---

setting where the project took place, as well as an explanation of the problem and the rationale for addressing it. As noted previously, supporting these points with other resources illustrates the need for the project, and a needs assessment or SWOT analysis (see Chapter 10 of this text) can be helpful during the planning phase of the project. Additionally, a review of supports and threats inherent in the setting allows one to approach the project realistically, and ultimately devise a feasible evidence-based practice question.

More details regarding the evidence-based practice setting are included because these projects, in contrast to ground-level research, are situated in real-life practice scenarios and involve application of existing research. Without a detailed description of the setting, the reader is unable to place the existing research into the current context. Also, when evidence-based practice is used for new program development or quality improvement, a strong rationale can aid in obtaining necessary funding or administrative approval for the project.

Chapter 2: Literature Review

In both research and evidence-based practice projects, Chapter 2 contains the literature review. The group of research articles selected for the literature review can be referred to collectively as the **research portfolio**. In-depth descriptions about the search methodology, key search terms used, as well as inclusion and exclusion criteria for the articles selected, is usually included. Reporting on the databases searched, search terms (and combinations of search terms) used, and any other parameters set (such as limiting the search to articles published within the last 5 years) allows the search to be replicated if necessary and lets the reader know how exhaustive the search was. Box 10-3 includes an example of what the search methodology section might look like.

Describing and Synthesizing the Literature

After the search methodology is sufficiently explained, the task of describing and synthesizing the research articles within the portfolio should be undertaken. The description of the portfolio is usually a straightforward review of the number of articles, study designs, time frame of the studies, where the studies took place, and the general topics. Box 10-4 contains an example of a portfolio description for a professional leadership project. Following description of the portfolio, one would expect a comprehensive narrative synthesis of all studies within the portfolio. This section is likely one of the most labor-intensive to write and will include multiple subsections individualized to the project being conducted. Subsections will be organized around common themes within the literature, with multiple citations from the referenced articles to support each theme. Remember that themes can only be identified when more than one study yields the same or similar findings.

In order to effectively synthesize studies in the portfolio, each one should be critically appraised, regardless of whether research or evidence-based practice is being conducted. When conducting research, existing literature on the topic needs to be appraised in order to ascertain gaps in the research that the new study aims to fill. This task also helps to situate the current study within the context of past studies in the field. In evidence-based practice, evaluating the scientific rigor and applicability of each study to the current practice situation allows the evidence-based practitioner to make decisions about if and how the research will be applied to practice. An individual template to appraise each study is included in Table 10-3 of this text.

Chapter 3: Methodology

Chapter 3 is very similar for the research study and the evidence-based practice project. It should include the detailed methodology as well as discussions of guiding frameworks and conceptual models, assumptions, and subject and participant information. In both cases, one should strive to sufficiently describe the procedures so that they can be replicated. This serves two purposes. First, it allows the reader to fully understand and apply the results of the project; second, it permits modification of specific aspects of the procedures if shortcomings are noted.

In describing the procedure, three elements need to be included. First, it is important to review any frameworks or models of practice used to guide or design the methodology. As noted in Chapter 5 of this text, conceptual frameworks, also known as models of practice, are theoretical explanations of functioning that can guide practitioners in client treatment or researchers in their approach to a study. Discussing these guiding principles helps the reader understand the perspective from which the evidence-based practitioner or researcher approached the project.

Second, operational definitions of all key terms and concepts should be included within the methodology. Recall from Chapter 5 of this text that operationalizing involves strictly defining terms so that their meaning cannot be misinterpreted. It is acceptable to use definitions from dictionaries, medical textbooks, authorities on the topic, or to create your own. As long as sufficient detail is provided, misunderstanding of concepts or inconsistent measurement of phenomena can be avoided.

Third, assumptions made when designing the methodology should be discussed. As noted in Chapter 5 of this text, assumptions are underlying principles that the researcher or evidence-based practitioner believes or accepts but that are difficult to prove in any concrete way. Assumptions can be made about the ideological principles upon which the project is based, or concerning the procedures used in the project. Assumptions can be discussed in narrative form, but are frequently enumerated in a bulleted list.

Subject or Participant Recruitment & Selection

Information about the subject or participant (client) recruitment and selection is also included in this chapter. To clarify, the term *subjects* is often employed when discussing research, whereas the terms *participants* or *clients* are used more commonly in the evidence-based practice literature. For a research study, a list of subject inclusion and exclusion criteria, as well as descriptions of subject recruitment and sampling methods, should be included. For an evidence-based practice project, participant inclusion and exclusion criteria are clarified as well as the approach to client-centeredness. Remember from Chapter 10 of this text that evidence-based practice involves the interweaving of three elements—evidence; practitioner skills and knowledge; and client goals, values, and circumstances. Care should be taken to delineate exactly how the methodology will be varied to meet each client's needs in an evidence-based practice project. This section is omitted in a research project, where the aim is to adhere to stricter procedures to generate new information.

Chapter 4: Implementation and Results

Whether you are conducting research or evidence-based practice, Chapter 4 will be used to elaborate on the course of the project as well as the results. For an evidence-based practice project, thorough descriptions of the actual participants, modifications to the original project plan, and a synopsis of the implementation are commonly provided. For a research project, it is usually not necessary to include lengthy discussions about these elements because little deviation in stringent procedures occurs. The descriptions of the participants and project progression are typically more in depth for evidence-based practice projects, because of the fact that procedures are commonly altered to accommodate real-life practice situations and participants' needs. In any case, if modifications in procedures are necessary, they should be presented and discussed.

Describing Subjects or Participants

The subjects or participants should be described numerically for research or evidence-based practice projects. From this information, it will be possible for readers to gain a clear picture of the study sample or participant group, so that later they may superimpose the findings of the project on that picture. It is customary to present descriptive statistics including frequencies, percentages, a range, and some sort of central tendency (such as the mean) for the data. This information will give readers solid information about what the subjects or participants looked like and how they performed during the project. The description can be in the narrative format or in the form of tables or figures. See Box 12-2 for an example.

Reporting Results

Research studies and evidence-based practice projects can yield quantitative data, qualitative data, or both, depending on the topic, setting, and goals of the venture. Results are typically included in this chapter

---

BOX 12-2 ■ **Example of Description of Subjects**

In Chiarello et al.'s (2010) study on family priorities for activity and participation of children with cerebral palsy, they described the subjects in a table as well as in the narrative that follows.

Table 1 provides demographic information on the participants and their children. The participants were primarily mothers (80%) and fathers (11%). Other participants included stepparents, foster parents, grandparents, and guardians. All will be referred to as parents throughout the article. Parents had a mean age of 40.3 years (SD = 9.3), 50% had education beyond high school, and 61% were employed. The children and youth were 2 to 21 years of age, with a mean age of 11.0 years (SD = 4.5); 56% were male, and 44% were female. Table 1 provides demographic information of the children and youth grouped by age: under 6 years, 6 to 12 years, and 13 to 21 years. Gross motor function varied across Gross Motor Function Classification System (GMFCS) levels. (p. 1256)

of the formal report (Chapter 4) and can be discussed in narrative format, or displayed in tables and figures. In the results section of an article, only the facts of the study or project are presented, with no interpretation. Authors must be careful not to include their own biases or conclusions in the results section. Rather, they must keep to a factual account of what actually happened and what was actually found.

All the results must be mentioned in the results section of a report, not just the ones that substantiate the hypotheses or suit the researcher's or practitioner's needs. Even though interpretations and conclusions will be presented later in the article, readers must be able to decide for themselves the efficacy of these conclusions by having all the data at hand. In a research report, it should be clearly stated which of the hypotheses were or were not supported. In the case of inferential statistical results, the reader should be told if the significance level established at the start of the project was reached.

Experimental, quasi-experimental, or correlational research will yield quantitative data, and inferential statistics may be used to determine if there are meaningful differences or similarities between groups. The probability ratios provide that information and indicate if the hypotheses have been substantiated. Each hypothesis should be reviewed and checked against the statistical results. For each hypothesis, readers should be informed if it was substantiated and then provided with the probability level and details of the findings. It is customary for results to be reported from the general to the specific. For example, in their study on the effects of virtual reality gaming on dynamic balance and strength in older adults, Rendon et al. (2012) reported "the Mann-Whitney test was used to determine significant differences ($P < 0.05$) between groups at baseline and change in outcome measures over time" (p. 551). Comparison of the statistical results with the chosen probability level reveals that the virtual reality group demonstrated significantly improved balance ($P = 0.038$) and self-confidence with balance ($P = 0.038$) when compared with the control group (Rendon et al., 2012).

Survey research, case studies, and evaluation research may likely garner descriptive quantitative data. The data should be reported in a manner similar to that used to describe the sample or participant group; that is, using descriptive statistics such as frequencies, percentages, ranges, and central tendencies. Presenting this data in narrative or visual form is appropriate.

In a nonexperimental study or a qualitative study, you may have subjected some data to one or more of the coding procedures. The results of the coding must be presented as clearly and simply as possible. In this type of presentation, the weight of the evidence will determine if the hypotheses have been substantiated—a judgment the researcher must make because it is not possible to subject the evidence to statistical significance testing.

Descriptive statistics or qualitative thematic analyses are most commonly used in evidence-based practice. Because these projects tend to be rooted in real-life clinical situations, and participant groups are smaller or restricted to one practice, clinic, or health system, inferential statistics are usually not appropriate. In addition, remember that the goal of evidence-based practice is to apply existing evidence to practice and then evaluate the success of the outcomes. Although standardized measures can be used to gather participant data, success of the intervention is not based on statistical outcomes, but rather clinical ones. Tables and figures are commonly used to display data in evidence-based practice projects as well.

Visual Displays of Data

Displaying data pictorially allows readers to gain an immediate and overall concept of the results and lets them make sense of quantities of data at a glance. As the old saying goes, "A picture is worth a thousand words," or in this case, a thousand numbers. Tables and figures can eliminate many complicated or boring narratives, but they should be used judiciously; too many can become confusing.

Data can be presented pictorially in one of two ways—tables and figures. **Tables** are the most common type of illustration, and can be used to present simple lists of frequencies and percentages, or to consolidate and present data, such as numbers of pounds squeezed on a dynamometer. For example, if scores are arranged in order from highest to lowest (rank ordering), readers can easily gain an overview of the responses. They can see the range of scores—the highest, lowest, and middle scores—and can compare one person's scores against the others.

Tables are especially useful for condensing large quantities of data so that the reader can understand the information more readily. Suppose a study yielded 50 scores of degrees of elbow flexion for a group of patients. Even presenting the 50 scores in order of magnitude would be difficult for a reader to digest and think about usefully. In this case, grouping the scores, say into units of 20, would reduce the data and allow the reader to grasp its implications more efficiently (see Table 12-1). From this table it is possible to understand quickly the spread of scores. Most patients had flexion in the midrange (60 degrees to 120 degrees), whereas few patients had flexion at the greater and smaller angles. Even though some detail is lost in this type of grouping, it is generally a useful and efficient representation of data.

Tables are commonly used to illustrate the findings from descriptive and inferential statistics. In this case, they can present detailed information more easily and in less space than would be required by narration. It is not necessary to repeat all the table data in the text. The researcher or evidence-based practitioner should merely highlight important points. Tables 12-2 and 12-3 present data generated from descriptive statistics and inferential statistics.

Although tables are invaluable for concisely communicating a large set of numbers, many people find

Table 12-1 ■ Degrees of Elbow Flexion Following Treatment (N = 50)

Degrees of Elbow Flexion	Frequency of Occurrence
20–40	2
41–60	4
61–80	9
81–100	10
101–120	12
121-140	9
141-160	3
161-180	1

Table 12-2 ■ Distribution of Demographic Characteristics of Healthcare Administrators and Clinicians (N = 385)

Demographic Characteristics	Administrators (N = 201)		Clinicians (N = 184)		Total Group	
	Frequency	Percentage	Frequency	Percentage	Frequency	Percentage
Age:						
20–25 years	0	0	2	1	2	0.5
26–30 years	17	9	46	25	63	16
31–35 years	56	28	52	28	108	28
36–40 years	33	16	26	14	59	15
41–50 years	53	26	40	22	93	24
51+ years	42	21	18	10	60	16
College degree:						
Associate	95	47	113	61	208	57

Table 12-2 ■ **Distribution of Demographic Characteristics of Healthcare Administrators and Clinicians (N = 385)—cont'd**

Demographic Characteristics	Administrators (N = 201)		Clinicians (N = 184)		Total Group	
	Frequency	Percentage	Frequency	Percentage	Frequency	Percentage
BA/BS	13	10	17	9	30	8
MA/MS	10	6	8	4	18	6
Certificate	21	11	4	2	25	7
Clinical doctorate	47	25	19	15	66	17
Research doctorate	4	2	0	0	4	1
Age when took first job:						
20–25 years	178	89	156	85	334	87
26–30 years	14	7	17	8	28	7
31–35 years	4	2	5	3	9	2
36–40 years	2	1	5	3	7	2
41+ years	5	2	4	2	9	2
Specialty of practice:						
Psychiatry	60	30	49	27	109	29
Pediatrics	31	15	59	32	90	24
Physical disabilities	95	47	63	35	158	41
Geriatrics	15	8	11	6	26	7

it difficult to get the "big picture" from a table. This is where we turn to figures. **Figures** are used to illustrate visual images of items or events, changes in numbers of items over time, or comparisons of multiple items. Figures can include bar graphs, line graphs, diagrams, flowcharts, pie charts, photographs, schematics, or drawings, to name a few. To further clarify, tables are best for presenting data, whereas figures are used to help the reader gain a clearer understanding of the outcomes and to propose relationships among key concepts in the study or project. Consult Table 12-4 to determine the most appropriate illustration for your goals.

Line graphs are used to show changes in a phenomenon over time. Measurements of some attribute are plotted at multiple points during the study, and all points are joined to form a continuous line on the graph. Line graphs can only present continuous data, and more than one line can be included on the same graph to reveal trends among two or more groups. An example of a line graph can be found in Figure 12-1; student test scores were plotted for 2000 and 2012. Examination of the graph reveals that scores improved in 2012, possibly because of changes in curriculum design, for example.

Bar graphs are similar, except that they are formed by drawing a vertical bar at each frequency gained

Table 12-3 ■ Differences Between Administrators and Clinicians on Demographic Characteristics (N = 385)

Role by Characteristic	Pearson Chi-Square	Significance Level
Role by age	31.22	0.00*
Role by degree	31.22	0.00*
Role by age when decided to enter the field	2.68	0.75
Role by age at taking first job	2.24	0.69
Role by specialty practice	18.20	0.00*
Role by mother's education	3.71	0.81
Role by father's education	7.73	0.36
Role by mentor	6.22	0.10

$*p < 0.001$

Table 12-4 ■ Choosing the Most Effective Type of Illustration for a Given Goal

To Accomplish this:	Choose one of these:
To present exact values, raw data, or data which do not fit into any simple pattern	Table, list
To summarize trends, show interactions between two or more variables, relate data to constants, or emphasize an overall pattern rather than specific measurements	Line graph
To dramatize differences or draw comparisons	Bar graph
To illustrate complex relationships, spatial configurations, pathways, processes, or interactions	Diagram
To show sequential processes	Flowchart
To classify information	Table, list, pictograph
To describe parts or electric circuits	Schematic
To describe a process, organization, or model	Pictograph, flowchart, block diagram
To compare and contrast	Pictograph, pie chart, bar graph
To describe a change of state	Line graph, bar graph
To describe proportions	Pie chart, bar graph
To describe relationships	Table, line graph, block diagram

Table 12-4 ■ Choosing the Most Effective Type of Illustration for a Given Goal—cont'd	
To Accomplish this:	**Choose one of these:**
To describe causation	Flowchart, pictograph
To describe an entire object	Schematic, drawing, photograph
To show the vertical and horizontal hierarchy within an object, idea, or organization	Flowchart, drawing tree, block diagram

Matthews, J. & Matthews, R. (2008). Successful scientific writing: A step-by-step guide for the biological and medical sciences. (3rd ed.) United Kingdom: Cambridge University Press. Reprinted with permission of Cambridge University Press.

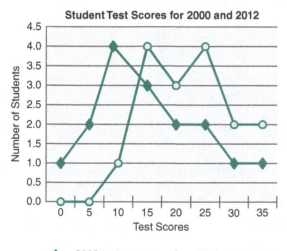

Figure 12-1 Line Graph Comparing Test Scores for Students at Two Different Points in Time

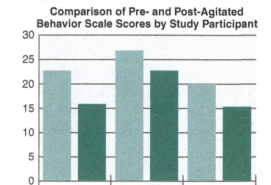

Figure 12-2 Bar Graph Comparing Pre- and Postscores for Study Participants

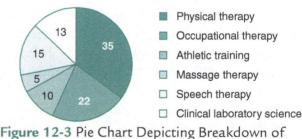

Figure 12-3 Pie Chart Depicting Breakdown of Employees

across the width of the score interval. This offers a strong visual impact and is often effective for comparing scores among all participants, or in comparing pre- and postscores among individuals or the study groups. See Figure 12-2 for an example of a bar graph. In this example, subjects were assessed using the *Agitated Behavior Scale* (Bognar, Corrigan, Bode, & Heinemann, 2000), before and after sensory based treatments. Because higher numbers on the scale indicate the presence of more behaviors, this graph reveals behaviors dropped following the treatment sessions.

A pie chart is often used to depict a breakdown of some quantity; for example, expenditures for a program or types of employees in a facility, as shown in Figure 12-3.

Flowcharts, schematics, drawings, and design trees are all ways of visually explaining processes, systems,

or phenomena. In designing these figures, the level of detail should match that required and understood by the reader. The example in Figure 12-4 depicts the three phases of a proposed research project on the impact of online and group activities in promoting healthy habits in obese adolescents. It clearly defines

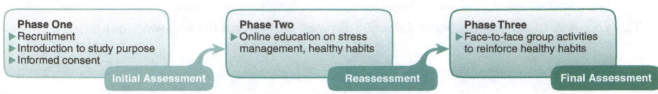

Figure 12-4 Flowchart Depicting the Phases in a Proposed Research Study

the steps in each phase of the intervention and at what points in the process formal assessments of the subjects will take place.

These are just a few of the possibilities for displaying data pictorially. For further ideas or descriptions of all types of figures, you may refer to *Successful Scientific Writing: A Step-by-Step Guide for the Biological and Medical Sciences* (Matthews & Matthews, 2008). If you use these visuals for presenting data, be sure to label them correctly—tables are called "tables," whereas graphs, charts, drawings, photographs, and so forth, are called "figures." Include accurate and complete titles, column headings, axes labels, and legends, so that tables and figures can be understood on their own, without text. In addition, always refer to each table and figure within the body of the formal report. Tell readers what to look for and be sure to point out salient features.

Chapter 5: Evaluation, Discussion and Conclusions

Up until this point, the results should be presented in a straightforward manner, without further discussion or interpretation. The discussion or conclusion sections of the formal report are where the analysis of results and the comparison of them to the literature review take place. In addition, limitations of the project, implications of the findings, and recommendations for the future are presented.

In both research and evidence-based practice, this last chapter is used by authors to evaluate the project and draw conclusions about what the results actually mean. Ideally, each new project should be contributing to a larger body of work, adding one more brick to the wall of knowledge about that topic and perhaps adding evidence that will tip the scales in one direction or the other concerning theory about a particular issue. The results are typically compared with the results of other studies on the topic, and

similarities and differences are acknowledged. If you note parallels between your literature review and your project's results, this lends support to prior findings. When dissimilar results are found, it is customary to speculate plausible reasons for the departure. Recognizing confounding results and suggesting plausible reasons for them allows readers to fully understand what happened in your project. These findings will add to the body of knowledge on the topic and provide implications for future studies.

What If Results Do Not Support the Project Question or Hypothesis?

This brings us to the topic of what to do about projects that generate limited data in support of the proposed hypothesis or evidence-based practice question, or those in which the hypotheses are not supported at all. Should these projects be reported and published? It is important that healthcare professionals be given access to the results of such projects for the following reasons:

- They may put to rest a popular myth that needs to be dispelled.
- They may show that a particular methodology or research design is not a useful way to investigate or approach a particular problem, thus saving others from making the same mistake.
- Others may learn from the flaws and problems in the project. The project can then be redesigned to achieve the original purpose.
- Ethical dilemmas exist when treatments are used that were shown to be ineffective. Reporting and publishing this information promotes evidence-based practice.

Limitations

A review of the limitations of the project is also customary. Acknowledging the shortcomings is respectable and allows readers to view the results in light of these concerns. Limitations may be related to an unreliable data collection instrument, a small sample size or participant group, an unforeseen interference to the project, faulty assumptions by the researcher or evidence-based practitioner, or any one of the forms of bias discussed in prior chapters. Some limitations may be unavoidable; however, giving readers the information will allow them to decide for themselves if the integrity of the project has been compromised.

Future Implications

Finally, the practical and clinical implications of the project, as well as suggestions for future practice, policy, education, or research, should be discussed. Specifically, you should review each of these questions:

- How does the project contribute to the body of knowledge on this topic?
- What are the clinical and practical implications of the project's findings? For example, the results of your research study might not be statistically significant, but what does this mean in regard to clinical application of the information? Or perhaps, results of your evidence-based practice project were overwhelmingly positive. What does this mean for future clinical scenarios that are similar?
- What are your suggestions for future work on this topic? For research projects, you might include suggestions for improvements to the study's design or procedures as well as proposals for new research, if applicable. For evidence-based practice, you might incorporate ideas for program development, modification, or expansion, as well as changes to healthcare policies or educational opportunities.

Thinking critically about your outcomes and the implications for the future can lead to a thought-provoking discussion. Although it is common for readers to skim the more technical sections of the project's report, such as the literature review or the statistical analyses, the discussion is usually reviewed in its entirety. This is where the summary of the results and the "take home message" are clearly delineated.

The Abstract

The abstract is a comprehensive summary of the information contained throughout the project's report (Chapters 1 through 5), with the purpose of providing a snapshot of the entire project. Readers frequently review the abstract to decide if the report warrants further inspection or is applicable to their purposes. Although the abstract is placed at the beginning of the formal report, it is typically written last after all the chapters have been completed. Abstracts are typically 150 to 250 words in length, use clear and concise language, and effectively summarize content in the chapters without the use of technical jargon.

Scientific Writing Styles

Now that we have addressed the content for each section of the report, let us turn to the topic of writing style. The style of writing is commonly dictated by the setting and purpose of the report. In academic settings, the accepted writing style is usually set forth by the instructor, whereas many clinical settings may not have specific requirements. For publication purposes, the writing style is specified in the author guidelines for the particular work. (See Appendices M and N for a sample of Author Guidelines for each of two publications.) A variety of writing styles exist; Table 12-5 includes some of the most popular style manuals applicable to the allied health professions.

Table 12-5 ■ Style Manuals

Writing Style	Manual Reference
APA	American Psychological Association. (2009). *Publication manual of the American Psychological Association* (6th ed.) Washington, DC: Author.
MLA	Modern Language Association. (2008). *MLA style manual and guide to scholarly publishing* (3rd ed.). New York: Author.
AMA	American Medical Association. (2007). *AMA manual of style: A guide for authors and editors* (10th ed.). New York: Oxford University Press.
The Chicago Manual of Style	University of Chicago Press Staff. (2010). *The Chicago manual of style* (16th ed.). Chicago, IL: Author.

Each style manual outlines specific methods for formatting headings, in-text citations, and reference lists, as well as for organizing the various sections of the report. The manuals also address plagiarism, grammar, and syntax. Although there are many online resources available for each style, having a hard copy of the appropriate style manual at your disposal will prove invaluable. Reviewing the manual before the start of writing allows you to become familiar with the overall content so that you know where to find the information when you need it. A well-worn, highlighted manual with dog-eared pages is a sign of a meticulous writer.

Becoming a Better Writer

Although basic writing skills are necessary in the allied health professions for documenting patient progress, recording program outcomes, or taking notes in education or meetings, many of us do not view ourselves as professional writers. However, with the emphasis on research and evidence-based practice, there is a push to disseminate information from these types of projects to other healthcare professionals. Whether it is a formalized report that is submitted to your facility administrator or a doctoral thesis submitted to your professor, the ability to clearly and concisely articulate the main points of your project is essential. Assuredly, everyone has completed courses in basic grammar and writing as part of earlier schooling, and that training can be applied to the scientific writing process. In addition, some other writing tips will be reviewed here.

Use of an Outline

Basic outlines for a research study or evidence-based practice project have been provided in Boxes 12-1 and 10-2, respectively. These outlines provide a good starting point where additional details individualized to your project can be inserted. Many writers prefer to begin with a detailed outline and progress to a draft of the formal report generated directly from it, whereas others do better starting into the writing immediately. It is a matter of personal preference, but either way, visualizing the writing plan, on paper or in your head, is essential to the process.

Grammar and Organization

The grammatical style and organization of the information sets the tone for the writing and ensures that it flows smoothly. Care should also be taken to ensure the level of writing is appropriate for the target audience. Considering the following can assist with these goals:

1. **Organization:** Present information in a logical order, building on each point to develop the next one. Beginning each paragraph with an effective topic sentence and then elaborating on those points as you progress through the paragraph can increase understanding of the information you are presenting.

2. **Concise Language:** Use clear and concise language, choosing words precisely. Avoid inserting extra words that do not add to the content. In scientific writing, more isn't always better. Brevity is a skill that requires diligent effort to achieve.

3. **Comprehension:** Limit use of technical jargon, acronyms, and abbreviations to aid in comprehension. Consider your audience and be sure the writing is geared to that group. Using layman's terms and writing out most words allows your work to be understood by a broader audience.

4. **Verb Tense:** Writing in past tense is customary, because the project has already been completed. Although you may have written some sections in future or present tenses when the project was initially being conceived, going back and revising everything into past tense at the end places your work in the appropriate context.

5. **Grammatical Person:** There is much debate regarding use of first-person versus third-person writing in scientific endeavors. For most academic programs and publications, the general rule of thumb is to use first-person sparingly, or only when it is absolutely necessary. Third-person professional writing is generally preferred for formalized reports and research publications. First-person writing may also be acceptable in clinic-based settings or when recording outcomes of evidence-based practice projects, as these situations warrant more personal connections with participants and procedures are not as stringent.

6. **Grammatical Voice:** Grammatical voice refers to the placement of the nouns and verbs in a sentence, and two types are active and passive voice. With active voice, the noun is performing the action indicated by the verb, whereas with passive voice the noun is being acted upon *passively* by the verb. See the following example:

   Active: The researcher conducted the study.

   Passive: The study was conducted by the researcher. There are cases when passive voice may be appropriate, but active voice is generally preferred because it is more direct and easier to understand.

7. **Use of Direct Quotations:** Reserve use of direct quotes for situations when you are unable to paraphrase the material effectively (i.e., when technical phrases or terms are used that cannot be stated another way or when the original authors stated the information in such a unique way that meaning would be lost with paraphrasing). Using too many direct quotes in one section or paragraph limits the flow of the writing and does not show that you understand the material and can effectively integrate it. A general rule of thumb is to limit direct quoting to no more than one quote per several pages of your own words. When using direct quotes, always be sure to follow the guidelines set forth in the style manual for proper formatting and citation. Remember that failure to cite appropriately can be considered plagiarism.

Use of Software Features

Consider use of a variety of features contained within your word processing program to increase the quality of your writing and to eliminate errors. These features can include spelling and grammar checks, readability formulas, a computerized thesaurus, document statistics, translators, and support for creating reference lists and a table of contents automatically. Although it might take some extra time to figure out how to activate these features, the benefits will long outweigh the initial effort. Each of these features is discussed here:

1. **Spelling and Grammar Checks:** This feature can typically be activated to check the document as you write or to check the entire document after you have finished. Most programs also provide suggestions as to how to correct the identified errors.

2. **Readability Formulas:** Readability formulas are used to analyze the average sentence and word length used in the document to determine the level of writing. Two of the most common tests are the Flesch Reading Ease Test and Flesch-Kincaid Grade Level Test. The Flesch Reading Ease Test rates reading ease on a 100-point scale (with a score of 90 to 100 easily understood by a fifth grader, 60 to 70 easily understood by eighth or ninth graders, and a score of 0 to 30 understood by college graduates) (Flesch, 1948; Kincaid, Fishburne, Rogers, & Chissom, 1975). Writing at the level of 60 to 70 is appropriate for most purposes; however, for doctoral level projects or education, one might expect levels to be closer to 30. The Flesch-Kincaid Grade Level Test transfers the readability score into a U.S. school grade level. So if the Flesch-Kincaid Grade Level score is 10.8, we would expect students in 10th to 11th grade to be able to understand it. These two tests are inversely proportional, so as the readability score increases (meaning it gets easier to understand) the grade level score gets lower (meaning those in a lower grade can understand it). Although these are just one measure of the level of writing, these tests provide a quick way for you to screen your writing to see if it is at the appropriate level. Most word processing programs will perform these calculations automatically (Microsoft, 2010) or a number of calculators are available online (ReadabilityForumulas.com). For example, in Microsoft Word this option can be activated by selecting "Word Options" under the Microsoft Office Button, then clicking "Proofing" and then ensuring that the following options are checked: "Check grammar with spelling" and "Show readability statistics." Results are shown once the entire document has been checked.

3. **Thesaurus:** Most word processing programs have a built-in thesaurus that allows you to highlight any word within a document to check for alternative choices. This is especially useful when

you are struggling with a word choice or if you seem to be using the same word repetitively. Using the thesaurus can add variety to your writing and may even help you choose a stronger word than what originally came to mind.

4. **Document Statistics:** Most programs are equipped with features to automatically calculate statistics of your document including the number of pages, words, characters, and lines. This can be useful if you are striving to meet the word limits set forth in the author's guidelines for a particular publication or trying to be clear and concise in a particular passage (for example, trying to limit the abstract to 150 to 250 words). Additionally, this feature can be used to verify the length of directly quoted material for proper citation. For instance, in APA style, direct quotes that are more than 40 words in length require special formatting (APA, 2009).

5. **Translators:** Translators can be used to convert text in one language to another language. Although opponents to these features argue that accuracy is somewhat limited, it is a viable option. It can be useful if your literature search turns up a quality piece of evidence in another language. Using the translate feature in your program or one of the many found online allows you to integrate this useful information into your report.

6. **Automatic Reference Lists and Table of Contents:** Creating each of these items manually is definitely an option, but utilizing the automated features of your program can help to ease the burden. Most programs allow you to create a database of references that you have used within the body of the formal report. This is accomplished by first selecting the writing style, say APA style, and then manually entering vital information, such as the authors, journal article, journal title, volume, and page numbers for each reference used. Once references are added to the database, they can be inserted within parenthetical citations, footnotes, or in the master reference list as appropriate. The table of contents feature works similarly. Headings are formatted according to the selected style guide via an automated heading feature in the software program. Doing so permits the author to insert the entire table of contents after the formal report is written with only a few key strokes.

Chapter Summary

This chapter provides a starting point for writing up your research study or evidence-based practice project, and the suggested outlines can be tailored to meet the needs of your setting or practice discipline. Paying close attention to the required writing style, the grammar and organization of your formal report, and the software features available to you will all help to strengthen your writing and ensure that the details of your project or study are accurately conveyed.

SKILL-BUILDING TIPS

■ Enlist the help of at least three proofreaders to review your writing. Select one person who is familiar with your topic and can proofread for actual content, one outside of your content area so that you will know if you are writing for a broader audience or if your content can be easily understood by those outside your field, and one that is skilled in grammar, writing, and formatting.

■ Avoid contractions in professional writing.

■ Never end a paragraph with a direct quote. Being able to sum up the paragraph in your own words creates ownership of the material that you are presenting.

■ Steer clear of absolutes in your writing. Using words such as *always* or *never* can create inaccuracies in your conclusions.

■ Congratulate yourself when you write something—a sentence or a paragraph can sometimes take an entire day, whereas other days you will write many pages.

■ Get in touch with your creative side, even if you never thought of yourself as a writer. Spend some time exploring your skills in this area. Participate in a writing workshop or use a book such as Reeves' (2010) *A Writer's Book of Days*, to get you started. This book is full of helpful tips about organizing your writing space, managing writer's block, improving the quality of your writing, and creating meaningful and articulate passages. Without effective writing skills, scientific writing can be tedious and boring. Perfecting the art of writing will allow you to create a factual and inspiring account of your research or evidence-based practice project.

LEARNING ACTIVITIES

1. Before you start to write, consider your audience and the goals of your writing. For example, do you need to write a report for formal academic coursework? Or will you be submitting your report to an administrator or supervisor? The goals and approach can be very different.

2. How would you rate your writing skills—below average, average, above average? Be honest with yourself; if you feel your writing is an area of weakness, brainstorm how you might improve these skills or where you might seek out additional supports to assist in this endeavor.

3. Begin with the appropriate outline from Boxes 12-1 or 10-2 (depending on whether you are engaging in evidence-based practice or research). Insert additional subsections into the outline as applicable to your project.

REFERENCES

American Psychological Association [APA]. (2009). *Publication manual of the American Psychological Association* (6th ed.). Washington, DC: Author.

Bognar, J., Corrigan, J., Bode, R., & Heinemann, A. (2000). Rating scale analysis of the agitated behavior scale. *Journal of Head Trauma Rehabilitation, 15*(1), 656–669.

Chiarello, L. A., Palisano, R. J., Maggs, J. M., Orlin, M. N., Almasri, N., Kang, L., & Chang, H. (2010). Family priorities for activity and participation of children and youth with cerebral palsy. *Physical Therapy, 90*(9), 1254–1264.

Flesch, R. (1948). A new readability yardstick. *Journal of Applied Psychology, 32,* 221–233.

Kincaid, J. P., Fishburne, R. P., Rogers, R. L., & Chissom, B. S. (1975). Derivation of new readability formulas (automated readability index, fog count, and Flesch Reading Ease formula) for navy enlisted personnel. Research Branch Report 8-75. Chief of Naval Technical Training: Naval Air Station Memphis.

Matthews, J., & Matthews, R. (2008). *Successful scientific writing: A step-by-step guide for the biological and medical sciences* (3rd ed.). United Kingdom: Cambridge University Press.

Microsoft. (2010). Microsoft Excel [computer software]. Redmond, WA: Author.

ReadabilityForumula.com. (n.d.). Welcome to readabilityforumulas.com. *Readability Formulas.* Retrieved from http://www.readabilityformulas.com/

Reeves, J. (2010). *A writer's book of days: A spirited companion & lively muse for the writing life* (Revised ed.). Novato, CA: New World Library.

Rendon, A. A., Lohman, E. B., Thorpe, D., Johnson, E. G., Medina, E., & Bradley, B. (2012). The effect of virtual reality gaming on dynamic balance in older adults. *Age and Aging, 41,* 549–552. doi:10.1093/ageing/afs053

ADDITIONAL WRITING RESOURCES

Day, R. A., & Sakaduski, N. (2011). *Scientific English: A guide for scientists and other professionals* (3rd ed.). Santa Barbara, CA: Greenwood.

Hofmann, A. H. (2009). *Scientific writing and communication: Papers, proposals, and presentations.* New York: Oxford University Press.

Katz, M. J. (2009). *From research to manuscript: A guide to scientific writing* (2nd ed.). New York: Springer Science + Business Media B.V.

LaRocque, P. (2003). *The book on writing: The ultimate guide to writing well.* Portland, OR: Marion Street Press, LLC.

Lindsay, D. (2011). *Scientific writing = Thinking in words.* Australia: CSIRO Publishing.

Matthews, J., & Matthews, R. (2008). *Successful scientific writing: A step-by-step guide for the biological and medical sciences* (3rd ed.). United Kingdom: Cambridge University Press.

Reeves, J. (2010). *A writer's book of days: A spirited companion & lively muse for the writing life* (Revised ed.). Novato, CA: New World Library.

Strunk Jr., W., & White, E. B. (1999). *The elements of style* (4th ed.). Upper Saddle River, NJ: Pearson.

Zinsser, W. (2006). *On writing well, 30th anniversary edition: The classic guide to writing nonfiction* (7th ed.). New York: HarperCollins.

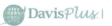 For additional materials, please visit **http://davisplus.fadavis.com, key word: Hissong.**

Chapter 13

The Art of Presenting the Research Study or Evidence-Based Practice Project

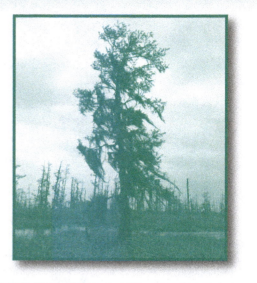

If you think in terms of a year, plant a seed; if in terms of ten years, plant trees; if in terms of 100 years, teach the people.
—*Confucius*

LEARNING OUTCOMES

The information provided in this chapter will assist the reader to:

- Understand the reasons for presenting a study or project.
- Evaluate how learning styles can impact presentation style.
- Choose an appropriate presentation method from those reviewed (oral presentations, poster presentations, and cyber presentations).
- Create a meaningful PowerPoint or other visual aides to support the presentation.
- Identify additional resources for creating effective presentations.

Presenting can be considered a form of art, as the skills required to successfully impart knowledge on others requires diligence, creativity, and attention to detail. The art of presenting is closely tied to the art of teaching. Consider the metaphor of a tree, with the roots symbolizing the foundation of your presentation—the content that you hope to bestow upon your audience. With proper planning and ingenuity, your knowledge is spread and the result is a tree that flourishes, perhaps bearing fruit or providing shade on a hot summer day. As the tree grows, branches split and the trunk expands, just as new professional connections are made with the aim of advancing the knowledge of your specialty or discipline. And similar to a tree withstanding the harsh wind or weather, your presentation can leave a lasting impression on your audience with ample care in design and delivery.

Presenting your research or evidence-based practice project is an effective way to disseminate details about the project and its outcomes in academic settings, clinical situations, and continuing education venues. A variety of presentation methods can be used depending on your goals for the presentation. In addition, presentations can occur locally, nationally, and even internationally. Reasons for presenting and several presentation methods, including oral presentations, poster presentations, and cyber presentations, will be discussed.

Why Present?

There are several reasons for presenting your research study or evidence-based practice project. They include:

- To increase the ability for others to understand your work
- To reach a variety of audiences, especially those that may not be easily reached by other methods
- To network and collaborate with others in your discipline or those that share an interest or passion in your topic area
- To expand your professional skills

First, presentations are used to refine and translate the information in your detailed project report so that it might be more easily understood by others. Although many in your audience may have little interest in reading a lengthy and detailed report or lack the skills or knowledge to understand it on their own, using a presentation tailored to the specific audience is an effective way to transmit the information. Presentations are often used in academic settings as part of formal coursework to ascertain a student's ability to succinctly summarize his or her work. Conducting a master's or doctoral thesis can take months or even years, yet a successful presentation recaps the entire project in significantly less time. Clinical presentations can be used to distribute information about projects whose results can impact practice. These presentations might take the form of an inservice, where treatment ideas are presented, discussed, and rehearsed. In addition, clinical presentations can address program development and outcomes, with the aim of gaining support from supervisors and administrators for practice changes.

The second reason for presenting is to reach audiences that may otherwise have been unavailable. Getting the word out about your project can allow others to use the information in practice (where applicable), or to design future research studies or evidence-based practice projects. Presenting your project is an effective way to reach fellow researchers, students, policy makers, administrators, or the general public, depending on the venue. For example, if you conducted a research project on the effectiveness of massage on joint pain in geriatric clients, you would be unlikely to reach potential clients themselves by presenting at a national conference or publishing in a professional journal. Although there are definite benefits to each of these actions, they are not appropriate if your goal is to convey the information to geriatric clients. In this case, a presentation at a local senior center, hospital, or gym might be more fitting.

Third, presentations at continuing education venues allow you to share your knowledge with others in your discipline or those interested in your topic. This is an excellent way to network and collaborate with others, and to advance the science of your discipline. The professional exchanges that often occur in continuing education workshops; state, national, and international conferences; or Web-based learning scenarios can lead to increased knowledge for you as well as your attendees. These professional connections can lead to other collaborative projects, publications, and friendships!

Finally, for some, presentations can be used to hone public speaking skills or to accrue required continuing education units for licensure or certification. Being able to clearly articulate details about your project and to field questions to a variety of audiences are worthy skills for many endeavors. Moreover, the addition of multiple presentations to your resume can emphasize your commitment to sharing your knowledge and expanding your professional skills.

What Is a Presentation?

The term *presentation* is used rather loosely, as the session might take the form of a lecture, where the presenter is dishing out information with little interaction from the audience. In another scenario, the presentation might be very interactive, offering hands-on experiences for the participants, or the opportunity to engage in lively discussions or question-and-answer periods. From a pedagogical standpoint, these examples focus on the "how" of presenting. **Pedagogy** is essentially the art of teaching based upon scientific research and subsequent learning theories. With any presentation, it is fundamental to consider your audience before determining the structure of the presentation. Reflecting on the developmental stages, memory and attention skills, learning styles, and cultural influences of your audience, as well as the goals of your presentation, can assist you.

Learning Styles

A vast array of learning theories exist; they include those rooted in classical conditioning, cognitive learning and information processing, developmental maturation, neuroscience, and motivation (Shunk, 2012). These theories attempt to explain how knowledge is conveyed and how learning takes place from a variety of perspectives; they can be used to tailor presentations of information for optimal learning experiences. Research supports the connection between learning theories and **how** the information is presented (University of Pennsylvania, 2009). Just as we all have different preferences for clothing, food, or vacation spots, each one of us has preferences for the way we take in and process new information.

One common model for classifying learning preferences is the VAK model. Learners are categorized by one of three sensory systems—visual, auditory, or kinesthetic—that predominates their ability to process and understand new information. Visual learners tend to prefer the written word, charts, diagrams, or videos, to name a few examples. Auditory learners respond best to verbal instructions or presentations, and kinesthetic learners learn better when they are provided with hands-on tactile experiences for learning. Even though all three systems are typically used, a learner may respond more favorably to one method over another, or the method may vary based upon the information and topic being presented (Fleming & Mills, 1992). Several free inventories are available online (http://www.brainboxx.co.uk/a3_aspects/pages/vak_quest.htm; http://www.business-balls.com/vaklearningstylestest.htm) or for purchase in print (Walsh, Willard, & Whiting, 2011) to determine your preferred learning style. The supplemental materials for this book also include additional links and information on learning inventories. Understanding your learning style can help you gain perspective on the styles of your audience. Infusing a variety of learning styles and techniques into your presentations

increases the likelihood that every attendee will walk away with valuable information.

Oral Presentations

An **oral presentation** is typically a live presentation to an audience that is physically present in the same location as the presenter. Oral presentations can follow a lecture format, but may also include demonstrations of techniques or equipment, individual or group learning activities, role-playing, question-and-answer periods, interactive discussions or brainstorming, case studies, hands-on learning experiences, or any combination of these strategies. **Lectures** are formal oral presentations in which there is little to no interaction between the presenter and the attendees. Lectures are commonly used with larger audiences where increased interaction is not practical, or when the goal is to merely share technical or straightforward information. Although this one-way communication may limit comprehension of the material being presented, it is an efficient use of time and allows the presenter to get through the necessary information as planned.

Although lectures definitely have their place, using a variety of strategies within one presentation is preferred in order to ensure optimum transfer of knowledge from the presenter to the attendees. Presentations that employ more interactive methods such as demonstrations, discussions, or hands-on learning experiences tend to be less formal and audiences are often smaller in size and more engaged. Although these types of presentations are generally preferred, they also have several disadvantages. They require more preparation time; presenters need to be prepared to field questions, give additional clarification when needed, and keep the presentation on track. With more interaction from the audience, a discussion or activity can easily derail the presentation if the presenter is not skilled in making adjustments or guiding the group appropriately. Gauging the time for a presentation with interactive elements requires much more planning and practice.

Visual Support for Oral Presentations

Oral presentations are often accompanied by handouts, overhead displays, or PowerPoint slides. Presenters need to be mindful of the fact that these visual elements should **support** or **enhance** the spoken word, but should not take the place of it. There is nothing worse than a presentation in which the presenter reads directly from the handouts or slide presentation. **Handouts** may be provided to the audience for ease of note taking, or when the presenter wishes to reference detailed or complex elements that would be difficult to see on a slide or overhead presentation. Handouts are also an effective method for sharing your references and contact information, in the event that attendees wish to learn more about the subject or have questions later on.

An **overhead projector** can be used to display slides developed ahead of time or to create other visuals or lists of information on the spot as the presentation progresses. **Flip charts**, **chalkboards**, **whiteboards**, or **Smart boards** are other options for creating a dynamic presentation. These options allow presenters and attendees to generate lists, figures, and other clarifying visuals during the presentation. These types of technology might be especially useful when additional examples are needed to clarify a complex concept or process or when group brainstorming or a discussion is planned as part of the presentation. In each case, the presenter needs to adjust the presentation as it progresses in order to ensure comprehension of the subject matter by attendees.

PowerPoint Presentations

PowerPoint presentations are currently the most popular type of visual media used to supplement oral presentations, yet much controversy exists over the effectiveness of this method. Although the purpose of this software is to enhance the presentation, without effective slide construction, the presentation becomes boring and the intended message may not be successfully conveyed to the audience. Constructing PowerPoint slides is just one part of the preparation for an oral presentation; the slides are for the audience and should **supplement** what the presenter has to say. Many presenters make the mistake of trying to include everything they want to say on the slides (see Figure 13-1), but this only serves to create a presentation devoid of spontaneity and interest. Presenters should develop the slides with their audience in mind, and then create a separate set of notes for themselves to be used as a guide during the actual presentation. See Figures 13-1 and 13-2 to compare two slides describing the increased incidence of Alzheimer's dementia and the need to consider alternative forms of behavior management. The first slide (Figure 13-1) is constructed based upon the presenter's needs and includes a significant amount of text. The second slide (Figure 13-2) is simplified and only includes guiding points that the presenter will expand upon during the presentation. Figure 13-2 is the preferred layout.

Slide Construction

As seen in the previous two examples, content and design are important considerations. In regard to content, the prevailing thought is "Less is more." The

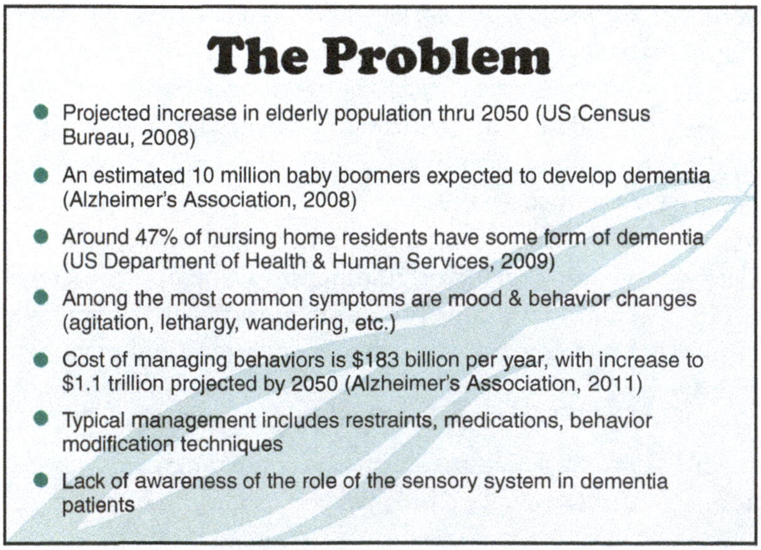

Figure 13-1 PowerPoint Slide Tailored to the Presenter With Too Much Text

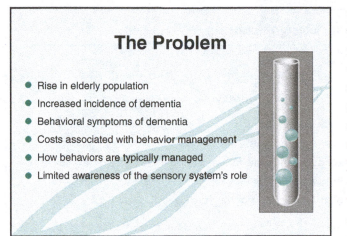

Figure 13-2 PowerPoint Slide Tailored to the Audience With Guiding Points

presentation should not be a replication of your formal project report; it should only summarize the most important details and outcomes of the project. Your time with the audience is limited, so it is critical to use the time efficiently. When considering whether or not to include a particular detail in the presentation, it is often effective to ask yourself "So what?" If you cannot come up with a strong reason for including the information, then leave it out. Although some details are important to you, they will really have no bearing on the audience's understanding of the project. After you have decided on the slide content, the focus turns to slide design. Table 13-1 includes some basic recommendations for designing your PowerPoint presentation.

Some proponents of PowerPoint presentations advocate for traditional slides with information arranged in bulleted lists, whereas others suggest more nontraditional layouts composed of less text, more graphics or other visuals, and increased time devoted to discussion of the content on each slide (Alley & Neeley, 2005). Although PowerPoint software makes creating the actual slides very easy, presenters need to consider the design, structure, and delivery of the presentation in order to be successful. Some additional resources regarding creation of effective PowerPoint presentations are included in the reference list for this chapter.

Table 13-1 ■ Recommendations for PowerPoint Design

Organization	■ Use a consistent theme and font. Frequent changes can distract the audience. ■ Arrange slides in chronological order, beginning with a title slide and topic introduction, and progressing through the various stages of your study or project. ■ Present only one topic or idea per slide.
Visual Appeal	■ Ensure the display is visually appealing and easy to read. ■ Dark text on a lighter background is generally preferred. Using very bright white or other vivid colors can be harsh on the eyes.
Language	■ Know your audience; Avoid technical jargon and terminology as well as abbreviations unless you are presenting to an audience that is sure to understand them.
Text	■ Use a minimum of 14 to 28 point font. ■ Headings should be at least 2 points larger than general content. ■ Avoid using all capitalized letters. ■ Reserve bold and italics for points that really need emphasis. ■ Use short phrases to summarize points, rather than whole sentences. General rule of thumb: No more than six words per line; no more than six lines per slide. ■ Use graphics, photos, and figures in place of text when possible. If you include everything you intend to say on the slides, there is no need for the presentation.

Continued

Table 13-1 ■ Recommendations for PowerPoint Design—cont'd

Tables	■ Simplify tables used in your project if you plan to include them in the presentation. ■ A table with too many numbers will be difficult to read. ■ If you need to use the table in its original form, distribute it in your handouts and skip putting it into the PowerPoint.
Graphics and Figures	■ Include a title and label all components and axes. ■ Choose colors wisely so that attendees can easily discern differences in the components, or understand the relationships or outcomes being illustrated. ■ Check the scale to eliminate distortion; the ratio of height to length is usually 1:2.
Pictures	■ Resolution should generally be set at 1024 pixels X 768 pixels for good quality when the image is portrayed on a larger screen. Often, graphics will look adequate on your computer screen, but will be very "grainy" when enlarged. Testing your presentation out on a larger screen ahead of time or zooming in on your computer screen to 100% to view each image are other ways to ensure the images are of adequate quality.
References	■ Always include citations for information, tables, and figures in your presentation, where applicable. Include the author's name and the year; using a smaller font for this information is acceptable. ■ Include full references in your handout rather than in the PowerPoint itself.

Oral Presentation Etiquette

Presenters should be familiar with some basic etiquette for conducting effective oral presentations. In addition to dressing appropriately for the venue, making good eye contact with attendees, and tailoring the presentation for the intended audience, presenters should always arrive early to the presentation. Arriving early allows extra time to check technical components, such as PowerPoint presentations, supporting videos, microphones, and laser pointers, and to resolve glitches before the start of the presentation. This is also a good time to connect with the presentation moderator, if one is provided. Many conferences use **moderators**, often volunteers, who are present during the presentations with the responsibility of assisting with technology issues, monitoring the time, introducing and thanking the presenter, facilitating question-and-answer sessions, and recording attendance for conference goers. Moderators might also help to prepare the session room by ensuring the lighting, temperature, and seating arrangement are adequate for the presentations. A presenter arriving early to the presentation location will have time to become acquainted with the moderator and to resolve any issues in a timely manner.

Practice

Presenters make many choices when creating an oral presentation. Will you decide on a lecture format or will you opt for a more interactive presentation? What will be the best way to get your message across and will you need to use additional visual supports to enhance the spoken word? Regardless of the methods that you choose, practicing your oral presentation ahead of time is very important. Practice allows you to become familiar with the content and flow of information and to gauge how much time it will take to get through the material. You want to be familiar enough with the material so that you will not need to read from the slides or your notes; however, practicing too much can lead to delivering a memorized speech.

A good oral presentation, if you have ever attended one, includes some level of spontaneity, confidence, and entertainment. Spontaneity allows you to make adjustments in the presentation as you go by offering additional examples or clarification when needed. Watching your audience will let you know if they are engaged (and if perhaps you should elaborate more on a point they are interested in) or if they are bored (in which case you may need to do something to gain their attention again). You should be confident in presenting your topic—after all, you know it better than anyone else! Practice can help to decrease nervousness, but some level of public speaking jitters is normal. Finally, adding some element of entertainment to the presentation will help to sustain the audience's attention. Although the focus should be on the main content of the presentation, starting out with a personal story, interactive activity, or another attention-getting technique, as well as wrapping up in a creative way, can really enhance the presentation. Giving examples, telling stories, or adding humor (when appropriate) increases the connection between the presenter and the audience and contributes to a greater understanding of the material.

As a final point, know that even if you practice and effectively deliver your presentation, the information your audience will remember afterwards is limited. Recall the Rule of Three, which Aristotle wrote about years ago. People are able to easily remember three things, and as the number of items increases beyond that, the ability to remember decreases. Consider what three take-home messages you want the audience to get from your presentation. Designing your presentation and supporting visuals around these three points will increase your chances of success.

Poster Presentations

Poster presentations involve creation of an eye-catching vertical display, which typically includes a combination of text and figures or graphics aimed at portraying the results of research or evidence-based practice. These presentations usually occur at professional conferences and meetings, where many posters are displayed together in one area for a set period of time. It is also common for the author(s) of the poster to be physically present to discuss the project.

Poster presentations are an effective means of getting the word out about your project, eliciting feedback from others before expanding the project or seeking publication, and networking with others (Plunkett, n.d.). In contrast to oral presentations, poster presentations allow you to connect with a large number of attendees, from more diverse backgrounds and interest areas, on an individual basis. They also provide an excellent opportunity for the first-time conference presenter, since the format is less formal and intimidating than an oral presentation.

Poster Design

Many of the techniques discussed previously in regard to PowerPoint design are also applicable to poster design. In fact, most professional posters are created using just one PowerPoint slide, which is scaled appropriately for the finished size of the poster. A template (36" × 56") is included in the supplemental materials of this book. A variety of other templates are available online that you can customize to suit your needs; the links are included here as well as in the supplemental materials.

1. http://www.posterpresentations.com/html/free_poster_templates.html
2. http://www.makesigns.com/SCiPosters_Templates.aspx
3. http://office.microsoft.com/en-us/templates/medical-poster-TC010021411.aspx)

Although using a single slide for poster construction is most common, another option is to create individual PowerPoint slides for each section of the poster (for example, methods, results, discussion, and so on) which are then assembled on a larger board for the presentation. The style and size of your poster will likely be dictated by the conference you are presenting at, and checking the specifications ahead of time will avoid last minute revisions to the poster's formatting or a stressful situation when you arrive at the conference.

The poster is commonly organized into various sections that summarize different phases of your project. For research projects, sections might include the introduction, methodology, results, limitations, and implications of findings. For evidence-based practice projects, sections may consist of setting or background, literature review, project design, outcomes, and significance of the project to the field or practice area. Each section can be customized to suit the needs of the author and the venue where the presentation will occur. A list of some of the common sections, as well as recommended content for these sections, is included in Table 13-2. Section titles and content can be adjusted for research or evidence-based practice presentations.

After selecting a template for poster construction and determining the sections and content that will be included, attention must be given to the visual layout and design. Remember that your poster should not be a duplication of your entire project report, but rather a striking visual representation of it. "Many people find it helpful to view the poster-writing process not as trying to condense a paper but rather as expanding and enriching the abstract" (Matthews & Matthews, 2008, p. 99).

A superior poster includes a balance of text and graphics, a visually-pleasing layout and color scheme, and adequate information about the project, such that it could be understood, even if the author is not present. Consolidating text and using photographs, tables, and figures in place of text, where possible, can add visual interest and attract more viewers. Moreover, a three-column format works best, and the material should flow from top to bottom and left to right. The majority of attendees will be most interested in the results and application of the project, so avoiding excess focus on the methodology,

---

Table 13-2 ■ Sections of a Poster

Section	Recommended Content Includes:
Title Box	■ A shortened project title ■ Author(s) names with credentials and affiliation (school or place of employment)
Introduction, Setting, or Background	■ A description of the problem that was addressed in the project. ■ Justification for the project. May include statistics or visuals that help to support the need for the project. ■ A description of the setting or other background information that led to the project.
Literature Review	■ A recap of the existing research on the topic that was reviewed before the start of the current project. It is common to review the number of studies, and to describe the portfolio in terms of levels of evidence and common themes.
Methodology or Project Design	■ A summary of the steps of the project. Using bulleted lists or figures can be an effective way to outline the various steps.
Results or Outcomes	■ The main findings of the project. Most often this is done visually, through the use of tables, graphs, or other figures.
Discussion or Implication of Findings	■ Correlations and comparisons of the current project's results with the literature review. ■ Implications of the findings for future practice or research.
Limitations	■ A review of limitations believed to have a significant impact on practical implications of the project. ■ Limitations may include those related to study design, instruments, or participants. ■ This section is typically omitted for evidence-based practice projects.
Significance of the Project to the Field of Study or Practice Area	■ An explanation of the importance of the project for the profession or practice area involved.

background, and literature review sections is appropriate. Table 13-3 provides some additional recommendations for poster design, and Figure 13-3 includes an example of a professional poster.

Printing and Transporting the Poster

Because of their size, posters require use of a specialized printer. Many local print shops or office stores have the capability to print them, as do many online sites. The advantage of online sites is that you can upload your poster from home, and they can usually e-mail you a proof of the poster before they print it. Posters can be printed on an array of paper with varying quality and finishes, depending on personal preference or the specifications of your institution or conference. Scoping out printing options in advance

---

Table 13-3 ■ **Recommendations for Poster Design**

Visual Appeal	■ Use a consistent theme and font.
	■ Information should flow from top to bottom and left to right.
	■ Do not use photographs as background. Instead, use photographs on the poster to illustrate a point or to add visual interest.
	■ Format section headings to draw attention to them and guide the attendees from one section to the next in a logical progression. Use thin borders around each section heading and a light-colored background to highlight the different sections and to emphasize which items are grouped together.
	■ Balance text and graphics. Placing all the graphics on one side of the poster will create visual imbalance.
	■ Strive for an organized, uncluttered representation of your work. White space can improve flow and balance.
	■ Limit text. Use short phrases to summarize points, rather than whole sentences. Use graphics, photos, and figures in place of text when possible.
Text	■ Use a minimum of 28 to 36 point font for all content; 48 point font for section headings, author(s) names, and affiliations; and 72 point font for the title.
	■ Dark text on a lighter background is generally preferred. Using very bright white or other vivid colors can be harsh on the eyes.
	■ Content should be readable from 4 feet away.
	■ Choose a simple font such as Times Roman or Arial, since more complex fonts are difficult to read from a distance.
	■ Avoid use of all capitalized letters.
	■ Reserve bold and italics for points that really need emphasis.
	■ Keep headings centered; Keep content text right justified.
Tables	■ Simplify tables used in your project if you plan to include them on the poster. A table with too many numbers will be difficult to read.
	■ Use a minimum of 28 point font for all tables.
Graphs and Figures	■ Include a title and label all components and axes.
	■ Choose colors wisely so that attendees can easily discern differences in the components, or understand the relationships or outcomes being illustrated.
	■ Check the scale to eliminate distortion; the ratio of height to length is usually 1:2.
	■ Use a minimum of 28 point font for all graphs.

Continued

Table 13-3 ■ Recommendations for Poster Design—cont'd

Pictures and Clip Art	■ Resolution should generally be set at 1024 pixels X 768 pixels for good quality when the image is enlarged, but check with your poster printer. They can give you specifics related to the size of your poster. Often, graphics will look adequate on your computer screen, but will be very "grainy" when enlarged. Zooming in on your computer screen to 100% to view each image is another way to test the quality of your images. ■ Be aware that images copied and pasted from the Internet are usually of poor quality when enlarged. ■ Use photos you have taken yourself or ones in the public domain to avoid copyright infringement. ■ Obtain informed consent if you plan to use photos of patients or subjects.
References	■ Always include references for information, tables, and figures on your poster, where applicable. Include the author's name and the year; using a smaller font for this information is acceptable. ■ Include full references on a handout for those that are interested.
Handouts	■ Craft a one-page handout on your project that you can offer to interested attendees. Some ideas for the handout include: 1. A miniature reproduction of your poster on one side of the paper, and some important references and additional information on the other side. 2. Using the abstract on one side of the handout, and references on the other side. 3. A handout with bullet points highlighting sections of your project. You may also want to include a graph or chart depicting the results. 4. Regardless of what format you choose, be sure to include your name and contact information.

---

will allow you to determine the best option for your needs, and to ensure adequate turnaround time.

There are a variety of ways to transport your poster to the presentation site. Carrying cases range from more expensive options with shoulder straps to less expensive cardboard tubes. If you are traveling by air, you will need to check with the airline to determine if you can take the poster with you as a carry-on item. From experience, some airlines will permit this free of charge, whereas others charge additional fees or insist that posters be checked. If you must pay a fee, consider coordinating poster transport with others in your area who are presenting posters at the same venue. Multiple posters can be placed in one carrying case and presenters can share the expense. Other options include shipping your poster to the hotel ahead of time, or arranging to have it printed near the conference site.

Poster Etiquette

As a final point, it is important to consider the etiquette required during poster presentations. Dressing professionally and wearing your name badge, arriving on time to the presentation, and ensuring you have an adequate number of handouts (or business cards) will portray a positive image to those in attendance. Aside from creating the poster itself and the accompanying handouts, you should also be prepared to field a variety of questions on your topic or project. That being said, if you do not know the answer to a question, you should not feel compelled to make one up. One of the purposes of presenting your poster is to network with others interested or experienced in your topic, and it is quite possible that you will make valuable connections and learn something new in the process. You should stay close to your poster during the entire session and greet attendees professionally.

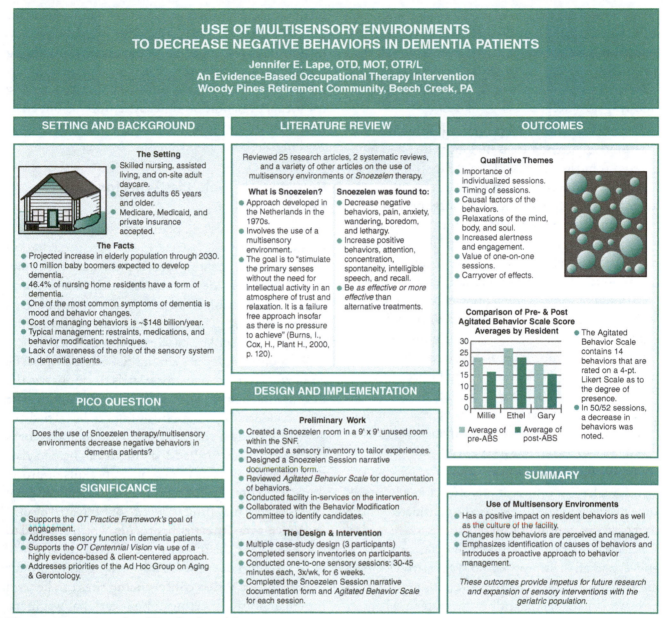

Figure 13-3 Example of Professional Poster

Give them time to view the poster on their own and offer to answer any questions when they are finished. Remember not to spend too much time with one attendee if others are waiting; connecting with all interested attendees is the goal and socializing with friends or colleagues should be reserved for after-conference hours. With adequate attention to style, design, and content of the poster, and adherence to proper etiquette during the poster session, you can expect to make professional connections, advance your skills and knowledge, and share valuable information about your project.

Cyber Presentations

Here, the term **cyber presentation** will be used to refer to any Web-based presentation delivered synchronously or asynchronously, in which the attendees are physically located in a different location or setting than the presenter. A **synchronous presentation** is one in which the presenter and attendees are online at the same time, whereas in an **asynchronous presentation** the presenter makes the presentation available online and attendees can access it whenever it is convenient for them. Cyber presentations offer the following advantages:

1. **The ability to reach a larger and more diverse audience**. Attendance is no longer dictated by geographic location, and the ability to connect with individuals across the globe is possible.
2. **Increased access to the latest advances and information in your field.** Information can be dispensed more efficiently and timely, which can impact research, medical advances, and practice.
3. **Financial.** Travel to conferences, especially national or international ones, could be cost-prohibitive. The ability to attend or provide presentations over the Internet can minimize the financial impact for all involved.
4. **Convenience.** Presentations can be accessed nearly anywhere on Earth via computers, laptops, or mobile devices such as iPods or smartphones. Asynchronous presentations offer an added convenience for attendees as they can view the presentation when it is most convenient for them.

Although cyber presentations offer clear advantages, some disadvantages should also be considered. Particularly with asynchronous presentations, there is a lack of personal interaction between the presenter and attendees and often little opportunity for attendees to ask questions. For this reason, asynchronous presentations are better suited for straightforward material where few questions might be anticipated. The presenter can also address this issue by providing his or her e-mail or a discussion forum where questions can be posted and responded to. Asynchronous presentations tend to be highly focused on topic content with little emphasis on collaboration or social support (Hrastinski, 2008).

Synchronous presentations allow more collaboration between attendees and the presenter; questions can be responded to immediately, and attendees are usually more committed to the learning experience (Hrastinski, 2008). However, since all attendees must participate simultaneously, synchronous presentations can be less convenient or present challenges if

technological glitches occur during the scheduled presentation time. To combat this problem, presentations could be made available online for viewing asynchronously after the formal presentation, for attendees who experienced technical problems during the actual presentation time. Synchronous presentations are most appropriate for complex topics, networking, and collaboration.

Presentation Tools/Platforms for Cyber Presentations

The variety of tools and platforms for cyber presentations is nearly endless. Creating a cyber presentation is very similar to creating an oral presentation; the presenter must consider the audience, the amount and level of information to include, and how the material will be presented. This can include use of visual aides to support the spoken or written word.

Web-based software similar to PowerPoint can be employed to create dynamic visuals to emphasize the information being discussed. These presentations are often conducted synchronously but can be carried out asynchronously if the presenter narrates and records the presentation. **Embedded videos** can help to clarify complex points or to demonstrate skills or procedures. Presenters can use programs to create original videos or they may utilize and cite ones created by others. **Voice-over-Internet protocols**, which are used to make calls over the Internet, are effective for synchronous meetings or conversations among small groups of individuals. **Video conferencing** sites can be used for collaborative meetings or educational webinars. These sites allow all attendees to gather virtually to view and hear presentations, and to converse verbally or via an instant messaging system. **Podcasts**, or short digital media presentations typically published in a series, can be created to disseminate information asynchronously. **Screencasts** are similar to podcasts, but use narration to accompany video of a computer screen (where a screenshot is a picture of a computer screen; a screencast is a video of what is actually happening on the screen). Table 13-4 includes descriptions of some of the most common tools for cyber presentations. Many other options are available; the intention here is to provide a brief overview.

Table 13-4 ■ **Tools for Effective Cyber Presentations**

Type of Tool	Name	Description
Web-based presentation software	SlideRocket (www.sliderocket.com)	Enhanced Web app with advanced text, graphics, and media integration. Presentations can be shared through social networking, and statistics on viewers and their comments can be collected.
Web-based presentation software	Prezi (http://prezi.com)	Web-based presentation and storytelling software. Instead of slides, it uses a dynamic canvas with zooming features.
Video sharing site	YouTube (http://www.youtube.com/)	Video sharing site that allows you to create, edit, and store your own videos as well as embed them into your dynamic presentation.
Voice-over-Internet protocol	Skype (http://www.skype.com/en/)	Software that employs VoIP (voice-over-Internet protocol) to make calls over the Internet. Can be used for conference calling, and callers can see each other if a webcam is used.
Video conferencing	GoToWebinar or GoToMeeting (http://www.gotomeeting.com/fec/)	Video conferencing sites used to conduct lectures, presentations, or meetings.
Podcast creation site	PodBean (http://www.podbean.com/)	Site for creating and sharing digital media arranged in an episodic series (podcasts). May include audio, video, and other related files.
Podcast creation site	Buzzsprout (http://www.buzzsprout.com/?source=gaw03&gclid=CPDEgZHwtrYCFY9DMgodBi8A0Q)	Site for creating podcasts. Can track statistics on your listeners.
Screencast creation site	Screenr (http://www.screenr.com/)	Site for creating screencasts. Can be shared through social media.

Chapter Summary

In summary, there are many elements to consider in designing and delivering your presentation. Carefully matching your presentation format with the learning styles and needs of your audience can ensure attendees walk away with the information you intended. With advances in technology, a variety of tools exist to increase understanding of your material and to add pizazz to your presentation. Beginning with an informal presentation to a small group of individuals and progressing to more formal or larger scale ones is the perfect way to hone your public speaking skills and promote expansion of your topic as well as your own professional growth.

SKILL-BUILDING TIPS

■ Know that you will likely need to submit a proposal for your presentation to the conference committee or venue that you have chosen. Proposals are usually peer-reviewed and scored based upon the quality, relevance, and innovation of the topic. Top scoring proposals are accepted for presentation, and lower scoring presentations are rejected. Each venue has a limited number of spots available, so if you are not successful initially, do not be afraid to try again. Poster presentations and shorter presentations (those 15 to 30 minutes in length) are a great way for the novice presenter to get started.

■ Be sure to practice enough. Not practicing enough can lead to limited time to cover all the information you had planned; as the presenter, you will appear rushed toward the end or need to skip important information to stay within the time limit. The opposite can also occur; the presentation will end very early, creating an awkward feeling about what to do with the excess time.

■ Know that slide and visual preparation is very different from presentation preparation. Preparing your PowerPoint, poster or other visual aids is just one part of the process. Actually rehearsing what you will say and how you will say it is the key to a smooth presentation.

■ Videotape yourself, practice in front of a mirror (for live presentations), or record your voice (for cyber presentations) to help you identify errors in speaking, posture, and hand gestures. Another alternative is to practice the presentation for a group of friends or colleagues ahead of time. Ask them to be brutally honest with you regarding the quality of the presentation and be willing to accept the constructive criticism.

■ Do not spend too much time addressing technology issues. However, be sure you are familiar with the technology that you will use during the presentation, if any. Practice ahead of time if you can, and do not spend more than 5 to 10 minutes trying to resolve the issue. Doing so will decrease your presentation time and it may be difficult to adjust the plan you have practiced. In case of technical difficulties, be sure you have a backup plan in mind.

■ Be sure to allow time for questions and answers and provide attendees with your contact information in case they have questions later.

■ Use storytelling, case studies, or personal and real-life examples to bring life and passion to your presentation. These elements often help gain the attention of your audience and establish a connection between you and the attendees.

■ Remember that even experienced presenters get nervous, and some degree of public speaking jitters creates positive energy for an enthusiastic presentation. Breathe deeply, maintain your composure, and remember that you are an expert on your topic.

■ Begin your presentation by telling your audience what you will tell them (review the objectives for the presentation); then tell them (give the presentation); then end by reminding them what you just told them (recap and summarize the presentation). Following these three steps, regardless of if the presentation is formal or informal, live or Web-based, can ensure your intended message is received.

● LEARNING ACTIVITIES

1. What are the three main points that you want your attendees to take away from your presentation?

2. How will the title or abstract of your presentation impact attendees? Using a highly descriptive, yet catchy title and succinct abstract can increase interest and attendance at your presentation. Brainstorm some possible titles and write a two to three sentence abstract, to share with others for feedback.

3. Consider your presentation from the viewpoint of your audience. What would you want to know? What organizational method would make the most sense? What techniques and visual aids would help you to understand the more complex relationships or concepts?

4. Are you a visual, auditory, or kinesthetic learner? Use one of the inventories mentioned earlier in the chapter to identify your learning style; then consider the style of your audience. What method of delivery will be most effective for your presentation and why?

REFERENCES

Alley, M., & Neeley, K. A. (2005). Discovering the power of PowerPoint: Rethinking the design of presentation slides from a skillful user's perspective. *Proceedings of the 2005 American Society for Engineering Education Annual Conference and Exposition*, ICME2005-2461.

Fleming, N. D., & Mills, C. (1992). Not another inventory, rather a catalyst for reflection. *To Improve the Academy, 11*, 137–155.

Hrastinski, S. (2008). Asynchronous & synchronous e-learning. *Educause Quarterly, 31*(4), 51–55.

Matthews, J., & Matthews, R. (2008). *Successful scientific writing: A step-by-step guide for the biological and medical sciences* (3rd ed.). United Kingdom: Cambridge University Press.

Plunkett, S. W. (n.d.). Tips of poster presentations at professional conference. Retrieved from https://www.csun.edu/plunk/documents/poster_presentation.pdf

Shunk, D. H. (2012). *Learning theories: An educational perspective.* Boston: Pearson Education, Inc.

University of Pennsylvania. (2009, March 28). Visual learners convert words to pictures in the brain and vice versa, says psychology study. *Science Daily*. Retrieved from http://www.sciencedaily.com/releases/2009/03/090325091834.htm

Walsh, B. E., Willard, R., & Whiting, A. (2011). *VAK self-audit: Visual, auditory, and kinesthetic communication and learning styles.* British Columbia, Canada: Walsh Seminars Publishing House.

ADDITIONAL RESOURCES FOR CREATING POWERPOINT PRESENTATIONS

Altman, R. (2012). *Why most PowerPoint presentations suck and how you can make them better* (3rd ed.). Pleasanton, CA: Harvest Books.

Atkinson, C. (2011). *Beyond bullet points: Using Microsoft® PowerPoint® to create presentations that inform, motivate, and inspire* (3rd ed.). Redmond, WA: Microsoft Press.

Galloway, R. (2011). *Rethinking PowerPoint: Designing & delivering presentations that engage the mind.* Method Content LLC.

Matthews, J., & Matthews, R. (2008). *Successful scientific writing: A step-by-step guide for the biological and medical sciences* (3rd ed.). United Kingdom: Cambridge University Press.

ADDITIONAL RESOURCES FOR CREATING POSTER PRESENTATIONS

Carter, M. (2013). *Designing science presentations: A visual guide to figures, papers, slides, posters, and more.* London: Academic Press.

Nicol, A. A., & Pexman, P. M. (2010). *Displaying your findings: A practical guide for creating figures, posters, and presentations* (6th ed.). Washington, DC: American Psychological Association.

ADDITIONAL RESOURCES FOR CREATING CYBER PRESENTATIONS

Clay, C. (2012). *Great webinars: Create interactive learning that is captivating, informative, and fun.* San Francisco, CA: Pfeiffer.

Gendelman, J. (2010). *Virtual presentations that work.* New York, NY: McGraw-Hill.

Handley, A., & Chapman, C. C. (2012). *Content rules: How to create killer blogs, podcasts, videos, ebooks, webinars (and more) that engage customers and ignite your business* (Revised ed.). Hoboken, NJ: John Wiley & Sons, Inc.

Turmel, W. (2011). *10 steps to successful virtual presentations.* Alexandria, VA: ASTD Press.

ADDITIONAL PRESENTATION RESOURCES

Kapterer, A. (2011). *Presentation secrets.* Hoboken, NJ: John Wiley & Sons, Inc.

Reynolds, G. (2008). *Presentation Zen: Simple ideas on presentation design and delivery.* Berkeley, CA: New Riders.

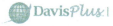 For additional materials, please visit **http://davisplus.fadavis.com, key word: Hissong.**

Chapter 14

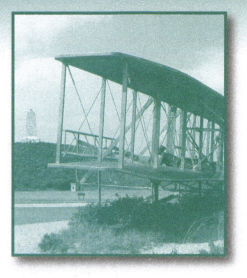

The Art of Publishing the Research Study or Evidence-Based Practice Project

Believe you can and you're half way there.
—*Theodore Roosevelt*

LEARNING OUTCOMES

The information provided in this chapter will assist the reader to:

- Explore the reasons for publishing a study or project.
- Determine publishing goals and consider how they impact publication style and approach.
- Differentiate between peer-reviewed and non–peer-reviewed publications.
- Choose an appropriate target publication for the identified publication goals.
- Use the formatting guidelines discussed to write an article for submission to the target publication.
- Identify additional resources and tips for composing a quality article.

material languishes in a drawer waiting to be written. Until colleagues, consumers, policy makers, or the general public are informed about the findings of the study or project, those findings are not useful. Specific reasons to pursue publication may include:

- To share knowledge gained via research or evidence-based practice efforts to allow informed decision-making by professionals and consumers
- To allow fellow researchers or practitioners to build on your work
- To enable others to avoid pitfalls noted in your study or project in their future endeavors
- To network and collaborate with others in your discipline or those interested in your topic area
- To expand your professional research and writing skills
- To build your resume for future employment or funding opportunities

Why Publish?

No research study or evidence-based practice project is complete until the results are shared. Unfortunately, this is often the point at which researchers and practitioners lose momentum; as a result, the

Defining Publishing Goals

Once you have decided to pursue publication, it is important to consider the goals you hope to achieve in this effort. For example, are you most interested in sharing your results with fellow professionals who could benefit from or build on your work? Might your work be appropriate to share with the general public who are consumers of your service? Or could your work impact the decisions of policy makers or administrators, in which case it really needs to be shared with them? Depending on the nature of your study or project, you may find one or more of these options to be fitting. There are usually multiple opportunities for publication within a single study or project. Boxes 14-1 and 14-2 show examples

---

BOX 14-1 ■ Example Research Study and Potential Publication Opportunities

A research study was conducted by three physical therapy students and their faculty advisor to explore the impact of a balance training program on the incidence of falls within one senior retirement community. Seventy-six subjects were randomized into one of two study groups: an experimental group that participated in the balance training program three times per week for 2 months and a control group that did not participate in the balance training program in the initial phase of the study. Results indicate that the experimental group had significantly fewer falls during the study compared with the control group. Publication opportunities might include:

- Publication in a professional peer-reviewed physical therapy journal to share the study's outcomes with others in the field who might want to expand on this research or apply the results to their practice
- Writing an article for a discipline-specific magazine on the steps involved in setting up a balance training program similar to that used by the researchers
- Composing a piece for a senior citizens' newsletter on the risk factors for falls, how physical therapy can help, and how to get more information or find a physical therapist in the area

---

BOX 14-2 ■ Example Evidence-Based Practice Project and Potential Publication Opportunities

An evidence-based practice project was undertaken by a school-based occupational therapist. She was interested in exploring the research related to the use of sensory-based activities to improve attention and emotional regulation in 5-year-olds with known sensory processing difficulties. She appraised 25 research articles on the use of sensory-based activities with similar populations. Then she designed and implemented a program based upon her findings from the research; her prior knowledge and experiences with the use of sensory-based treatments; and consideration of the goals, values, and circumstances of the 5-year-olds on her caseload. She collected data throughout her treatments to compare information before and after implementation of this new program to determine if her outcomes matched that of the literature that she searched. Publication opportunities might include:

- Publication in a discipline-specific journal or magazine (may be peer-reviewed or non–peer-reviewed, depending on the journal) to share her experiences or the procedures she used in conducting the evidence-based project as well as the outcomes from the project
- Writing an article for a parenting magazine on how to recognize signs of sensory-processing difficulties, tips for managing behaviors, and where to locate additional resources if needed
- Publication in an education journal or magazine focusing on collaboration between teachers and other professionals to address sensory processing difficulties with children

of a research study and an evidence-based practice project, respectively, with some potential publication avenues for each.

Although these examples are not exhaustive, they illustrate the variety of opportunities that exist in any given situation. The goals of publication can vary greatly and thus will impact the publication style and approach. Some key elements to consider when establishing your publication goals are:

1. **Who is your audience?** Identifying your potential audience can help you choose an appropriate publication, and will often dictate the approach and style of writing. For example, if you hope to reach consumers of your service, publishing in a discipline-specific peer-reviewed journal is unlikely to accomplish this goal. Similarly, the style of writing and choice of language for an article geared toward other professionals may not be easily understood by the general public. Some publications are discipline specific; others span multiple disciplines or practice groups. Still others are appropriate for specific groups of people, for example, those older than 65 years of age, or those caring for a child with disabilities. Identifying your audience can guide your publishing decisions.

2. **What is your message?** Considering the main points that you want to convey to your audience is a foundational step in publication. Publications vary in their purpose. Some aim to disseminate research, whereas others are geared toward evidence-based practice. Moreover, publications appropriate for the general public tend to be less formal and not as scientific. Comparing your intended message with the goals of your target publication can help you determine if the chosen publication is a good fit.

3. **What are your personal and professional goals?** Your personal and professional goals can impact your publication decisions. For example, if you are looking to connect with other researchers interested in your topic, then a more formal publication in a peer-reviewed journal is a good choice. If your priority is to disseminate your study's or project's outcomes to consumers or practitioners who might find it useful, a less formal publication

accessible to the public or others in your field is appropriate. Publishing allows you to contribute to the body of knowledge within your discipline, and the potential for personal and professional growth is great. Contemplating your personal and professional goals will ensure that your publication decisions support them.

Choosing a Publication

After outlining your publishing goals, you must decide the type of publication you want to pursue. There are generally two options: peer-reviewed journals and non–peer-reviewed publications. Both are explored in more detail here.

Peer-Reviewed Journals

Peer-reviewed journals (sometimes called scholarly or refereed publications) are publications that contain articles authored by one or more experts in a particular field or topic area, which are reviewed by other experts in the field or topic area to confirm each article's quality before acceptance for publication. To minimize biased reviews of the articles, the reviewers are usually unaware of who the authors of an article are when they are reviewing it. In this way, the reviewers must assess the value and quality of the article itself without being influenced by the reputation of the authors.

The publication process for peer-reviewed journals is often very rigorous with multiple revisions required over long periods of time. The aim of most peer-reviewed journals is to disseminate quality research or evidence-based practice. Peer-reviewed journals are not appropriate for informational-type articles or articles geared toward the general public. Some features of peer-reviewed articles include:

- Evidence of completion of a research study or formal evidence-based practice project. Keep in mind that some journals may *only* publish research, but others will consider high-quality evidence-based practice projects.
- Approval by an Institutional Review Board (IRB) to conduct the study or project. See Chapter 11 for additional information on the IRB process.

- Possible use of complex statistical methods, graphs, or tables to support outcomes.
- Highly structured format, with required sections specified in the author guidelines.
- Inclusion of multiple references from other scientific or professional journals to support the work.
- Use of complex professional language and terms that may not be easily understood by those outside the profession or unfamiliar with the topic.

Peer-reviewed journals typically appear very plain, with black and white photos or illustrations and little or no advertisements. Publication in these journals is highly respected among academicians, who are often required to publish for continued employment. Others may seek publication in peer-reviewed journals to gain professional respect and recognition for future employment or funding opportunities.

Most peer-reviewed journals publish accepted articles free of charge; nonetheless, **pay-to-publish journals**, which require authors to subsidize publishing fees, are increasing in number. There is no guarantee of publication with pay-to-publish journals, and articles submitted still undergo rigorous review. Authors submitting to pay-to-publish journals may have to pay review costs as well as per-page charges if the article is accepted.

Some examples of peer-reviewed journals include *The Journal of the American Medical Association*, *The British Journal of Occupational Therapy*, *The American Journal of Physical Medicine & Rehabilitation*, and the *Journal of Athletic Training*, to name a few. Most professional organizations publish discipline-specific journals, and there are many multidisciplinary or subject-specific journals that you might consider. A list of some common health-related journals is included in Appendix I to get you started.

Non–Peer-Reviewed Publications

Non–peer-reviewed publications include magazines, books, pamphlets, or other works that publish articles intended to provide more general information. Authors are usually professionals with some advanced level of experience in the subject area; however, conducting research or evidence-based practice in the subject area is usually not a requirement. In contrast to peer-reviewed articles, non–peer-reviewed articles are typically reviewed only by the editor(s) of the publication, who are not necessarily experts in the field or subject area. Non–peer-reviewed articles must be appraised by the individual readers to determine the quality and applicability of the information contained within it.

The publication process for non–peer-reviewed publications is less demanding than that of peer-reviewed publications, although some revisions are usually necessary. Non–peer-reviewed articles are usually less scientific, intended for general audiences, and aim to publicize information on a focused topic. Some features of non–peer-reviewed articles include:

- Less structured organization, with sections designed and arranged by the authors
- Provision of news or other general information to the public or other professionals
- Possible use of anecdotal evidence, photographs, simplified charts and figures, or personal or procedural narratives to illustrate the main points of the article
- Limited to no inclusion of references from other sources to support the work
- Use of layman's terms that can be easily understood by those outside the profession or unfamiliar with the topic

Author Guidelines

Most publications include specific **author guidelines**, available either in the print version of the publication or online, that outline the specific requirements for submitting your work. Author guidelines can include information about the writing style used by the publication (for example, APA style); the number of manuscript pages or words that are acceptable; and any specific requirements regarding photographs, drawings, figures, and so forth. Some publications have distinct guidelines for different types of articles, meaning that the requirements may vary depending on whether you are submitting a case study or an editorial. Submission requirements, including the need to provide additional items such as a cover letter, author biography, financial disclosure forms, copyright forms, or any associated publication or review fees, are also specified in the author guidelines.

It is essential to strictly adhere to the guidelines set forth by the chosen publication. Your work may be rejected simply because of improper formatting or failure to provide all the necessary forms and information, regardless of the content or quality of your work. Additional information on author guidelines, as well as some samples, can be found in Appendices L, M, and N.

In addition, looking at past issues of a publication you are considering can be an effective way to determine if it is a good fit for your work. Key elements to review and consider include:

- What organization is responsible for publishing the journal?
- Is the publication discipline-specific, multidisciplinary, or geared toward the general public?
- What is the aim and purpose of the publication?
- What topics are typically covered in the publication?
- Does the publication include specific columns or features, such as editorials, book reviews, personal anecdotes, or other topic-based columns?
- What is the review process for submissions (for example, editorial review or peer-reviewed, how many people will review the submission, and how long will it take to hear if an article is accepted)?
- What is the typical circulation of the publication? This can help you clarify how many professionals or other individuals your work will reach.

Answering each of these questions and then comparing this information with your publication goals and specific study or project content will help you to choose the most appropriate publication.

Format of the Article

The format and amount of detail for an article can vary depending on the chosen publication, the intended audience, and the topic being discussed. It is important to note that the approach and content for an article will differ significantly from the formal research or evidence-based practice report discussed in Chapter 12. Articles are considerably shorter in length and often written for alternative audiences, depending on the publication goals. For these reasons, merely copying and pasting content from the original research study or project report will be ineffective. Considering the content and organization of your article separate from the formal report is an essential step in the publication process.

Peer-Reviewed Articles

The format for research or evidence-based practice articles in peer-reviewed journals is highly structured, with required sections laid out in the author guidelines. A sample outline with sections typically included in a peer-reviewed article is contained in Table 14-1. In addition to the sections described in Table 14-1, authors typically submit an abstract. The abstract is a comprehensive summary of the research study or evidence-based practice project. Authors most often condense the main objective, methods, results, and conclusion of the project into 150 to 250 words. Readers frequently review the abstract to decide if the article warrants further inspection or is applicable to their purposes. Although the abstract is placed at the beginning of the article, it is typically written last after the article is completed.

Although most peer-reviewed articles follow a format similar to that included in Table 14-1, you may need to modify this outline, depending on the nature of your project. Articles based upon quantitative research should closely resemble this outline, whereas those based upon qualitative research will require more narrative description.

Format for Qualitative Research Articles

Qualitative articles are often ethnographically based, meaning they are specialized commentaries about a narrowly defined project that has been conducted using naturalistic methods. Qualitative articles are typically of greater length because of the more subjective methods and the subsequent need for richer description of procedures and outcomes. Fetterman (1998) feels that ethnographic writing is difficult, yet satisfying:

> *From simple notes about small events . . . to efforts to describe an experience or explain a sudden insight, ethnographic writing requires an eye for detail, an ability to express that detail in its proper context, and the language skills to weave small details and bits of meaning into a textured social fabric. The ethnographic writer must recreate the varied forms of social organization and interaction that months of observation*

Table 14-1 ■ Sample Peer-Reviewed Article Outline

Suggested Research Article Sections	What to Include in Each Section
Description of the Problem and Background	■ Clearly describe the major issue addressed in the study. ■ Most of the background section will come from the literature review you conducted. ■ Discuss the literature, but do not include an exhaustive historical review. This is the section that will be most condensed, given the amount of material you have amassed. Because of space constraints, most journals will not accept more than a few paragraphs concerning the background. ■ State the purpose of the study and the hypotheses.
Method ■ **Subjects or Participants** ■ **Interventions or Procedures** ■ **Outcome Measures** ■ **Data Collection** ■ **Data Analysis**	■ Describe how the study was conducted in sufficient detail to allow other researchers to replicate the study and readers to assess the appropriateness of your methods and the reliability and validity of the study. The method section may be divided into subsections covering subjects, procedures, outcome measures, data collection, and analysis. ■ *Subjects or Participants.* Describe criteria used to determine the population for the study, stating the literature that indicates that these criteria are necessary or desirable. Then, describe the method of sample selection (i.e., random or nonrandom). If nonrandom selection was used, was convenience sampling or some other technique used? The method of assigning subjects to groups should be addressed, if relevant. State the number of subjects in the study and how many were included in each group. If there was any subject attrition during the study, this should also be mentioned. ■ *Interventions or Procedures*. If any intervention or treatment was provided, this should be described in detail, including who provided the treatment, where it was provided and under what conditions, and specifically how it was provided. ■ *Outcome Measures (Testing Instruments)*. Identify all measures used with information on reliability and validity of the tools, if available. If you devised the measure specifically for the study, this should be mentioned, and it may be useful to include a copy of the instrument in the article. ■ *Data Collection*. Describe how the data were collected, including whether a pretest and posttest were used, who administered the tests, whether the tests were administered in a group or individually, the environmental conditions, and how long the data collection took. ■ *Data Analysis.* Report on specific statistical methods or software used, if applicable.
Results	■ Summarize the main findings (do not include interpretation of findings in this section). ■ Use figures and tables, if necessary, to illustrate results. ■ When reporting the findings from inferential statistics such as *t* tests or chi-squares, include information about the significance level and the degrees of freedom. Style manuals give information on how to type statistical results.

Table 14-1 ■ Sample Peer-Reviewed Article Outline–cont'd

Suggested Research Article Sections	What to Include in Each Section
Discussion ■ **Limitations** ■ **Implications of Findings** ■ **Future Research**	■ State whether the hypotheses were supported or the research question was answered. ■ Discuss similarities and differences in the findings of your study and the studies mentioned in the literature review. ■ Be sure to state findings that do not support your hypotheses and briefly speculate on why they might have come about and what they might mean. ■ *Limitations.* Review limitations within the study's procedures. ■ *Implications*. Explain implications of the study's findings to practice. ■ *Future Research*. Review recommendations for future research or evidence-based practice.
References	■ Include a full reference list (in the style specified in the author guidelines) for any references used in the article. ■ Include only references used in the article. You should not include references used in the study or project but not mentioned in the article.

and study have revealed. The manifold symbolism every culture displays and the adaptiveness of people to their environment must somehow come to life on the page. (p. 111)

The outline in Table 14-1 will still prove useful, but qualitative articles typically have limited focus on strict procedures and statistical methods. More of the article will be devoted to descriptions of the participants and their experiences and specific data collection techniques such as participant observation, in-depth interviewing, or document review. More detail is also included regarding data analysis and discussion of identified themes than in quantitative research articles. Specific methods of data analysis need to be explained, including how the data were obtained and if any checks were imposed to confirm the findings. If sufficient detail is omitted, it will be unclear if the findings come from your own knowledge of the culture, direct personal experiences of the activities studied, other people's theoretical frameworks, or actual fieldwork and interviewing.

Tips for Peer-Reviewed Articles

Whether the content is research or evidence-based practice, composing and submitting a peer-reviewed article can be challenging. Following these suggestions can assist you in getting your article accepted for publication.

1. Clearly identify the focus of your article.
2. Ensure that the aim of the chosen publication aligns with the focus of your article.
3. Follow the author guidelines for the chosen publication explicitly.
4. Use the reference style outlined in the author guidelines, and credit all sources appropriately.
5. Select a concise, descriptive title.
6. Include all required sections of the article, typically an abstract, introduction, body, and conclusion.
7. Use clearly designed and labeled figures and tables, where appropriate, to support the written word. (Refer to Chapter 12 for support in creating visual displays of data.)
8. Be prepared to receive constructive criticism and endure the rigors of multiple edits. The purpose is only to make your work stronger (PHC RIS et al., 2009).

Non–Peer-Reviewed Articles

In contrast to the structured format for peer-reviewed articles, the format for non–peer-reviewed articles allows for greater flexibility and creativity. The possibilities of how to organize and approach these articles is nearly endless, and the decision will be based largely on the chosen publication and audience.

Because many non–peer-reviewed publications are designed for the general population, the approach taken is usually a less formal, more conversational one. Layman's terms and explanations are more appropriate, as are color photos, diagrams, and attention-getting facts, stories, and titles. Although the purpose is still to inform or share scientific information based upon research or evidence-based practice, the information is tailored to a specific audience and organized as deemed appropriate by the author.

From the sample study in Box 14-1, one of the possible publications included composing a piece for a senior citizens' newsletter on the risk factors for falls, how physical therapy can help, and how to get more information or find a physical therapist in the area. Box 14-3 includes a possible outline for this article, to illustrate how the organization of a non–peer-reviewed article contrasts with that of the peer-reviewed article outline included in Table 14-1. This example reveals that the sections of the article are unique and are organized in a logical manner. Goals of the article are to grab the senior citizens' attention about falls, provide them with background information on fall risks in layman's terms, enable them to assess their fall risk via a short questionnaire, and explain that help is available for them if they need it.

Publication Procedures

Once you have selected an appropriate publication and written your article, you are ready to submit it. The author guidelines typically outline the submission procedure, with most publications requiring electronic submission now. Many publications require potential authors to sign a copyright form attesting that their work is not under consideration by any other publication. For this reason, you should submit your article to only one publication at a time. If and when you find out that your article has been rejected by one publication, then and only then is it acceptable to submit it elsewhere.

Authors are notified if their articles are accepted for review or publication; however, the length of time it takes to receive notification can vary greatly depending on the publication. If a peer-reviewed

---

BOX 14-3 ■ Outline for Non–Peer-Reviewed Article on Fall Risk in a Senior Citizens' Newsletter

Introduction
■ Attention-getting statistics on falls

What Are the Risk Factors for Falls?
■ Intrinsic Factors: Decreased strength, vision, reflexes, cognitive changes, disease-related changes (dementia, cardiovascular disorders, osteoporosis), fear of falling
■ Extrinsic Factors: Environment, medication, time of day, staff and caregivers

Am I at Risk for Falls?
■ Plan to include a short 10-item self-questionnaire that readers can use to identify their risk for falls as minimal, moderate, or maximum

What Physical Therapy Can Do If You Are at Risk for Falls
■ Environmental modifications
■ Strengthening and coordination activities
■ Balance retraining
■ Set up a home program

How to Get More Information
■ Consult your MD
■ How to find a physical therapist near you
■ How to learn more about falls

---

article is accepted for review, this means that the article passed the first evaluation and is being sent to multiple experts on the topic who will review it and provide feedback on whether or not it should be accepted for publication. Considerations include whether the topic is relevant to the readership, if it has been adequately covered, and if the study or project is of good quality. Once the expert reviews are complete, the editor will determine whether or not the article is appropriate for publication. Non–peer-reviewed articles are usually appraised by *only* the editor(s) of the publication and then rejected, accepted with revisions, or accepted as submitted.

Revising

Often editors accept an article but require the author to make revisions. These requests should be viewed positively because this means that the editor is interested in the work and wants to help the author polish it and share it with others (Day, n.d.). Reviewers or editors may request revisions to clarify confusing points, to simplify the information for better readability, or to more clearly align an article with the publication's aims or current research. Nevertheless, it is important to respond promptly to an editor's request for revisions and to make the necessary changes to the article. Do not be surprised if your article goes back and forth between you and the editor a few times before it is acceptable. Above all, do not become so discouraged that you stop revising and resubmitting. If the editor considers the material suitable for publication, it is merely a matter of time before you have it in publishable form.

What If My Article Is Rejected?

If your article is rejected for publication, you will usually be given the reason for rejection. Some common reasons that an article might be rejected are:

1. **Submission to the wrong publication**. If the topic and the purpose of your article do not mesh well with the aims of the chosen publication, your work could be rejected (Day, n.d.).
2. **Poor organization.** As noted in the discussion of formatting earlier in this chapter, the article should flow logically with later points building on earlier ones. Without good organization, readers will not understand your work.
3. **Lack of purpose or focus**. Although you could discuss many aspects of your study or project, consider the chief message you want to convey. Ask yourself what your paper is about and why this information is important. To gain focus, Day (n.d.) suggests trying to write in 20 words or less the main objective for writing your article (p. 9). Although you likely will not include this in the actual work, the exercise can be clarifying and

you can refer to it during the writing process to see if you are staying true to your purpose.
4. **Poor writing**. It is quite possible to have a quality project, but to have your work rejected based upon the quality of the writing. Day (n.d.) advises authors to avoid verbosity and jargon by writing clearly and concisely and avoiding technical terms that could confuse readers. She also recommends writing "to express—not impress," meaning that authors should avoid use of long impressive terms (pp. 23–24). In addition, articles should always be reviewed for proper grammar and spelling before submission.
5. **Failure to consider the audience.** Remember to consider the intended audience and how you will tailor the message to them. There is a clear difference between writing and communicating; altering your writing style and approach will ensure that the audience receives the message you intended (Day, n.d.).

Research articles might also be rejected based upon flaws with the research design, data collection, data analysis, or interpretation of results. Although you cannot erase these mistakes, you have several options. You might resubmit your article to a non–peer-reviewed publication, or alter the way you approached the article. For example, instead of writing a traditional research article, you could focus on summarizing your literature review or highlighting the topic via a case study. Both approaches may be beneficial to readers interested in your topic and still allow you to share what you have learned. Another option is to conduct another study, perhaps a pilot or case series, controlling for the previously identified flaws. The quality of the research upon which an article is based can definitely impact acceptance for publication.

If your work is rejected, you should not be discouraged. Even experienced authors can experience rejection or be asked to make substantial revisions. It is a learning experience and part of the writing process. Remember that you have valuable information to share with others—it is just a matter of finding the right publication, format, and approach to do so. With a little hard work, your publication goals are achievable.

Article Acceptance

Once your article has been accepted, it will be copy edited to clarify any uncertainties, to polish the writing and flow of the work, and to finalize the layout. This process will likely involve multiple revisions and collaboration with the editor. Your editor may send you one or more proofs to review and can let you know the anticipated publication date of your article. Depending on your topic and the publication, it could take a while for your article to appear in print. During this time, it is perfectly acceptable for you to list this publication on your resume, noting that the publication is "in press."

Chapter Summary

Focusing on your publication goals and reviewing the author guidelines for your chosen publication can guide you to write a meaningful article on your topic. The opportunities and benefits associated with publishing far outweigh the challenges along the way. In the end, you should be proud of your accomplishment and the contribution you made to your profession and area of study.

SKILL-BUILDING TIPS

■ Know your publications. Which publications are for a more generalized audience versus a more specific one? What are the acceptance rates for the publication you are considering? Review a copy of the publication you are considering. What are the styles of the articles within it?

■ How and where is the best place to disseminate your information? Who is your intended audience? Is a discipline-specific publication appropriate, or would another venue suit just as well or better?

■ Ponder some of the top reasons that papers are rejected: no clear focus identified; poor organization; and information is not current.

■ Contemplate the title. This is often what "sells" your paper initially. For peer-reviewed articles, you should consider something concise that clearly articulates the focus of your article. Considering a creative or catchy title might be more appropriate for a non–peer-reviewed article.

■ Remember your goal is to communicate information, not to write for self-recognition, although that may be a secondary gain. The most difficult part of the writing process is writing enough to be informative, but being clear and concise, so as not to bore the reader.

■ Consider use of photos, graphs, or charts to supplement or emphasize information in the text. Remember to secure permission for photos if they include participants.

■ Remember to include your references in the style specified in the author guidelines (often APA style). Be sure to include *only* those references that you used in the article, not all the references for your entire research study or evidence-based practice project.

■ Pay close attention to page, spacing, and style requirements. Often your article can be rejected if you did not adhere to these specifications.

⌣ LEARNING ACTIVITIES

1. Consider that there are likely multiple opportunities for publication within a single study or project (as illustrated in Boxes 14-1 and 14-2). Brainstorm and make a list of at least five publication opportunities for your study or project.

2. What is the main objective of your article? Try writing this down in 20 words or less.

3. What supplemental materials, such as tables, figures, or photographs, could be used to support or enhance the text of your article?

REFERENCES

Day, A. (n.d.). *How to write publishable papers.* Retrieved from http://sigma.poligran.edu.co/politecnico/apoyo/Decisiones/curso/howtowriteclean.pdf

Fetterman, D. M. (1998). *Ethnography: Step by step* (2nd ed.). Thousand Oaks, CA: Sage Publications, Inc.

PHC RIS, McIntyre, E., Nisbet, S., Magarey, A., Keane, M., & Roeger, L. (2009). *Fact sheet: Publishing in peer review journals: Criteria for success* (2nd ed.). Adelaide: Primary Health Care Research & Information Service.

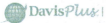 DavisPlus. For additional materials, please visit **http://davisplus.fadavis.com, key word: Hissong.**

Chapter 15

Grant Funding: Insights and Approaches

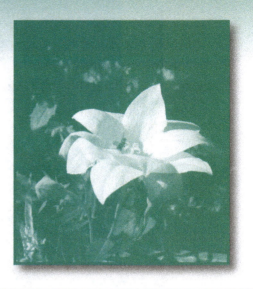

*Often when you think you're at the end of something,
you're at the beginning of something else.*
—Mr. Rogers

*Oh, it's delightful to have ambitions . . . and there never
seems to be any end to them—that's the best of it! Just as
soon as you attain one ambition you see another one glitter-
ing higher up still. It does make life so interesting.*
—Anne Shirley (L.M. Montgomery)

LEARNING OUTCOMES

The information provided in this chapter will assist the reader to:

- Gain knowledge in how to locate, write, and obtain grant funding.
- Identify the pros and cons to developing and implementing a program based on grant funding.
- Build skills in seeking out funding sources to ascertain as much information as possible before writing a grant.
- Acknowledge the need to celebrate and accept challenges during the grant-writing process.

Charge to Engage in Grant Writing

Acquiring money is a helpful, and often mandatory, task to help with the processes involved in a research or evidence-based practice venture. Key factors when searching for grants are identifying your skills and knowledge to carry out the inquiry, finding supporting evidence, enlisting people to help you with the project, and maintaining persistence and persever-ance. Grant writing involves a combination of the following:

- A well-thought-out and written work plan
- A collaborative and cooperative team
- An exhaustive search of your resources (in-house and out-of-house)
- A plan to network and check in with key support-ers of the grant project (i.e., letters of support, ad-ministrative assistant time, work-study student)
- A keen knowledge and insight into the client's needs for the program or product you are proposing
- A simple, yet inclusive mission statement as to why you need money (Figure 15-1)

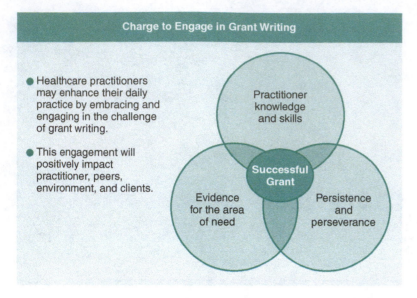

Charge to Engage in Grant Writing

- Healthcare practitioners may enhance their daily practice by embracing and engaging in the challenge of grant writing.
- This engagement will positively impact practitioner, peers, environment, and clients.

Practitioner knowledge and skills

Successful Grant

Evidence for the area of need

Persistence and perseverance

Figure 15-1 Charge to Engage in Grant Writing

When going through the process of grant writing, a helpful saying to recall is, "It is amazing how much you can accomplish when it doesn't matter who gets the credit" (unknown source).

Every single grant is different, yet the application process puts similar demands on your time and resources. The first priority is to recognize the mission of your project's targeted funding source. Determine upfront if their mission and requirements align with those of your project. Do not apply for a grant that is going to compromise the process or outcomes of what you want to accomplish.

When gathering information to support the components of the grant, start by utilizing what you have already written in your thesis, dissertation, or evidence-based practice plan. Start with your abstract and then look at your literature review. You will find that many of the answers to the questions asked in the grant application can be copied and pasted or simply tweaked from the work you have already done. You will more than likely need information from multiple people or sources within the institution or community housing your project. Keep detailed notes of who is giving you the information and where you are obtaining information to support the mission of the grant. This seems like a commonsense comment, but you will forget points and people if you do not write things down. Networking is a must when you are writing a grant, particularly a large grant. It often takes a village to write a grant. If this is your first attempt at writing a

grant, start small—but think big! You don't want to get yourself into a position where you take people's money, but then can't sustain the journey by fulfilling all the proposal's demands at the end of your project.

Grant Writer's Skills and Knowledge

If you are reading this, you are most likely planning to write or prepare a grant, so take three deep breaths and be confident in your ability to properly write and submit a grant on time! There are a few things to consider in relation to your skills and knowledge when you commence writing a grant:

- Trust yourself!
- Remember who you are doing this for and why . . . the process can get lonely, so if you can keep the original intent of securing funding at the forefront, it helps.
- You will be constantly gaining new skills and knowledge as you move through the process. Although you will not know every step of the way upfront and there will be bumps in the road, you must keep going. Every time you write a new grant or a renewal it is a new learning experience. The rules change constantly.
- Hence, be constant and consistent in keeping the pace. Although it is a time of learning, there is [always] a deadline for the grant to be submitted and it isn't optional. Grant funders give no extensions.

In addition to understanding your skills and knowledge, it is also important to glean when you need to enlist the help of others. Therefore, consider how your clients, students, and peers can help you write your grant. Ask them for answers—how do they feel, what do they need or want, and how can they assist you in accomplishing the task of writing a grant to improve upon a treatment intervention, modality, or piece of equipment? Dovetail your everyday experiences in practice into the grant-writing process. Consider interventions and programming that have been working or those components that need modification. Now that we have covered your skills and knowledge as a grant writer, the next section will review some grant-writing basics.

Grant Writing 101

The following list features pieces that you should pull together before you even start searching for a grant:

- Find out if there is a key person in your organization who assists with grant writing.
- Subscribe to as many grant and foundation listservs and e-mail alerts as possible.
- If the grant you are looking at is offering a workshop to review the application process, sign up and attend the workshop.
- Bookmark key grant websites and check them often.
- Remember that grant writing can become a 40+ hour per week occupation all unto itself! Take care of yourself!
- Write a background of the entities that will be involved with the grant. Look to mission statements, philosophies of education, and business plans.
- Find and secure a minimum of one partnership entity.
- Write down a brief description of the issue you wish to address with grant funding.
- Do a literature search on the issue you wish to address with the scholarly and general public domains.
- Write a one-page statement on why you are the most deserving entity to receive the foundation or grant source's money.
- Find someone who is efficient at designing budgets, even if you think you are good at this. If you

are the grant's primary investigator or coinvestigator, you will want someone else to do the budget. It typically accounts for 25% of the score on the application.

- Write a statement of how the grant will not only assist the individuals directly involved in the process, but the larger community as well.
- Consider and build in the outcome measures as early on as possible, using criteria and actual process measures.
- Seek out someone in your organization or circle who is proficient at quantitative statistics. Find another who excels in qualitative stats–narratives, themes, and stories are quickly becoming of interest to funding agencies.
- If the grant source states, *"Submit a four-page preliminary proposal,"* get on the Web and pull down some samples to follow. The sources are endless! You will find one to match your needs and style.
- Get sleep while you can. Once the window for state and federal grants opens, you have 6 to 8 weeks to upload all supporting materials to the site. Remember, most educational and business organizations have someone who will want to review the grant 2 weeks before it goes to the grant source; therefore, back your deadline up by a minimum of 10 days. *Unfortunately, when you are in the thick of writing the grant there is no minimum time for sleep . . . especially if you are the primary writer.* Again, take care of yourself!
- Utilize focus groups to assist with brainstorming. Client groups, boards of directors, and water cooler mates are great people to pull into the process.
- Finally, stay calm throughout the process. We've witnessed people melt down hard! Grants may be important to your organization; however, they are not worth risking your health or relationships.

Enablers and Barriers

There are many ways to empower yourself and others when you are thinking about writing a grant or when engaged in the post-grant funding process. First and foremost, facilitate and lead by example. We promise that if you keep a smile on your face and a light heart through the sometimes stifling process of grant writing, others around you will be intrigued and motivated to keep working. Be a trend setter and start a weekly grant e-mail update on the strengths and needs of the project. Start a grant-writing mentor program. Seek out others who have been successful in your setting with securing grants and have lunch with them to pick their brains. Incorporate grant writing into your professional development plan. Start a focus group with clients, students, and peers to brainstorm what is needed in your setting and make a top 10 list of possible projects and grant-funding sources.

The common barriers that are typically associated with grant writing are as follows:

■ No time is available to find or read grant application requirements.
■ No time is available to write up a proposal, as it takes an immense amount of time.
■ No time is available to carry out every component of the project that the funders may want included in the project.
■ Limited support is given from administration or peers.
■ A change in practice can be difficult and sometimes the status quo just seems too safe to move away from for some individuals, groups, or communities.
■ Some people on your team will not value securing a grant. They just do not feel a grant-funded program will add value to their or their clients' experience (Box 15-1).

In response to the enablers and barriers of grant writing, just remember: Breathe, *seriously*, breathe! Muster up the unshakable confidence and move forward in your skills and knowledge as a healthcare practitioner. By embracing the enablers and downplaying the barriers you will move forward in the grant-writing process and succeed in the following:

■ Gain new skills
■ Recognize what you already know
■ Believe more in your knowledge and skills
■ Learn from the positives and negatives that you encounter
■ Elicit and gain support from your peers
■ Assist in the skill and knowledge development of others

BOX 15-1 ■ Ten Reasons Proposals Get Rejected

1. Program activities are not based on best practices.
2. Proposals are unclear or missing required information.
3. Need has not been adequately identified in the proposal.
4. Programs are not well thought out. Portions are inconsistent with one another.
5. Proposals are too ambitious for the amount of time and money requested or proposals are not ambitious enough for the amount of time and money requested.
6. Budget is vague, inconsistent, or unrealistic.
7. Staff expertise is not conducive to program activities.
8. Program has a bad track record for completing activities.
9. Proposals are submitted after the due date (a deadline is a deadline).
10. Proposal submitter has good ideas but the proposal is written poorly.
http://www.cippp.org/pubs/granttip.pdf

■ Become more confident in your everyday practice
■ Take ownership in your mission to engage in best practice

Given all of this insight, there is one final point about grant making: Do exactly what the grant funders tell you to do—*exactly*! Follow the directions of the application exactly—do no more, no less! This is not the time to be creative with fonts or graphics. It is smart to have only a few writers; however, use many readers to proof the narrative with the application directions. Finally, have an expert do the budget. Seek out the best money manager within your organization or group and have him or her set up the budget and recheck it three times before hitting the submit button. Congratulations! You have engaged in the very meaningful process of grant writing. *See Appendix O for an outline of a grant proposal.*

Chapter Summary

As you can see by the comments and suggestions in this chapter, grant writing can be time-consuming and somewhat of a challenge; however, know that thousands of people every year find it is worth their time and effort. There are two overriding challenges in the grant process. The first is finding a grant source that aligns with your mission and the needs of your practice. The second is allocating the time and resources to write and submit the grant. Most importantly, throughout all phases of the grant-writing and implementation process, stay organized and ask for help when the tasks become too overwhelming.

SKILL-BUILDING TIPS

■ Remember to breathe—it is SO very important!

■ Congratulate yourself when you read or write something. Some days a sentence or a paragraph can take a day to write, whereas other days you will write pages.

■ Keep a 5 x 7 notebook with you all the time or use your phone to keep notes. As you dive deep into the grant-writing process, you will be amazed where and when thoughts pop into your mind. If need be, write thoughts down on napkins or old receipts, or ask your waitress or waiter for a piece of paper. At all costs, don't allow the thought to get lost!

■ It is essential to make a reading and writing space for yourself. Whatever you have to do, get your space organized! If you don't have a file cabinet drawer to organize the mass amounts of literature and information you will be collecting, buy a two-drawer file cabinet or get yourself a three-pack of cardboard file boxes.

■ When engaging in grant writing, you will generate a lot of paper. Another option is scanning and keeping files on your computer, as this will save a tree!

■ Own the passion of writing and reading as an occupation; it will be your primary means of communicating what you are doing with the money.

■ Embrace the ever-evolving organic arousal of your mind, body, and spirit in this process; we promise it is a journey to cherish! A great deal of the grant-writing process comes from within. . . you have to keep your momentum going. One way to do so is to allow the writing process to just wash over you! It is a grand thing—embrace it!

🌑 LEARNING ACTIVITIES

1. Identify at least five potential grant sources that address the needs of your project.

2. Write a draft of the components of a typical grant proposal:
   ■ Statement of need or rationale
   ■ Implementation strategies (i.e., goals, objectives, activities, time line)
   ■ Outcomes
   ■ Personnel
   ■ Evaluation
   ■ Budget

3. Do you need a one-time grant or is your program going to need ongoing funding?

   Consider and describe how you plan to sustain the program once funding from your first grant is complete.

4. Identify three people or institutions who can write a letter of support for your project. Write a draft of the support letter they can use as an example.

GRANT AND FOUNDATION FUNDING RESOURCES

Grants.Gov
http://www.grants.gov/
Grants.Net
www.grantsnet.org
Pages and pages of grant opportunities
National Collegiate Inventors and Innovators Alliance
http://www.nciia.org/grants.html
National Endowment for the Arts
http://www.nea.gov/grants/index.html
National Institutes of Health
http://grants.nih.gov/grants/grant_basics.htm
National Science Foundation
http://www.nsf.gov/about/glance.jsp

Population Research Institute

http://cairo.pop.psu.edu/allen/Agencies.cfm

This database is updated weekly by PRI staff and includes funding opportunity announcements targeting researchers in population science and related fields. For help on conducting your own funding search, please see the Population Research Institute Library's Funding Resources Links.

Sloan Grants

http://www.sloan.org/main.shtml

Small Business Administration

http://www.sba.gov/services/financialassistance/grants/index.html

Overwhelming amount of funding links

U.S. Department of Agriculture

http://www.csrees.usda.gov/fo/funding.cfm

U.S. Department of Health and Human Services

http://www.hhs.gov/grants/index.shtml

U.S. Department of Justice

http://www.usdoj.gov/10grants/

FOUNDATION OPPORTUNITIES

Foundation Center—One Stop Shop!

http://www.foundationcenter.org/

Top 100 Foundation Funders

http://foundationcenter.org/findfunders/topfunders/top100assets.html

DavisPlus | For additional materials, please visit **http://davisplus.fadavis.com, key word: Hissong.**

Appendix A

Example of Mixed Quantitative–Qualitative Study

The intent of providing you with the outline of this study is for you to glean insight from the structure and description of the inquiry.

The Effects of Massage Therapy on Pain Management in the Acute Care Setting

Background

Pain management remains a critical issue for hospitals and is receiving the attention of hospital accreditation organizations. The acute care setting of the hospital provides an excellent opportunity for the integration of massage therapy for pain management into the team-centered approach of patient care.

Purpose and Setting

This preliminary study evaluated the effect of the use of massage therapy on inpatient pain levels in the acute care setting. The study was conducted at Flagstaff Medical Center in Flagstaff, Arizona—a nonprofit community hospital serving a large rural area of northern Arizona.

Method

A convenience sample was used to identify research participants. Pain levels before and after massage therapy were recorded using a 0–10 visual analog scale. Quantitative and qualitative methods were used for analysis of this descriptive study.

Participants

Hospital inpatients ($n = 53$) from medical, surgical, and obstetrics units participated in the current research by each receiving one or more massage therapy sessions averaging 30 minutes each. The number of sessions received depended on the length of the hospital stay.

Result

Before massage, the mean pain level recorded by the patients was 5.18 [standard deviation (SD): 2.01]. After massage, the mean pain level was 2.33 (SD: 2.10). The observed reduction in pain was statistically significant: paired samples $t_{52} = 12.43$, $r = .67$, $d = 1.38$,

Continued

The Effects of Massage Therapy on Pain Management in the Acute Care Setting—cont'd

$p < .001$. Qualitative data illustrated improvement in all areas, with the most significant areas of impact reported being overall pain level, emotional well-being, relaxation, and ability to sleep.

Conclusions

This study shows that integration of massage therapy into the acute care setting creates overall positive results in the patient's ability to deal with the challenging physical and psychological aspects of their health condition. The study demonstrated not only significant reduction in pain levels, but also the interrelatedness of pain, relaxation, sleep, emotions, recovery, and finally, the healing process.

KEYWORDS: Massage therapy, acute care, hospital, pain management, research, inpatients, patient care management, postoperative pain, anxiety, reflexology, craniosacral, acupressure, Swedish effleurage, pregnancy, cancer, fibromyalgia, relaxation

Introduction

Pain management within the acute care setting is a concern that is being carefully examined not only by individual hospitals, but also by accreditation organizations across the United States (1). Massage therapy is one of the complementary and integrative medicine (CIM) therapies most often prescribed by physicians, and it is noted to be the most likely to be beneficial and the least likely to be harmful (2). Studies have examined the experience of hospitalized patients and found that high levels of stress and anxiety can increase pain (3,4) and slow a patient's recovery by limiting "physical functioning, including the ability to cough and breathe deeply, move, sleep, and perform self-care activities" (5).

The Mayo Clinic of Rochester, Minnesota, conducted a systematic evaluation of the patient hospital experience and found that "tension, stress, pain, and anxiety were key challenges for patients" (6). The integration of massage therapy into the team approach in patient care constitutes a move forward that recognizes pain as the fifth vital sign after pulse, blood pressure, temperature, and respiratory rate (5). Although each patient's healing process is unique (7), common themes of healing recognized in the present study underlie the significance of a holistic approach to patient care.

Research has documented the use of massage therapy as an effective tool for pain management (8–10), with the added benefit of producing few adverse reactions (11–13). When, with cardiac surgery patients, opioid medications are initially necessary, the continued use of large doses can delay the recovery process and lead to prolonged hospitalization (11). Patients with increased blood pressure because of stress may also benefit from massage therapy (14,15). A study at the Mayo Clinic, in which 58 cardiac surgery patients postoperatively received 1–3 massage therapy sessions of 20 minutes each, created evidence compelling enough for the Mayo Clinic to hire a full-time massage therapist to be available on the inpatient unit (6).

Cardiac surgery patients often complain of back, shoulder, and neck pain from manipulation of the body during the surgical procedure and from physical manifestations of tension and stress (11). When massage therapy is incorporated as part of the postsurgical protocol, fewer medications may be needed, providing an added advantage of fewer adverse side effects and acting as an effective adjunct or alternative to pharmaceuticals (10).

The gate-control theory of pain postulates that massage may be effective in "closing the gate"—that is, inhibiting the transmission of noxious stimuli by stimulating large nerve fibers

The Effects of Massage Therapy on Pain Management in the Acute Care Setting—cont'd

that have been shown to alter pain perception (13). In the acute care setting, health care professionals have a tendency to touch patients only when performing procedures, which can be uncomfortable and even painful. As White wrote, "Touch is often the most neglected or assaulted sense of the hospitalized patient" (16).

The relaxation response (RR) is the body's mechanism to decrease the level of psychophysiologic arousal produced by stress (17). Massage therapy can produce a RR that creates a calm state and enhances the ability to rest, qualities that are so essential for healing to occur (4). In addition, the RR elicits physiological changes, including lower blood pressure and heart rate, decreased oxygen consumption and muscle tension, and lower levels of cortisol and noradrenaline (15). "The majority of studies show that back massage induces a physiological or psychological relaxation response and that it is not injurious for critically ill patients with heart disease" (17).

Stressors experienced by hospital patients include excessive noise, lack of sleep, social isolation, enforced immobility, and pain from procedures. Anxiety and stress during cardiac catheterization can lengthen the hospital stay and increase the use of sedative medication before and during the procedure (3). Hamel's research using a randomized clinical trial design with 46 participants demonstrated that a 20-minute back massage successfully reduced blood pressure before cardiac catheterization (3). Studies note that fear and anxiety are common emotions felt by cardiac surgery patients (6), and as Moyer suggests, "There is much agreement that how a person feels, emotionally, is at least partly a function of that person's bodily state" (18). When patients have higher postoperative mobility, they may also have fewer serious postoperative complications, as demonstrated by Mitchinson and his colleagues in a randomized controlled trial of 605 veterans undergoing major surgery at Department of Veterans Affairs hospitals (5).

Lack of sleep in the hospital environment is a well-known phenomenon and can delay a patient's recovery (4,9,17). Hospital-induced sleep deprivation is generally remedied with medications (17). Critically ill and elderly patients are a vulnerable population and may benefit from non-pharmacologic methods to promote sleep (17). By studying the amount of REM and NREM sleep in 69 elderly men, Richards found that sleep efficiency was 14.7% higher in patients who received a 6-minute back massage than in a control group (17). That study is comparable with another that followed 30 patients with fibromyalgia who received 30 minutes of massage therapy twice weekly for 5 weeks. The patients experienced decreased depression, improved sleep (a greater number of sleep hours and fewer sleep movements) and decreased symptoms, including pain, fatigue, and stiffness (8). Another study of 41 hospitalized oncology patients illustrated that sleep quality, pain, symptom distress, and anxiety all improved when massage therapy was given during the hospital stay (19).

Egnew concludes that healing may be defined as "the personal experience of the transcendence of suffering" (7), and therefore each individual will have a personal concept of what "healing" means to them. Some aspects of healing are subjective and intensely personal, with different meanings for each person (7). Integration of massage therapy may improve the healing environment for the patient, thus allowing the deeper aspects of psychological healing to occur along with physical healing.

As authors, we felt that it was important to include both quantitative and qualitative investigation. The value of including qualitative

Continued

The Effects of Massage Therapy on Pain Management in the Acute Care Setting—cont'd

research is reflected by Kania and her colleagues in an article that describes how the use of the mixed methods approach "can provide highly valuable insights and a more complete understanding of the effectiveness of an intervention" (20). Using the mixed methods approach, the present study tests the research hypothesis "Does the use of massage therapy in an inpatient setting improve patient perception of pain management?"

Participants and Methods

This preliminary study enrolled a convenience sample of 65 inpatients admitted between October 1, 2006, and March 31, 2007, at a nonprofit community hospital serving a large rural area in the southwestern region of the United States. Criteria for inclusion in the study were a physician order for massage therapy, the patient's (or a family member's) ability to complete and sign a consent form, and willingness on the part of the patient to give feedback on the experience of hospital massage therapy and to return the qualitative survey after hospital discharge. Table A-1 presents demographic data for the research participants.

The plan for the current study was submitted and approved by the hospital's institutional review board. Participation in the research project was voluntary. Informed consent, including confidentiality and the right to withdraw from the study at any time, was obtained, and forms were completed before the initiation of any session for the research project. Participants were told that, whether they chose to partake or not to partake in the research, their regular treatment would continue unaffected. Standardization was assured by having each of the massage therapists use the same scripted dialogue when approaching potential subjects for the study. Visual analog scale (VAS) scores were obtained by the therapists before and after therapy.

Table A-1 ■ Demographic Data of Research Participants

Characteristic	Value
Participants (*n*)	65
Mean age (years)	45
Sex [% (women/men)]	87/13
Ethnicity (%)	
White	82
Native American	12
African American	2.3
Hispanic	1
Asian	1
Hospital unit (%)	
Medical	42
Surgical	31
Obstetrics	26

Participants were given the post-hospitalization survey at the end of their last session.

Three licensed massage therapists employed by the hospital provided the therapy sessions. The experience in massage therapy of the therapists (all female) ranged from 2 years to more than 20 years. Each had received additional training for working with hospitalized or medically frail patients, and all had worked in the acute care setting for 1 to 3 years.

Massage interventions consisted of 15-minute to 45-minute therapeutic massage sessions given at the bedside. Because of the disruptive nature of the hospital environment, the length of the sessions varied based on each participant's energy level and availability. Treatments included gentle Swedish effleurage or petrissage,

The Effects of Massage Therapy on Pain Management in the Acute Care Setting—cont'd

acupressure, craniosacral therapy, or cross-fiber myotherapy with light-pressure effleurage and pressure points being the most commonly used modalities. The treatment area on the body varied according to participant need or concern, taking into consideration any contraindications, including but not limited to areas of acute injury and surgical and intravenous sites. Head, neck, shoulders, back, and feet were the areas most commonly chosen, with participants in either supine or side-lying positions. Participants were given a choice of unscented or lightly scented oils, and relaxing music was offered.

The survey used in this research project (Patient Survey for Massage Therapy Research) was adapted from a survey used by Motsinger in her Capstone Project, titled Development of an Inpatient Massage Therapy Program in an Allopathic Hospital.[a] The survey asked about length of hospital stay, number of massages received, and whether massage therapy had improved, had had no effect, or had worsened the participant's overall pain levels, emotional well-being, ability to move, ability to participate in therapies, relaxation, ability to sleep, and recovery. Additionally, participants were asked if they felt that massage therapy had had an effect on their need for pain medication, how long the effects of the massage had lasted, and whether they planned to continue using massage therapy as part of their healing process. An open-ended inquiry at the end of the survey encouraged participants to comment freely about massage.

Quantitative and qualitative methods were used for analysis of this descriptive study. Demographic data, number of massage sessions, before-and-after pain levels using the VAS scale, survey data, and nursing comments were analyzed. Inferential statistical analysis was conducted using the paired t-test, with the significance level preset at $p < .05$.

Qualitative data drawn from nursing comments in a retrospective chart review and participant comments from the post-hospitalization survey were analyzed using the grounded theory method to code and label categories. "Grounded theory" can be described as a method of analysis that aims to develop middle-range theories from qualitative data. The founders of grounded theory, Glaser and Strauss, not only intended to conceptualize qualitative data, but also planned to demonstrate relationships between conceptual categories and to specify conditions within which theoretical relationships emerge (21) (pp. 311–312). We used the grounded theory method to group qualitative responses into several categories to guide the analysis. These categories reflected responses by the participants and nurses regarding reactions to the massage therapy session or sessions the participant received while hospitalized. The themes generated demonstrate an interrelationship between categories and an overall theoretical sensitivity that supports the overriding theme that "massage therapy promotes recovery." Finally, all data were triangulated to determine whether massage therapy improves patient perception of pain management while in hospital.

Results

Quantitative Data

From the initial sample of 65 participants, 53 completed the research project. Pain levels reported by the participants using the VAS ranged from 0–10. The mean score before massage was 5.18 [standard deviation (SD): 2.01]. The mean score after massage was 2.33 (SD: 2.10). A comparison of pain levels before and after massage shows the individual responses by massage session (Fig. A-1). The observed reduction in pain was statistically significant: paired samples t_{52} = 12.43, r = .67, d = 1.38, $p < .001$ (Table A-2).

Continued

The Effects of Massage Therapy on Pain Management in the Acute Care Setting—cont'd

Table A-2 ■ Analysis of Pain Level Before and After Massage Therapy

Variable	Value
Mean pain score (±SD)	
Before	5.18 (2.01)
After	2.33 (2.10)
Correlation	.67
Standard mean error	0.23
95% confidence limits	(1.88, 2.78)[a]
Significance (2-tailed)	<.001[a]
Cohen's d	1.38

[a] Statistically significant.
SD = standard deviation.

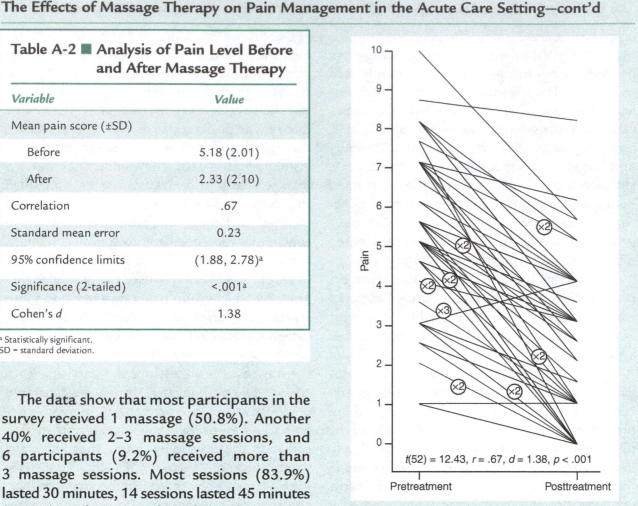

$t(52) = 12.43$, $r = .67$, $d = 1.38$, $p < .001$

Pretreatment   Posttreatment

Figure A-1 Pain level on a 1 – 10 visual analog scale before and after massage therapy in 65 inpatient research participants. Of the 65 charts reviewed, 53 charts contained complete data (before/after pain levels) and are shown here.

The data show that most participants in the survey received 1 massage (50.8%). Another 40% received 2–3 massage sessions, and 6 participants (9.2%) received more than 3 massage sessions. Most sessions (83.9%) lasted 30 minutes, 14 sessions lasted 45 minutes (14.9%), and 1 session lasted 15 minutes.

The effects of massage therapy were felt to last 1–4 hours by 34 participants (53.1%), and 4–8 hours, by 13 participants (20.3%). According to 9 participants (14.1%), the effects lasted 8–24 hours, and according to 7 (10.9%), more than 24 hours. One person felt no effect. The response to the question "Do you plan to continue using massage therapy in your healing process?" was yes in an impressive 67.2% of participants. Another 14.1% responded no, and 18.8% didn't know if they would continue with massage therapy after their hospitalization.

The survey reported participant perceptions concerning the effects of massage therapy on overall pain level, emotional well-being, ability to move, ability to participate in therapies,

relaxation after massage, ability to sleep, contribution to faster recovery, and less need for pain medication after massage. Participants were asked if there was improvement, no change, or a worsening in the foregoing factors because of the massage. In all areas surveyed, a majority of participants reported an improvement, although some participants stated that they could not remember. Notably, no participant indicated a negative effect from massage therapy. The most significant areas of reported effect were overall

The Effects of Massage Therapy on Pain Management in the Acute Care Setting—cont'd

pain level, emotional well-being, relaxation, and ability to sleep (Fig. A-2).

Findings from the current preliminary study parallel existing research showing that pain levels significantly improved with a massage intervention as an adjunct to conventional treatments (5,19). Other noteworthy observations included improved relaxation, emotional well-being, ability to sleep, and a reduction in the perception of use of pain medications.

Qualitative Data

Using the grounded theory method, "massage therapy promotes recovery" was the main theme identified. Within that theme, several subthemes emerged, including pain management (Table A-3), ability to sleep, relaxation, emotional well-being, and healing. Each category is represented with comments from nurses or participants or both. Of the 65 participants in the study, 45 (72.3%) returned surveys. At the end of the survey, an open-ended question encouraged participants to comment freely

Table A-3 ■ Qualitative Theme of Pain Management With Massage for Hospitalized Patients

Hospital inpatient	"After three days in the hospital I was suffering a migraine, nausea, and a lot of body pain. After the massage my headache was lessened and my body pain was greatly reduced."
Nurse	"Patient reports relaxation and pain relief after massage—slept for three hours"
Cancer patient in ICU	"I looked forward to the massages I received while in ICU—each helped to reduce the pain."

ICU = intensive care unit.

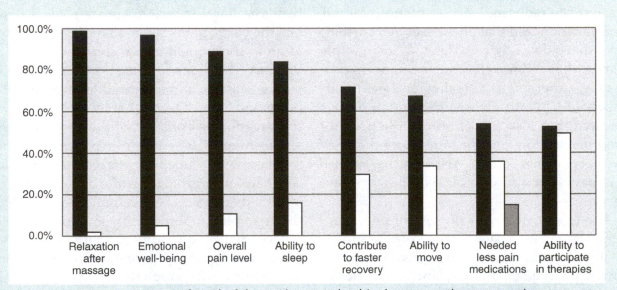

Figure A-2 Patient survey results. Black bars = improved; white bars = no change; gray bar = cannot remember.

Continued

The Effects of Massage Therapy on Pain Management in the Acute Care Setting—cont'd

about their experience of massage therapy. Qualitative responses were received from 33 participants.

In the medical charts of participants, 25 nursing comments relevant to the research project were found. All comments were categorized into themes and subthemes. Interrelating themes were also acknowledged.

Pain Management

Of the 33 qualitative responses from participants, 16 were related directly to pain management. Participants mentioned improved pain levels after surgery ($n = 9$), lessening of breast engorgement after a cesarean section ($n = 1$), decreased body and headache pain and intensity ($n = 4$), and decreased pain associated with cancer ($n = 2$). One cancer patient commented, "I looked forward to the massages I received while in ICU—each helped to reduce the pain." Another patient commented, "After three days in the hospital I was suffering a migraine, nausea, and a lot of body pain. After the massage my headache was lessened and my body pain was greatly reduced." While still hospitalized, one patient noted that "I've never had anything take this pain away completely." Still another noted that "I'm very much supportive of massage therapy as a healing and pain relief procedure." Not only was perception of pain lowered, but also perception of the need for pain medication. Significantly, more than half the participants (52.7%) felt that they needed less pain medication after receiving massage therapy.

The responsibility of nurses for pain management plays a significant role in quality health care. Managing pain is a team effort between physicians, nurses, and other health care providers. Of the 25 comments by nursing staff, 16 referred to decreased pain levels or decreased necessity for pain medications after

massage therapy. Nursing comments included "Patient states his neck pain lessened with massage," "Denies pain or needs . . . had massage therapy this am, in no apparent distress," and "Massage therapy ordered and given with good relief."

Sleep

Comments about ability to sleep were often associated with pain relief. One patient noted that "massage brought dramatic pain relief and ability to sleep and an overall sense of well-being in a stressful environment." Another commented that "I fell asleep almost immediately after [the massage therapist] left." Nursing observations confirmed what patients stated on the survey. Nursing comments included "Patient reports relaxation and pain relief after massage—slept for three hours" and "Patient stated the massage was a big help in decreasing his pain and allowed him to relax enough to get a good nap today."

Relaxation

Relaxation can play a significant role in a patient's healing and recovery process. More than half the participants surveyed mentioned relaxation in their qualitative responses ($n = 17$). Patients mentioned relaxation, relief from muscle tension, and increased feelings of well-being and calm. Overall nervous tension and the stressful environment of the hospital were also mentioned. Remarks from patients relating to relaxation included "[massage therapy] was very helpful, soothing, comforting, and relaxing," and "this was very helpful to me, in that this is so pleasurable during an unpleasurable experience." A quadriplegic patient who received massage therapy commented that "overall well-being (emotional, physical, spiritual, patience, decreased anxiety, and decreased pain and spasticity) was improved immeasurably by massage therapy and subsequent relaxation."

The Effects of Massage Therapy on Pain Management in the Acute Care Setting—cont'd

In 10 comments from the nursing staff, the benefits of relaxation for their patients were mentioned. Nursing notes reflecting the benefits included "Patient seemed calmer tonight," "Patient reports improved muscle relaxation post massage therapy," and "Massage made her relaxed, resting comfortably, no distress."

Emotional Well-Being

The interrelatedness of themes becomes apparent in how patient and nursing comments alike reflect the connection between emotional well-being and relaxation, pain relief, and ability to sleep. Participants mentioned emotional well-being 8 times in connection with decreased anxiety, state of mind, attitude improvement, and human contact. One patient commented "[massage therapy] was one of the few times I could look forward to human contact without the potential for pain (as opposed to shots, IV's . . .)." Another patient described her experience with massage therapy this way: "I was so relieved and grateful. I was no longer crying and felt much better. I was so grateful for the body and mind relief." One of the participants in the research project was in advanced stages of cancer. Although she died, her husband returned the survey, commenting that his "wife appreciated the pain relief, and that 'the massage brought a smile to her face,'" also noting his own appreciation of the therapy.

Although nursing comments focused mainly on pain management and relaxation, 2 nursing notes articulated improved emotional well-being. A nurse in the Women's and Infant Center noted that "patient has been teary about infant in special care nursery, had a massage, now coping a little better." Another nurse commented "Patient seemed calmer tonight, not agitated, or hostile."

Healing

References to healing and subthemes of healing including spirituality, recovery, and therapeutic benefits were found in responses from 10 participants. One participant noted that "I feel massage is very important to helping patients heal, in so many ways," and another commented that "[massage therapy] was a very healing experience emotionally and physically." Other participant comments included "Reduction of stress also was very helpful in recovery," "It was very therapeutic," and "It is such a healing process and definitely relaxing." No nursing comments on the theme of healing were found.

Discussion

The experience of hospitalization creates pain and anxiety for many people, regardless of their underlying medical condition. The goal of the present study was to explore how massage therapy would affect a patient's perception of pain in the acute care setting. Previous studies have established the benefits of massage therapy for patients suffering from particular illnesses—for example, cancer (19)—and cardiac surgery or procedures (3,6,17). Other studies have focused on patient experiences within particular hospital units including transplantation, neuroscience, and rehabilitation (4). By selecting research participants in units throughout the hospital, with a wide variety of diagnoses and reasons for hospitalization, our project provides a unique picture of how massage therapy may benefit any patient coping with the pain and stress associated with hospitalization, offering a strong argument that massage is an effective adjunct therapy for pain management.

The primary findings of this preliminary study show a strong correlation between reduction of pain levels after massage therapy and statistically significant differences in pain scores before

Continued

The Effects of Massage Therapy on Pain Management in the Acute Care Setting—cont'd

and after massage. The perception among participants of improved pain levels and less need for pain medication underscore the promise of massage therapy's positive effect on pain management protocols. In addition, a majority of patients felt that massage therapy contributed to increased relaxation, emotional well-being, ability to sleep, ability to move and to participate in other therapies, and faster recovery. For most patients, the effects of the session lasted 1–4 hours, with some participants experiencing benefits for more than 24 hours.

Reports of improved levels of relaxation after massage therapy were received from 98% of the research study participants. The fact that patients throughout the various hospital units, with a wide variety of pre-massage pain levels, experienced relaxation through massage therapy indicates the true potential for massage to support healing for hospitalized patients. This finding was reiterated in comments from patients and nurses alike. By accessing a patient's ability to relax, massage therapy addresses a variety of needs. Indeed, the RR may be the most profound mechanism through which massage therapy helps the hospitalized patient.

In addition to relaxation, massage therapy also counters another fundamental aspect of hospitalization, the sense of isolation experienced by many patients. In the present research study, participants reported an improvement in emotional well-being—an aspect of healing that may speak to the need for human touch. More and more hospitals are recognizing the importance of touch for the hospitalized patient (4,6). As the face of health care changes in the coming years, it is a hopeful sign that safe, skillful touch is being recognized as a mechanism of healing for patients in the acute care setting.

Participation in our research study was limited to adults whose medical circumstances allowed them to receive massage therapy and to complete the study paperwork. The study does not reflect the perceptions of patients whose energy or pain levels precluded them from participation. Patients whose level of pain did not allow for participation may have found less benefit from massage therapy, revealing the need for fully integrative services in which massage is merely one component of a comprehensive pain management protocol.

Another limitation of the present study is the lack of collection of physiological data, including heart rate, blood pressure, and oxygen levels. The absence of data on the physiological indicators of pain and the RR means that the study relied on participant perceptions without additional external measures to verify participant responses to massage therapy. Pain is an inherently subjective experience that includes physical and emotional elements. Within the hospital environment, health care workers rely on patient perceptions for pain management. The present study thus reflects current standards for assessing the effectiveness of various interventions to address pain in patients.

The current project, designed to gather preliminary data on the research hypothesis, did not use a control group. The selection of additional patients in units throughout the hospital, combined with randomization to groups, would have required substantial additional resources. However, future studies on massage therapy in an acute care setting may benefit from the addition of a control group. Such research may also help to identify specific types of massage therapy that are most effective in the acute care setting.

The Effects of Massage Therapy on Pain Management in the Acute Care Setting—cont'd

Conclusions

Evidence-based research continues to confirm the importance of human touch to balance the high technology of today's health care practices. The further integration of CIM therapies such as massage into the hospital offers the possibility to improve the experience for patients who face physical, psychological, and social challenges in an unfamiliar environment. A large and growing body of research, including the current project, justifies the use of massage therapy for pain management in the acute care setting. Massage therapy can provide pain relief and relaxation, can support a patient's emotional well-being and recovery, and can ultimately aid in the healing process for hospitalized patients.

REFERENCES

1. Pearson Education. American Academy of Pain Management accreditation helps pain organizations meet JCAHO standards. Pearson Education, Bridging the Gap website. http://test.pearsonassessments.com/bridginggap/fall2001-p1.htm. Published Fall 2001. Updated n.d. Accessed July 12, 2007.
2. Ezzo J. What can be learned from Cochrane systematic reviews of massage that can guide future research? *J Altern Complement Med* 2007; 13(2): 291–295.
3. McCaffrey R, Taylor N. Effective anxiety treatment prior to diagnostic cardiac catheterization. *Holist Nurs Pract* 2005; 19(2): 70–73.
4. Smith MC, Stallings MA, Mariner S, Burrall M. Benefits of massage therapy for hospitalized patients: a descriptive and qualitative evaluation. *Altern Ther Health Med* 1999; 5(4): 64–71.
5. Mitchinson AR, Kim HM, Rosenberg JM, Geisser M, Kirsh M, Cikrit D, et al. Acute postoperative pain management using massage as an adjuvant therapy: a randomized trial. *Arch Surg* 2007; 142(12): 1158–1167.
6. Cutshall SM, Fenske LL, Kelly RF, Phillips BR, Sundt TM, Bauer BA. Creation of a healing enhancement program at an academic medical center. *Complement Ther Clin Pract* 2007; 13(4): 217–223.
7. Egnew TR. The meaning of healing: transcending suffering. *Ann Family Med* 2005; 3(3): 255–262.
8. Field T, Diego M, Cullen C, Hernandez-Reif M, Sunshine W, Douglas S. Fibromyalgia pain and substance P decrease and sleep improves after massage therapy. *J Clin Rheumatol* 2002; 8(2): 72–76.
9. Hernandez-Reif M, Field T, Krasnegor J, Theakston H. Lower back pain is reduced and range of motion increased after massage therapy. *Int J Neurosci* 2001; 106(3–4): 131–145.
10. Melancon B, Miller LH. Massage therapy versus traditional therapy for low back pain relief: implications for holistic nursing practice. *Holist Nurs Pract* 2005; 19(3): 116-121.
11. Anderson PG, Cutshall SM. Massage therapy: a comfort intervention for cardiac surgery patients. *Clin Nurse Spec* 2007; 21(3): 161–165.
12. Cassileth B, Trevisan C, Gubili J. Complementary therapies for cancer pain. *Curr Pain Headache Rep* 2007; 11(4): 265–269.
13. Ferrell-Torry AT, Glick OJ. The use of therapeutic massage as a nursing intervention to modify anxiety and the perception of cancer pain. *Cancer Nurs* 1993; 16(2): 93–101.
14. Aourell M, Skoog M, Carleson J. Effects of Swedish massage on blood pressure. *Complement Ther Clin Pract* 2005; 11(4): 242–246.
15. Benson H. *The Relaxation Response*. New York, NY: William Morrow and Company; 1975: 99–110.
16. White JA. Touching with intent: therapeutic massage. *Holist Nurs Prac* 1988; 2(3): 63–67.
17. Richards KC. Effect of a back massage and relaxation intervention on sleep in critically ill patients. *Am J Crit Care* 1998; 7(4): 288–299.
18. Moyer CA. Affective massage therapy. *Int J Ther Massage Bodyw* 2009; 1(2): 4.
19. Smith MC, Kemp J, Hemphill L, Vojir CP. Outcomes of therapeutic massage for hospitalized cancer patients. *J Nurs Scholarsh* 2002; 34(3): 257–262.
20. Kania A, Porcino A, Vehoef MJ. Value of qualitative research in the study of massage therapy. *Int J Ther Massage Bodyw* 2008; 1(2): 6–10.
21. Charmaz K. Qualitative interviewing and grounded theory analysis. In: Holstein A, Gubrium JF, eds. *Inside Interviewing: New Lenses, New Concerns*. Thousand Oaks, CA: Sage Publications; 2003: 311–330.

ACKNOWLEDGMENTS

This research was conducted at Flagstaff Medical Center, Flagstaff, Arizona, from October 2006 to March 2007.

The authors thank Alisha Witcomb, LMT, for her contribution as one of the three massage therapists involved in this study and as an integral collaborator in the data collection process. The authors also express their gratitude to Lori Pearlmutter, PT, MPH. Lori was inspirational and supportive throughout the process, as a co-investigator and a mentor.

Continued

The Effects of Massage Therapy on Pain Management in the Acute Care Setting—cont'd

CONFLICT OF INTEREST NOTIFICATION

The authors declare that no conflicts of interest are associated with this research project or publication of findings.

[a] Motsinger S. Unpublished report for the Capstone Project for DPT. Flagstaff, AZ: Northern Arizona University; 2003.

Adams, R., White, B., and Beckett, C. The Effects of Massage Therapy on Pain Management in the Acute Care Setting. *International Journal of Therapeutic Massage & Bodywork: Research, Education, & Practice*, North America, 3, Mar. 2010. Available at:http://www.ijtmb.org/index.php/ijtmb/article/view/54/101. Date accessed: 26 Jul. 2013. Reprinted with permission.

Appendix B

Example of Qualitative Study

The intent of providing you with Chapter 1 from a qualitative study is for you to glean insight from the structure and description of the entire inquiry.

Chapter 1 of Qualitative Study

Introduction

The shape of one's knowing becomes the shape of one's doing, being and becoming.

—*Author Unknown*

This chapter provides an overview of a narrative inquiry that sought to glean a more informed and in-depth understanding from stories of four working mothers of school-age children and how they pursued and engaged in self-nurturance within a rural, religiously conservative, and historically patriarchal-driven context. The chapter includes the background of the study, need for the study, a purpose statement, guiding research questions, an overview of the theoretical framework undergirding the study, an overview of the research methodology, an identification of the study's significance, and a delineation of the assumptions and limitations associated with the study.

Background of the Study

My interest in facilitating a narrative inquiry with mothers of school-age children living within a rural, religiously conservative, historically patriarchal-driven environment and their subsequent journey to situate self-nurturance within their daily living stems from my experience as a woman, a mother, and an occupational therapist interested in women's wellness education within rural communities. Clandinin and Connelly (2000) note, "Narrative inquiries are always strongly autobiographical. Our research interests come out of our own narratives of experience and shape our narrative inquiry plotlines" (p. 121). As a woman living within this contextual environment I have consistently received nonconstructive messages about how much time and effort I should put forth nurturing self. The majority of the messages I have

Continued

Chapter 1 of Qualitative Study—cont'd

received over the years questioned whether I should, as a wife and mother, take time away from my household, husband, and children to facilitate and maintain my own personal health and well-being. One of my closest and dearest friends, who happens to be a woman, has posed this thought to me numerous times throughout the years, "Is it really appropriate for you to take time away from your children and husband to have a facial or sign up for a painting class—what if the boys need you and you aren't available because you are doing something for yourself—what if all mothers spent time taking care of themselves—who is going to cook, clean, and help the children with their home-work?" A religiously conservative man within the community, who has always been slightly irritated with my independent nature, once told me "Your place is in the home—you don't need time for yourself—your children and husband *always* come first!" These and similar messages from my sociocultural environment have facilitated my confused narrative about the worthiness of my identity as it relates to a mother who nurtures self. As an occupational therapist I have struggled for nearly a decade to conceptualize and move forward with an educational program focused on facilitating mothers' engagement in nurturing self within this sociocultural environment.

At this juncture, it is important to explain what self-nurturance means to this inquiry, which is focused on in-depth narratives. For the purpose of this study, self-nurturance refers to the invaluable and precious time required to refuel a mother's mind, body, and spirit—those moments of time that mothers capture to take walks, engage in gourmet cooking classes, write in journals, or join a book club. Additionally, as a function of this study, *self-nurturance* is defined as a meaningful occupation that supports and enhances mothers' overall health and well-being. In occupational therapy, *meaningful occupation* is defined as those experiences that promote, enhance, or maintain an individual's state of well-being (Christiansen, 1999). It has been further defined by Pierce (2001) as being personally constructed within perceived temporal, spatial, and sociocultural conditions. Wilcock (1998) describes engagement in meaningful occupation as, "[T]he synthesis of doing, being and becoming" (p. 249). Consequently, in the field of adult education, Parker Palmer's (2000) perspective of coming to know self enough to allow one's life to speak of its needs is closely related to Wilcock's interpretations of doing, being, and becoming (Hasselkus, 2002).

During the past decade as a mother, woman, and an occupational therapist, I have heard other mothers wanting to engage in self-nurturance; however, because of both time constraints and sociocultural influences that told them their needs are less important than husband and children, they had left the meaningful occupation of self-nurturance unexplored, untouched, and unattained. Nurturing self and taking care of one's emotional, physical, intellectual, and spiritual needs is important to women's overall development; thus, the conceptualization of this study was that self-nurturance and women's development of self must be dealt with simultaneously. It would be impossible to address nurturing self without the parallel notion of women's formation of self. Therefore, the focus of this inquiry was to deconstruct mothers' lived stories around nurturing self within their contextual environment and how their identities shifted over time as they attempted to or successfully engaged in self-nurturance.

As will be discussed later, key assumptions of the study were grounded in the feminist poststructuralist notions of constantly shifting identity and non-unitary self. The notion of

Chapter 1 of Qualitative Study—cont'd

non-unitary self is defined by Clark (1999) as a self that is consistently challenged by society and split between an experience and the interpretation of the experience. What one thinks and feels about one's self is not totally in that individual's control; rather, it is largely shaped by ideas and experiences within many different contexts in light of gender, race, class, religion, geographical location, and so on. The conjecture is that as an individual's knowing and understanding of how these factors influence his or her constantly shifting identity, a conscious raising is developed; hence, individuals have an enhanced understanding and management over their doing, being, and becoming.

This narrative analysis served as a means of focusing on the mothers' ownership and investment in self-nurturance as a positive determinant of their health and well-being. I was hopeful that by the conclusion of this study, the mothers had a deeper understanding of their constantly shifting identities and the impact discourse and power had within their environment on their learning, knowledge, and participation in self-nurturance. In addition, I was certain this narrative study would assist me in understanding how to more efficiently and effectively organize wellness education for mothers within this specific cultural context.

Need for the Study: Situating the Problem

In light of insights from my personal life and professional practice, it was my impression that there was a preponderance of women, more specifically mothers with school-age children living within this environment, who did not consider or engage in self-nurturance primarily for three reasons. First, they had a limited awareness of its value in relationship to their overall health and well-being. Second, they found the contextual and sociocultural barriers of engagement too great to overcome. Third,

these women did not feel they have the right to engage in self-nurturance. Throughout my years of living within this sociocultural context, I had noted nurturance of self was not generally highly regarded; therefore, it was rarely thought of or even talked about as a facilitator of women's health and well-being.

Again, I must note that I had heard mothers tell stories over and over again about not engaging in self-nurturance which revealed the basic fact of these women having limited amounts of time and energy; however, this fact appeared to be compounded by an overwhelming feeling of guilt and responsibility to make those around them content and comfortable above and before nurturing self. These mothers shared an unspoken truth with me—they knew they were neglecting and sacrificing self-nurturance; however, they had been unable to resolve key barriers in their path toward this important component of mothers' personal health and well-being.

As a researcher, I wanted to further explore mothers' stories of negotiating self-nurturance, in relation to their culturally defined roles and responsibilities as mothers with school-age children. By engaging in this narrative inquiry, it was hoped that both the researcher and participants would construct an expanded understanding of women's identity and, more importantly, their role in nurturing self. My agenda was to find four mothers willing to participate in the study and then glean insight from their stories. I then planned to narrate their stories in an effort to afford them the opportunity to reflect upon their constantly shifting identities within their cultural surroundings and determine how this impacts their balance of self-nurturance, health, and well-being. As Tisdell states (2001):

> It is the unpacking of the story around issues of positionality, and the critical reflection, both on the story and on the story's unpacking that

Continued

Chapter 1 of Qualitative Study—cont'd

helps us understand our constantly shifting identity around systems of power, privilege and oppression that inform our lives. It raises our consciousness, it changes our behavior, it does indeed, move us to action. (p. 283)

By affording these mothers the opportunity to share their stories around the cultural paradigms of motherhood, rural living, conservative religious beliefs and value systems, and patriarchy, I suspected that they would better understand the state of their constantly shifting identities and how this negatively or positively impacted their ability to nurture self.

Within the field of women's studies, Carol Ryff (1985) has argued that research needs to focus on combinations of identity, experience, and development as they specifically address lived experience. While conceptualizing the study, I felt that many mothers were unable to validate and put worth on the learning they incurred while engaging in meaningful occupations that were focused on self. As an occupational therapist, I conceived this lack of importance and negotiation of self to other's needs on a consistent basis was having a negative impact on mother's health and well-being.

Studies have been completed about women's inability to care for self; however, these studies are fueled by issues such as eating disorders, posttraumatic stress disorder, and older women's life experiences of well-being (Morris, 2000; Rashotte, 1997; Sherwood, 2000). Recently, Nemcek (2003) reviewed 19 research studies conducted within the past 8 years specifically related to self-nurturance. The research topics focused on eating disorder studies, ways of living (i.e., surviving grief and living with HIV or AIDS), and well adults (i.e., employees and college students). The research methodology for these studies included phenomenology, grounded theory, concept analysis, descriptive, and quasi-experimental inquiries.

There is a substantial amount of literature that consistently heralds women as being nurturers of others; however, none of the literature addresses why mothers consistently do not find the time, the privilege, or learning experiences aimed at nurturing self (Bateson, 1990; Chodorow, 1978; Duffy, 1991; Esdalie & Olsen, 2004; Gilligan, 1987; Ruddick, 1989). In addition, literature from the field of psychology implies that women have been socially constructed to take care of others, which consequently informs the basis of their identity of self (Duffy, 1992; Gilligan, 1987; Kegan, 1994; Miller, 1986, 1990; Rogers, 1961). Throughout my review of the literature on women's construction of self and nurturance of self, it became increasingly evident that the voices and experiences of mothers nurturing self, no matter what sociocultural environment they are living in, are absent.

Several research and conceptual pieces focused on women consistently advocate for inquiries that will offer a greater understanding of women's learning and knowing (Bateson, 1996; Collins, 1990; Hayes & Flannery, 2000; Hooks, 1994). From a narrative inquiry perspective Clandinin and Connelly (2000) state, "We need to continually ask questions about the way narrative inquiry illuminates the social and theoretical contexts in which we position our inquiries" (p. 124). By engaging in narrative analysis inquiry guided by the theoretical perspectives of feminist poststructuralism and non-unitary self, whereby women's voices and stories were heard firsthand, I hoped to contribute to the acknowledgement that this type of inquiry is important enough to put time, faith, and effort into as a woman, mother, and researcher. I feel this contribution has constructed new knowledge that will inform the way women teach, learn, and engage in self-nurturance.

Chapter 1 of Qualitative Study—cont'd

Purpose of the Study

The purpose of this narrative analysis study was to glean insight from and illuminate personal stories of four working mothers of school-age children living in a defined cultural context and to explore how the cultural realities impacted their engagement in self-nurturance. The study took place in a rural northeastern community, which was defined by the following characteristics: Ninety-five percent White or Caucasian, with 51% of the population being female. Seventy-two percent of the households are two parent households, with 64% of these households having both parents in the labor force. Seventy-six percent of the business industry within the community is owned and operated by men. Of the 20 religious faiths in the community, the largest percentage is identified as conservative Christian (i.e., Bible Brethren, Pentecostal, and Mennonite).

The narrative inquiry was completed in an effort to gain a greater understanding of the complexities and multiplicities that influence four mothers' lived experiences of self-nurturance. With the previously described context, as DuPlessis (1985) states, "Women need to make the conflicts that emerge from their marginalized status and their rebellions against marginalization *central* to their stories" (p. 67). It was the purpose of this narrative inquiry to provide an opportunity where four mothers' gendered perspectives and subjectivities, within their specific sociocultural context, are created into narratives as they related to self-nurturance (Bloom, 1998).

Guiding Research Questions

The goal of this narrative analysis inquiry was to concentrate on the sociocultural contextual issues that influenced engagement in self-nurturance for the mothers who participated in this study. Specific questions that I was concerned with were as follows:

1. How do these women explain their identity as a mother living within a rural, religiously conservative, and historically patriarchal-driven environment?
2. What positive or negative messages have these mothers received within their contextual environment about engaging in self-nurturance?
3. How have these mothers renegotiated aspects of their identity over time in order to nurture self within their cultural environment?
4. What aspects of self-nurturance are these women still struggling with at this point in time, secondary to perspectives and notions of the cultural environment?
5. How has past and present engagement of self-nurturance been simple or complex in relation to gender within this cultural environment?
6. How has past and present engagement of self-nurturance been simple or complex in light of living in a rural environment of conservative religious beliefs or values and patriarchal-driven systems?

Overview of Theoretical Framework

After considering many theoretical perspectives and insights gleaned from everyday experience, the theoretical perspective of feminist poststructuralism and the notion of non-unitary self were most appropriate as the guiding framework for this study. Feminist poststructuralism considers the positionality of women within society and offers a lens to address the intersections of gender, rural living, and conservative religious beliefs of the women who will be engaged in this narrative inquiry. Weedon (1997) broadly describes the relationships among the different aspects of positionality as discourse,

Continued

Chapter 1 of Qualitative Study—cont'd

knowledge, and power, with positionality being the intersections of social structures such as race, class, sexual orientation, geographical location, and so on (Tisdell, 2000). Furthermore, St. Peirre and Pillow (1998) state, "the representation of positionality is always in crisis, knowledge is constitutive of power, and agency is the constitutive effect, and not the originator, of situated practices and histories" (p. 5). The mothers engaged in this study were and still are deeply embedded and situated within a sociocultural context that for the most part does not understand or promote the discourse and active engagement of mothers nurturing self.

For this reason, the premises of non-unitary self were an integral part of the study. Actually, it is difficult to understand the notions of feminist poststructuralism without considering the notions of non-unitary self. Non-unitary self is defined by Robinson (1999) as, "the active and continual process of production of self within historical, social, and cultural boundaries . . . non-unitary subjectivity is an ongoing process of production and transformation [and] . . . a *doing* rather than *being*" (p. 11). Non-unitary subjectivity is a compatible venue for narrative inquiry because the participant usually feels more open to exploring multiple layers of self. The experience most often opens up the self-reflective nature of the participant (Bloom, 1998). Furthermore, it is extremely constructive to combine social appraisal with the theoretical perspectives of non-unitary self. This approach encourages the clarification of the cultural norms, power issues, and dominant ideologies that individuals must navigate and negotiate throughout their daily lives (Bloom, 2002). In this light, the notion of non-unitary self just made sense from my perspective as a woman, mother, and researcher.

By utilizing feminist poststructuralism and the notion of non-unitary self as the theoretical lens guiding these mothers' narratives related to self-nurturance, it was anticipated that cultural norms would be challenged and their participation in nurturing self would be facilitated by the insights gained in relation to the deconstruction and construction of their constantly shifting identity among the intersections of gender, rural living, conservative religious beliefs or value systems, and patriarchy.

Significance of the Study

Specifically, this narrative inquiry sought to tell the stories of four mothers who kindly gave of their time, among already overwhelming schedules, during a 5-month period as a means to open up dialogue in relation to their personal health and well-being. To this end, the four mothers who participated in this study presented narrative accounts of nurturing self around the cultural realities of motherhood, rural living, conservative religious beliefs and values, and patriarchy.

This study is significant to rural community health and well-being research in that it considered women's learning outside of academic structures utilizing deconstructed narratives. Stories from women about their lives and learning continue to be voices that need to be considered within the field of adult education (Hayes & Flannery, 2000). Consequently, at the recent Mid-Atlantic Women's Studies Associations Annual Conference, Mary Catherine Bateson (2004) noted the need for adult educators to actively pursue inquiries focusing on women's lived experiences and stories in rural communities.

Furthermore, there continues to be a need for the employment of feminist methodologies focusing on the diverse frameworks of women's learning within the field of adult education (Bloom, 1998; Brooks, 2000; Clark, 2001). The significance of this study utilizing the

Chapter 1 of Qualitative Study—cont'd

feminist poststructuralist philosophy was that it facilitated a collective group of women to question the circumstances of various oppressive forces alongside their routines of health and well-being. This philosophical standpoint appeared to give these mothers more of an opportunity to question what had been facilitating or squelching their collective health and well-being. A narrative study of mother's nurturance of self guided by feminist poststructuralist philosophy afforded the opportunity to dive deep into the societal norms and thoughts about how the four mothers did or did not nurture self on a daily basis. It moved them to question, challenge, and critique society's minimalist notion of women's health and well-being (World Health Organization, 2002).

Lastly, this study is significant for occupational therapy theory and practice. Yerxa (1998) purports that occupational therapists must develop a better understanding of how to assist individuals in learning how to promote their own status of health and well-being. She states, "Occupational therapists need to learn much, much more about how human beings develop adaptive skills, rules, and habits that enable competence . . . such knowledge of 'coaching' could benefit all persons who need to develop skills in order to survive, contribute, and achieve satisfaction in their daily life occupations . . . " (p. 418). In addition, it is gleaned from a wide range of literature on women's learning that women who have a greater understanding of their own learning and knowing can more effectively and efficiently promote the positive aspects of self (Belenky et al., 1986; Goldberger et al., 1996; Hayes & Flannery, 2000; Hooks, 1994). The outcome of this study provides occupational therapists with a greater understanding of how mothers, who were up against socioculturally prescribed issues of power and discourse, successfully engaged in the meaningful occupation of nurturing self.

Overview of Research Design and Methodology

Narrative analysis or narratology was utilized as the methodology for this inquiry in an attempt to understand the mothers' process of nurturing self and how this plays out in their everyday lives. The narratives focused around the cultural realities of motherhood, rural community living, religious values or belief systems, and patriarchy, and it was guided by feminist poststructualism and the notion of non-unitary self. As Bloom (1998) states, "Personal narratives provide primary data through which we can explore ways that different dominant ideologies and power relations are maintained and reproduced, or subverted in the discourses of the respondent's narratives" (p. 145).

Reissman (1993) describes narrative analysis as the investigation of a story, in order to discern how individuals telling the story make sense of their actions and the surrounding contexts of the story. Mishler (1995) feels there are many methods of approaching, defining, and studying narrative analysis. He feels the researcher should be clear in the design and methodological premises under which they will conduct their study. Denzin (1989) provides insight to the notion of narratives in the following statement:

> A narrative is a *story* that tells a sequence of events that are significant for the narrator and his or her audience. A narrative as a story has a plot, a beginning, a middle and an end. It has an internal logic that makes sense to the narrator. A narrative relates events in a temporal, causal sequence. Every narrative describes a sequence of events that have happened. (p. 37)

Continued

Chapter 1 of Qualitative Study—cont'd

As noted earlier, this narrative analysis inquiry was informed by feminist poststructuralism. Bloom (1998) contends there are three core objectives that theoretically structure a feminist poststructuralist approach to narrative research: (a) the study focuses on individual life stories of women as the primary source of data; (b) narratives of *self* as a location from which the researcher can generate social critique and advocacy is necessary; and (c) deconstruction of self as a humanist conception, allowing for non-unitary conceptions of self by women, is a primary goal for narrative inquiry. The challenge for me, as stated by Polkinghorne (1995), was to, "Construct a display of the complex, interwoven character of human experience as it unfolds through time" (p. 18). As a researcher, I planned to focus on Bloom's charge that poststructuralist feminist researchers engaged in narrative analysis inquiries must, "Embrace the idea that an understanding of non-unitary subjectivity in women's lives is critical" (p. 3). The concept of non-unitary self was critical to this study because it was utilized as the grounding by which these mothers explore the multifaceted, multilayered, complexity and fragmentation of self within this specific sociocultural context and how this notion of self impacts their past, present, and future nurturance of self.

Bloom (1998) further suggests that any narrative that utilizes the notion of non-unitary self as a theoretical lens is a solid grounding for studies that wish to get to the heart of women's stories. Narratives are indispensable resources for occupational therapists because they are individual interpretations and perspectives of their engagement in meaningful occupation (Wicks & Whiteford, 2003). To this end, it was the goal of this narrative study to gain a deeper understanding of how working mothers with school-age children living in a rural, religiously conservative, and historically patriarchal-driven environment nurture self, while at the same time deconstructing the foundations on which their daily living is constructed and experienced (Bloom, 1998). Within this inquiry, four mothers elaborated and offered extensive accounts of nurturing self as related to the realities of their sociocultural context. It involved my careful interpretation as I completed an in-depth analysis of and reflected upon the experiences that these women recalled in relation to their personal stories of health and well-being (Grbich, 1999; Rice & Ezzy, 1999).

The data collection consisted of two semistructured interviews, participant journaling, a creative synthesis project, and a dinner gathering after all other data collection. The first interview utilized a semistructured interview guide and the second interview was led by questions gleaned by the reading of the first interview and journal. Both interviews were audiotaped and transcribed. The women kept a self-nurturance journal for 3 months focusing on the cultural components of motherhood, conservative religious beliefs and values, patriarchal-driven implicit and explicit dynamics, and rural community living. In addition to completing two interviews and journals, each woman completed a creative synthesis project focusing around the following themes: (a) How does it feel when you are not engaged in self-nurturance? (b) What are the obstacles to self-nurturance? and (c) How do you feel when you are engaged in self-nurturance? The creative synthesis projects were completed after the second interview and were to be brought to the dinner gathering where the women met one another. Following the completion of their creative synthesis projects, three of the four women attended the dinner gathering to discuss their overall participation in the project and to share their creative synthesis projects

Chapter 1 of Qualitative Study—cont'd

with one another. The interview transcripts, journal entries, creative synthesis projects, and the dinner gathering provided the data for which the findings of this study were based and are explained in more detail in Chapter 3.

Consequently, feminist poststructuralism demands that researchers be more responsive and attentive to women's everyday life contexts (Bloom, 1998). I discerned it was my responsibility as a researcher to listen to the lives of women in relation to their needs and strengths of nurturing self as a unique dovetailing into their personal health and well-being. Throughout the study I felt comfort in Bloom's (2002) sentiment, "For feminist researchers, the need to know is based on a need to understand the forces that shape women's lives and a need to discover ways for women to transform and have authority over their own lives" (p. 147). The research environment provided the lens of feminist poststructuralism to initiate and enlighten these four mothers' understanding of the oppressive and sometimes overpowering sociocultural realities of their lives. As Hooks (1989) notes, women need to learn to resist sexism in the home—"That special place in which there should be care for others . . . the need for transformation of the self, of relationships, so that [women] might be better able to act in a revolutionary manner, challenging and resisting domination, transforming the world outside the self" (p. 22). The central objective of this narrative inquiry was to offer these mothers an opportunity to deepen their understanding of their self-nurturance routines within their sociocultural environment.

Assumptions

The following were the major assumptions that I held as I entered into this inquiry from a feminist poststructuralist lens:

1. For research to be valid and useful in the everyday lives of individuals, those individuals must actively participate and be actively represented in all aspects of the research process.
2. The feminist poststructuralist perspective of constantly shifting identity (non-unitary self) is an empowering notion for women living in the 21st century.
3. The process of motherhood has not been researched adequately in terms of the overall positive and negative effects it has on the health and well-being of women.
4. The feminist poststructuralist theory is a powerful and meaningful lens to view the deconstruction of power and discourse within women's lives.
5. Individual understanding of, and the engagement in, meaningful occupation is a positive aspect of personal health and well-being.
6. The primary researcher is always present in the inquiry and the final product.
7. Attending to my feminist poststructuralist sense of being, I am entering into this research project thinking and feeling that the participants will want to speak for themselves in the data collection and data analysis section of this dissertation.
8. The unique relationship that exists between researcher and coresearchers in a narrative inquiry present a unique set of ethical considerations that reflect the unique relationship between researcher and coresearchers.
9. An inquiry should challenge beliefs of *truth* that have held some women in bondage for generations–knowledge production outside of the box is empowering and emancipating.

Limitations

The following are the major limitations that I felt were relevant as I entered into this inquiry:

1. I was a novice researcher; therefore, this was my first attempt at conducting a narrative analysis inquiry.

Continued

Chapter 1 of Qualitative Study—cont'd

2. This study was conducted within a small geographical area with the characteristics of being religiously conservative, patriarchal-driven, and in a rural defined area of the United States. It may or may not be pertinent or useful to other mothers of school-age children living in different contextual environments.

3. A potential limitation was the loss of data outside of the narrative structure; however, I made every attempt to conduct a global analysis of the entire transcript, as well as specifically focusing on intact stories.

Summary

To date, insights from feminist perspectives have not been addressed adequately within the field of occupational therapy and occupational science. This may be why the occupational therapy profession continues to struggle with finding its place in providing preventative and holistic education for women; more specifically, mothers of school-age children. Most importantly, the outcome of this research is for the women involved in the study and for those lives that are touched by the extensions of this research. I hold the overwhelming belief that a large majority of working mothers of school-age children living in rural environments are in eminent need of a starting point of conversation for learning more about their constantly shifting identity and how this relates to their constructive engagement in self-nurturance as a facilitator of their everyday health and well-being.

This narrative analysis inquiry situated from a feminist poststructuralist lens will assist healthcare practitioners in understanding more about research outside of formal academic and work structures. Specifically, it will assist them in understanding the unique wellness education needs of the mothers in rural communities. In addition, on a broader scale, I am hopeful that this inquiry will serve as a facilitator for healthcare practitioners to consider how they may incorporate concepts of women's learning and knowing into their daily practice.

Definition of Terms

In order for the reader to understand, with more clarity, I have defined the following terms that will be frequently utilized throughout this dissertation.

Constantly shifting identity—based on the ongoing development of women's understanding of their positionality (see definition below), which encumbers their historical, political, and cultural lives.

Feminist poststructuralism—notions of deconstruction and reconstruction of power, discourse, and knowledge as related to the everyday lives of women.

Health and well-being—includes elements of choice, meaning, balance, satisfaction, opportunity, and self-actualization (Wilcock, 1998).

Meaningful occupation—meaningful work, play, or daily living tasks in the stream of time and in the contexts of one's physical and social world (Kielhofner, 2002). Wilcock (1998) describes engagement in meaningful occupation as, "the synthesis of doing, being and becoming" (p. 249).

Non-unitary self—active and continual process of production of self within historical, social, and cultural boundaries . . . non-unitary subjectivity is an ongoing process of production and transformation [and] . . . a *doing* rather than *being*" (Robinson, 1999, p. 11).

Occupation—activities, tasks, and roles for the purpose of productive pursuit, maintaining oneself in the environment, and for purposes of relaxation, entertainment, creativity, and

Chapter 1 of Qualitative Study—cont'd

celebration; activities in which individuals are engaged to support their roles and needs (Christiansen & Baum, 1997, p. 60). [A]ctivities . . . of everyday life, named, organized, and given value and meaning by individuals and a culture. Occupation is everything people do to occupy themselves, including looking after themselves (self-care) . . . enjoying life (leisure) . . . and contributing to the social and economic fabric of their communities (productivity) (Law, Polatajko, Baptiste, & Townsend, 1997, p. 32).

Positionality—An understanding of "particular structures" such as racism, sexism, or eurocentrism. A form of theorizing with first knowing where you are positioned. Locating the self in relation to others within social structures (Maher & Thompson Tetreault, 1994, p. 202).

Self-nurturance—the acts of engaging in meaningful occupations which promote, enhance, or maintain one's state of health and well-being (Nemeck, 2003).

Synopsis of Research Inquiry

The following is a *picture in preview* of the remaining chapters of the qualitative research inquiry. Chapter 2 includes a review of the literature, both research and conceptual, deemed relevant to this study. Chapter 3 of the study provides a detailed explanation of, and the rationale for, the methodology utilized to conduct the inquiry. Chapters 4 to 7 is the presentation of *narratives in motion* for each mother who participated in the study. Chapter 8 will present the *intersecting narratives in motion,* which is collective theme interpretation of the *narratives in motion.* Chapter 9 offers an in-depth analysis of the findings, which represents the insights gleaned from this narrative inquiry and recommendations for future research.

Appendix C

Example of Evidence-Based Practice Project

An example of the first chapter from an evidence-based practice project is provided for you to gain insight into the purpose as well as the process of engaging in evidence-based practice.

Introduction

This chapter describes the geographical location and the practice setting in which the evidence-based practice project was conducted. It provides background information related to managing problematic negative behaviors in patients with dementia within the skilled nursing facility and the rationale for considering use of a multisensory environment as a viable solution. Potential opportunities and threats to implementation of the project as well as its impact on the field of occupational therapy are also discussed.

Description of Evidence-Based Practice Setting

Woody Pines, located in a rural community in southwestern Pennsylvania, is a geriatric care center that includes a 109-bed skilled nursing facility, a 70-bed assisted living facility, and an on-site adult day care. The rustic log home, built in the early 1900s, originally served as a private family home, but was purchased in 1988 by a management services company and renovated to function as it does today. The facility offers pharmacy, medical supply, hospice care, and rehabilitation services primarily to adults over the age of 65 years.

A brief statistical description of the population and geographical location serves to set the scene for this intervention. The rural community, nestled in the foothills of the Laurel Highlands in southwestern Pennsylvania, boasts a population of just over 11,000, with approximately 17% of the population over the age of 65 according to the 2000 U.S. Census. The borough itself has a population of 4,728, with the remainder of the population residing in primarily single-family dwellings within its more rural township. The U.S. Census Bureau projects a significant increase in the population of those 65 and older from the year 2000 to 2030. Statistical projections for the state of Pennsylvania suggest an increase from 4% to 50.6% in the elderly population during this period (U.S. Census Bureau, 2007).

Background Supporting the Evidence-Based Practice Intervention

Dementia is the significant loss of intellectual abilities, such as memory capacity, which is severe enough to interfere with social or occupational functioning (MedicineNet). The Alzheimer's Association (2007) reports Alzheimer's disease is the primary form of dementia, affecting over 5 million Americans. It is the seventh-leading cause of death and limits cognitive and behavioral abilities, thereby affecting one's ability to engage in meaningful work, self-care, leisure, and social activities. In the skilled nursing facility, these residents often exhibit inappropriate behaviors including "severe mood swings, verbal or physical aggression, combativeness, repetition of words and wandering" (Alzheimer's Association, 2007). Staff often become frustrated and respond by raising their voices, trying to reason with the residents, requesting medication changes from the doctor, and physically restraining the residents; however, many of these responses only stand to exacerbate the symptoms of dementia.

The complex interaction of the senses of audition, vision, taste, smell, movement, touch, and body position is necessary for an individual to interpret information in his or her environment and make appropriate behavioral responses to the stimuli (Kremer, Hildeman, Lape, & Miller, 1998). The integration of all of these sensations promotes adaptive behaviors (Fisher, Murry, & Bundy, 1991). In addition, the importance of sensory function is highlighted in the Occupational Therapy Practice Framework under the client factors area. Vision, hearing, vestibular function, taste, smell, proprioception, touch, pain, temperature, and pressure are all areas to consider when viewing the dementia resident holistically (AOTA, 2008). In the skilled nursing facility, where the regulations of Medicare and third-party payers often reign, little attention is given to this vital area. Review of a typical occupational therapy evaluation includes a short section on vision, hearing, and touch sensation, but does a poor job of investigating other areas of sensory processing, despite the fact that it can significantly impact moods, behaviors, and the ability to participate in meaningful occupations.

The intent of this evidence-based occupational therapy program is to explore current literature on the use of *Snoezelen* or multisensory environments to manage negative behaviors in clients with dementia who reside within a skilled nursing facility. The project requires creation of a multisensory environment within the skilled nursing facility, identification of residents exhibiting negative behaviors

related to dementia, and implementation of sensory-based treatments in an attempt to curtail unwanted behaviors and increase engagement in meaningful occupations.

Rationale for Evidence-Based Practice Intervention

Caregivers, staff, and families of patients with dementia often find the behavioral changes that accompany the disease most challenging to manage. Damage to the brain cells as a result of disease progression can cause agitation, aggression, anxiety, and sleep disorders. Other explanations for the onset of these behaviors include medication side effects, other medical conditions or diagnoses, and environmental factors. Environmental factors can loom high on the list of causes for nursing home residents because of the inability to manage the transition to a new living situation, changes in routine, absence of familiar surroundings and individuals, and perceived fears (Alzheimer's Association, 2005).

Yet another plausible explanation for negative behaviors is occupational deprivation, which is a lack of involvement in required or meaningful occupations, because of factors that are uncontrollable by the individual (Whiteford, 2000). This concept can be seen in the typical nursing home resident, but two other occupational terms are also discussed in the literature that accurately describe the occupational dilemmas of residents with dementia. The first is *occupational dysfunction*, which is explained as a consequence of unresolved deprivation related to a lack of adequate occupational capacities (Whiteford, 2000). The second is *occupational alienation*, which describes situations where occupations may be available, but they may not be meaningful. Townsend and Wilcock (2004) note that this concept is associated with "prolonged experiences of disconnectedness, isolation, emptiness, lack of a sense of identity, a limited or confined expression of spirit, or a sense of meaninglessness" (p. 80).

A visit to a typical skilled nursing facility could allow one to view the following:

Several residents are seated in various wheelchairs and recliner chairs around the nurses' station. One balding gentleman smiles gently at passersby and repeatedly asks, "Where can I get the bus to Chicago?" Another emaciated woman with needle-straight gray hair beckons with one outstretched finger, "Come here" over and over to anyone that glances in her direction. A small-featured woman clutches a baby doll and cries uncontrollably, so much so that the words she utters are not discernible. Another African-American man stands repeatedly from his wheelchair and the alarm sounds its familiar tune, while the nurses nearby repeat, "Sit down; Sit down."

Some residents are found in the dining room participating in bingo or beauty spot, whereas others seldom leave the confines of their rooms. Some residents are able to bathe and dress themselves, whereas others have nurse aides who complete the chore because of sheer convenience or increased speed. A lack of appropriate socialization skills seems to prevail because of worsening symptoms of dementia and increased frustrations by family members and staff. You can see it in the furrowed brow of a tired spouse unable to make the connection with a loved one, or in the hurried pace of a nurse's aide who apparently has too much to do in too little time. Televisions blare in various rooms and lounges, but no one really appears to be watching. Many residents are put to bed when the staff feels that it is time. Many are not given the choice of clothing or when they will get up or get washed. They are told what to eat and when to eat. The facility has an assortment of activities scheduled daily, but at times the schedule seems to lack variation. Some activities are appropriate for either sex, but many are geared more toward the women, who make up the majority of the residents residing there.

The philosophy is quality of care, but closer examination reveals a facility full of elderly people, most with some form of dementia, who are no longer able to make decisions about their care or to participate in meaningful occupations. These frustrations become apparent in the cries, aggressive behaviors, wanderings, and lethargy of the residents.

In a study by Christianson, he comments on the "positive relationship between time spent engaging in meaningful occupation and perceived wellbeing" (Whiteford, 2000, p. 203). For the resident with dementia in a skilled nursing facility, time is irrelevant. Often the days run into the nights. There are no discernible differences between weekends and weekdays. Often there are few meaningful events to look forward to. A familiar yet inappropriate response to this situation is sleep. Whiteford (2000) reports the same response in inmates who are occupationally deprived.

Focusing on increasing awareness of sensory processing in relation to function in dementia residents within the skilled nursing facility could provide a more holistic approach to therapy and nursing care, help to decrease physical and chemical restraints, and increase the staffs' understanding of dementia and effective interventions to create a positive and meaningful experience for residents and caregivers alike. A concentration on occupations and the environment is most appropriate with dementia residents, who often exhibit symptoms that cannot be changed, but rather need to be managed.

Patricia Wilbarger lays claim to the term *sensory diet*, which involves a usually unconscious modification of sensory activities throughout the day to calm, alert, and organize behaviors (Occupational Therapy Innovations, 2008). With disease, illness, or injury, as in the case of the dementia residents, this ability may be missing or ineffective. The *Snoezelen* approach, which originated in the Netherlands in the 1970s, is one approach to coping with poor sensory modulation. The term comes from the combining of the Dutch words *sniffing* and *dozing*. The goal of this approach is to provide environments and sensory experiences "that stimulate the primary senses without the need for intellectual activity in an atmosphere of trust and relaxation. It is a failure free approach insofar as there is no pressure to achieve" (Burns, Cox, & Plant, 2000, p. 120). Much of the literature available presents *Snoezelen* as more of a philosophy of care that infiltrates all aspects of care with the elderly, rather than a single therapy modality (Achterberg, 2004; Burns et al., 2000). Application of this philosophy can range from whole rooms devoted to the sensory experience to mobile carts or bags with more portable items that can be used in other areas of the building including the residents' rooms (Ball &

Haight, 2005). Moreover, this approach comprises many of the tenets of occupational therapy laid out in *The Occupational Therapy Practice Framework: Domain and Process* (AOTA, 2008). *Snoezelen* "requires a resident-oriented attitude, knowledge and skills, allowing care-givers to incorporate personal circumstances such as lifestyle, preferences, desires, and cultural diversity to achieve or maintain a state of well-being" (van Weert, van Dulmen, Spreeuwenberg, Ribbe, & Bensing, 2005, pp. 24-25). The overwhelming reason that this project might be beneficial to the skilled nursing facility setting is to "overcome the expectation on confused people to function in 'our world' and instead understand the meaning of their world" (Burns et al., 2000, p. 120).

Identification of Support and Barriers in the Setting

Support

As with any good project, the support of numerous individuals was required to bring this evidence-based intervention to fruition. As the manager of the rehab department, the project coordinator had a great deal of flexibility with how things operated on a day-to-day basis and the program initiatives implemented, so getting "buy in" from the rehab staff was not an issue. Facility administration was usually receptive to proposals from the rehab department, provided that solid justification for the service was provided and the therapy staff was willing and motivated to allocate time for accomplishment of the initiative. The support from administration was believed to be critical because this project had the potential to affect the entire philosophy of care within the facility.

In regards to physical space, a small unused room—formerly an office—existed within the therapy department, which was to be transformed into a multisensory environment. Use of this space enabled initiation of the project with the possibility of expansion at some point, as the long-range goal was to infuse a more sensory-based assessment into the occupational therapy evaluation, to educate and train all facility staff in this approach, and to have items available for them to use on a routine basis in the common resident areas.

Finally, but probably most importantly, was the need for financial support. Financial support was deemed necessary to provide any needed equipment and to allow work time to educate and train nursing and rehab staff. Strong organizational and clinical skills of the project coordinator and fellow rehab staff facilitated development of a structured presentation to justify the need for the project as well as the expected outcomes. Describing the marketing and customer service advantages to the facility were used to gain approval for purchase of the necessary supplies.

Barriers

Initially, the most common foreseeable threats to this project were lack of financial support and time constraints. It was believed that the greater the financial support given, the more expansive the project could become. Ultimately, this evidence-based project was conceptualized with many possibilities, perhaps being viewed in phases, with each phase providing the support for further expansion into the subsequent phases. The entire project was designed to be undertaken with little financial support initially, if necessary.

With the current climate of health care, staff retention and productivity are highly scrutinized factors that threatened this project. Use of creative scheduling and teamwork were essential to allow ample time to educate and train facility staff. During education, the information was presented in innovative and fun ways so as to excite the staff about the program's possibilities and help them recognize the benefits to using the equipment and techniques.

Significance of the Evidence-Based Project

The Occupational Therapy Practice Framework: Domain and Process highlights the overarching goal of the field of occupational therapy as "supporting health and participation in life through engagement in occupation" (AOTA, 2008, p. 626). Use of multisensory environments, in which neither performance nor independence are essential, support this objective. Sensory-based approaches "stimulate the primary senses without the need for intellectual activity in an atmosphere of trust and relaxation. It is a failure free approach insofar as there is no pressure to achieve" (Burns et al., 2000, p. 120).

Sensory functions and pain appear under the *Client Factors* area in *Occupational Therapy Practice Framework*

(AOTA, 2008). Review of typical evaluations used in the skilled nursing facility reveals a lack of attention to this vital area. Honing in on one's sensory modulation abilities can provide insight into behavioral issues and activities that derive pleasure and meaning. Considering sensory functions can also increase use of a truly holistic approach to treatment.

As this sensory program is based highly on current literature and evidence, the project provides a model for others to engage in evidence-based practice. Synthesis of critically appraised research articles for design of this program adds to the existing body of evidence on use of sensory approaches in clients with dementia. Education of the public is also an important facet of this evidence-based project. Use of the sensory approach involves collaboration with the resident, families, nurse aides, nurses, social service, case management, and facility administration. This project provides a perfect platform to accentuate occupational therapy's niche in our ever-changing healthcare system.

Occupational therapists, as well as other healthcare providers, are charged with the following priorities:

- Assisting the elderly to age in place when possible
- Supporting caregivers
- Promoting increased quality of life for those living in institutional settings (AOTA, 2007).

The goals of this evidence-based project support these priorities. Attention to quality-of-life issues has grown in recent years with the corresponding growth of the elderly population. Carlson, Clark, and Young (1998) propose that "if we cannot couple the addition of years to our life with the infusion of life to our years, then the recent longevity revolution may merely translate into a sickness revolution" (p. 107). This evidence-based practice project has the potential to impact the provision of services within the facility and the quality of life of clients with dementia via use of a unique approach to management of negative behaviors.

Synopsis of This Evidence-Based Practice Project

The following is a preview of the remaining chapters of this evidence-based practice project. **Chapter 2** (of this project) includes a review of 25 research articles on the use of sensory-based treatments and describes common themes in the literature. **Chapter 3** (of this project) discusses the project's methodology, including a description of any models of practice used to guide the project and how the procedures will be altered to meet each client's needs. **Chapter 4** (of this project) reports the outcomes, both quantitative and qualitative, of the project after it was implemented. Finally, **Chapter 5** (of this project) offers an evaluation of the entire evidence-based practice project as well as a correlation of the outcomes with the literature described earlier in Chapter 2 of this project. Limitations as well as recommendations for future policy, practice, and education are also presented in this closing chapter.

Please note that a sample chapter outline for an evidence-based practice project is provided in Chapter 10.

Appendix D

Outline for an Informed Consent

Title:

Principal Investigator:

Advisor:

1. **Purpose:**
2. **Procedures:**
3. **Discomforts and Risks:**
4. **Benefits:**
5. **Duration or Time:**
6. **Statement of Confidentiality:**
7. **Right to Ask Questions:** You have the right to ask questions and to have questions answered.
8. **Compensation:** You will not receive monetary compensation for participating in this study.
9. **Voluntary Participation:** You do not have to participate in this study. You can end your participation at any time by telling the person in charge. You do not have to answer any questions that you do not want to answer.

You must be 18 years of age or older to consent to participate in this study. If you consent to participate in this study and to the terms above, please sign your name and indicate the date below. You will be given a copy of this form to keep for your records.

_____   _____

Participant Signature   Date

I, the undersigned, verify that the above informed consent procedure has been followed.

_____   _____

Investigator Signature   Date

Appendix E

Guidelines for Informed Consent for Human Subjects in a Study

One of the most important components of research involving human subjects is that of informed consent.

For the purpose of these guidelines, *informed consent* will be defined as: *Consent freely given by a participant in a research project based upon full disclosure of the procedures that the individual will undergo.*

General Information

The consent form should be written in terms comprehensible to the lay person and should include all information about the study that any reasonable person would need and want to know. It should, realistically and honestly, express what a participant may expect, and should avoid persuasion by raising false hopes.

Informed consent forms used for research programs are not legal documents, although there have been adverse legal decisions in cases where informed consent was felt to be sufficiently lacking.

Informed consent is to be obtained from every person who agrees to participate in any program falling under the jurisdiction of the Consent Committee. The consent form for each study is to be submitted to the Committee with the approved protocol before the beginning of any part of the investigation.

All efforts should be made so that the participant fully understands the information obtained in the informed consent, despite any complicating factors, such as mental incompetence, language difficulties, illiteracy, age, and so forth. If it appears that patients,

parents, or guardians are incapable of comprehending this information, the executive officers should be notified and a member of the Consent Committee will be made available. In cases of a language barrier, the executive officer will obtain the assistance of a knowledgeable person in that language to translate the informed consent or interpret during the explanation. Should the participant have questions, and so forth, regarding the research once it has begun, the participant will again be provided with an interpreter.

A. Written Informed Consent

A standardized format has been devised in order to facilitate writing of informed consent.

Using the standardized format, the following elements should be included:

- Description and explanation of procedure
- Risks and discomforts
- Potential benefits
- Alternatives
- Consent

1. Description and Explanation of Procedure

The basic procedures of the research should be stated clearly and concisely in nontechnical terms. Special note must be made of any part of these procedures that are experimental. The purpose of the study should be described, and the reason this person is being asked to participate should be explained.

2. Risks and Discomforts

List in simple terms the most serious risks and those most likely to occur. For each risk or hazard, whenever applicable, answer such questions as:

- How much will it hurt?
- How long will it take?
- What danger will the patient be in?
- What will be done to counteract adverse effects?
- Are the side effects reversible?
- What will be done beforehand to minimize risk or discomfort?
- Is there inconvenience to the patient regarding time or cost?
- Could there be psychological harm, invasion of privacy, loss of confidentiality, embarrassment, or social injury?

It is important to state whether risks of experimental procedures or side effects are known.

3. Potential Benefits

Potential benefits are considered to be either (a) of direct benefit to the subject or (b) of value to future patients or society as a whole. If physical or emotional problems might be uncovered during a study, it might be desirable to state that professional services would be offered to help the problem. If appropriate, results of testing, questionnaires, or interviews might be offered to the subject's school or physician if the parent or subject requests it.

4. Alternative

There are sometimes alternative procedures or medications to the ones described, and these should be listed to give the subject a clear choice. The risks and benefits of each alternative also should be stated. Where there are no alternatives to a particular treatment, this should be noted. If the only alternative is nonparticipation, the section can be omitted. This section has to be carefully worded so as not to make a patient feel pressured into participating because the alternatives are made to sound much less desirable.

5. Consent

The following additional items must be contained in every consent form.

- The assurance that full information regarding the study has been given to the subject.
- The fact that the physician or investigator is available to answer any inquiries concerning the study.
- The option of subjects to withdraw from the project at any time without any effect on their treatment or, if hospital employees, their employment.

The following paragraphs are part of the standard format and should be included at the end of the consent document:

I have fully explained to_____ (insert participant's/patient's/guardian's name) the nature and purpose of the above-described procedure and the risks involved in participation. I have answered and will answer all questions to the best of my ability. I will inform the participant of any changes in the procedure or the risks and benefits if any should occur during or after the course of the study. _____ Primary Investigator's signature and date

I have been satisfactorily informed of the above-described procedure with its possible risks and benefits. I consent to participation in this study. I know that _____ (Insert primary investigator's name or contact) will be available to answer any questions I may have. I understand that I am free to withdraw this consent and discontinue participation in this project at any time and it will not affect my care. I have been offered a copy of this form.

_____   Date:_____

Participant Signature

_____   Date:_____

Witness Signature

_____   Date:_____

Parent or Guardian signature (if applicable)

Modification of the wording in these paragraphs may be made in certain cases, depending on the nature of the study.

The parent or legal guardian must sign the document, as well as the physician or investigator, and witness. The witness is to the signatures only. In cases where witnesses to the explanation are required, a member of the Consent Committee will fulfill this function.

The consent form containing the original signatures must be placed in the medical record. If there is no medical record—as for volunteers, students, and so forth—then the signed copy must be kept in the investigator's files. A copy of the consent form should always be offered to the participant.

If new information occurs during the course of a study, the investigator has the obligation to inform the subject. The consent form should then be revised accordingly and the changes communicated to the executive officer.

B. Other Types of Consent

■ Letter or e-mail. In some instances, the Committee will approve consents in letter or e-mail form, particularly when they involve questionnaires or other low-risk studies. These generally occur in school populations or retrospective studies of former patients when mailings are sent out to individuals not likely to be at the facility.

■ Short form. Occasionally, because of a study's complexity, it is not possible to write a concise consent form. In such instances, the investigator may explain the procedure orally and at length, but present the patients with only a short form to sign. The short form will indicate that all the requirements for informed consent have been met by means of the oral explanation and will include the standard closing paragraphs of written consents. If such form of consent is used, a written summary of what is told to the patient should be part of the protocol and must receive Committee approval.

C. Participation of Children in Consent Process

Children should be involved in the consent process whenever appropriate or feasible. They should be as fully informed about the research project as is appropriate for the child's age and should be given the right to refuse participation. It is recommended that a child not be used as a subject in research if there is a conflict between parent and child regarding participation.

It is recommended that children younger than 18 years of age who are capable of understanding a procedure and its ramifications and who agree to participate sign a separate consent form, often referred to as an assent form along with the parent or guardian's consent form. This process is left to the investigator's discretion.

Appendix F

Example of Informed Consent—Practitioner Study

Electromechanical Games and Exploration Behavior in Adults With Moderate Developmental Disabilities

Name(s) of Investigator:_____
Name of Participant: _____

The Participant, with permission of the Parent or Guardian, has been selected to take part in a research study on the effect of electromechanical games on exploration behavior. The purpose of the study is to see if electromechanical games will encourage the Participants who have diminished interest in their surroundings to explore and interact with the game.

The Participant, with permission of the Parent or Guardian, will be given a battery-powered game for 15 minutes, 3 days per week for 6 weeks at his or her group home. His or her behavior will be recorded in writing by the Investigator of this study to see if his or her exploration behavior changes and if the game interests him or her. Behavior will be videotaped on two separate occasions.

The Participant, with permission of the Parent or Guardian, will have the choice whether or not to interact with the game. Participation is entirely voluntary and Participant or Parent or Guardian has the right to withdraw consent and discontinue participation in the study at any time without prejudice to present or future care. There is no cost for any part of the study.

No discomfort or risks are anticipated for this intervention. It is hoped that the Participant, with permission of the Parent or Guardian, will enjoy interacting with the game and may benefit from doing so by learning more about his or her environment. Information from this study will be anonymously coded to ensure confidentiality and the Participant will not be personally identified in any publication containing the results of this study.

The videotapes and written material from the study will be kept in a locked cabinet. The videotape recordings will be viewed solely by investigator(s) of the study and will be destroyed upon completion of data analysis.

The Parent or Guardian may view any videotape of the Participant which is filmed for the study.

_____,
primary investigator of this study, may be reached at_____/_____
(phone number/e-mail), anytime and will be available to answer any questions the Parent or Guardian may have concerning the study, the procedures, and any risks or benefits that may arise from participating in the study.

As Parent or Guardian of the previously named Participant, I give permission for him or her to participate in the research study described.

A copy of this consent form has been given to me.

Signed:

_____   Date:_____

Parent or Guardian

_____   Date:_____

Principal Investigator's Signature

_____   Date:_____

Witness Signature

Appendix G

Example of Informed Consent—Student Thesis

Massage Therapy Patients' or Clients' Compliance With Treatment From the Therapists' Perspective

_____ (Hereafter known as the "Investigator") has asked _____ (Hereafter known as the "Participant Therapist") to take part in a study regarding massage therapy patients and their compliance with treatment.

The Participant Therapist will be asked to tell the Investigator two stories, one about a patient or client the Participant Therapist perceived as successful and one about a patient or client the Participant Therapist perceived as unsuccessful. He or she will also be asked to discuss what elements he or she thinks make a patient or client successful or unsuccessful. The Investigator will audiotape the stories and all questions and answers.

Participation in the study is voluntary and the Participant Therapist has the right to discontinue participation at any time without repercussions. There are no discomforts or risks associated with the study.

Information from the study will be coded to ensure confidentiality, and the Participant Therapist will not be identified in any publication that may result from the study. The audiotapes will be heard by the Investigator, a transcriber, and possibly by another occupational therapy student (who will aid in selecting relevant portions of the tape for transcribing), and the three faculty advisers to the investigator.

The transcribed stories will not be printed for public use, but short excerpts will be taken from them and included in the Investigator's thesis and in possible future publications.

The Investigator will be available to answer further questions regarding any aspect of the study or participation therein _____/_____ (phone/e-mail).

I understand that members of the Human Subjects Committee of the _____are also available to answer questions and their names, phone numbers, and e-mails are as follows:

I agree to participate in the study described above. I have been given a copy of this form.
Signed:

_____ Date:_____
Participant Therapist

_____ Date:_____
Investigator

_____ Date:_____
Witness

Example of a Permission Form for Photographs and Other Media Materials

I give permission to _____.

(Name of facility)

to use materials identifying_____
in the following situations: (Name of client)

_____External publications (e.g., professional journals, newspapers, magazines)
_____Radio programs
_____Television programs
_____Internal publications (e.g., facility publications)
_____Internal/residential building displays (e.g., bulletin boards, photo albums)
_____Conference materials (e.g., slides, overheads)
_____Other_____

(Specify)

In many cases, the use of the patient's (client's) first and last name is not necessary, but can add to the completion of the story or photo. If you do not want the last name used, please indicate below:

_____NO, the use of first and last name is *not* permissible
_____YES, the first and last names may be used
_____Only the first name and last initial may be used

I give consent on the condition that the material be used only for the above purpose(s). It is my understanding that I may see the materials before confirming consent or before the material is released. Also, it is my understanding that I will receive verbal notification before any material is used, and that I may place the following restrictions on the material or its use, including time limits:

I give this consent voluntarily, without threat of punishment or promise of special reward. I have been given an opportunity to fully discuss the release and to have my questions answered. I understand that I may withdraw consent at any time prior to release without fear or punishment.

Signature: _____ Date:_____

(Client)

Signature: _____ Date:_____

(Parent or Guardian, if applicable)

I have fully explained the information above and answered all questions to the best of my ability. It is my opinion that consent has been given knowingly and freely.

Signature: _____ Date:_____

(Person obtaining consent)

_____

(Title or position)

Appendix I

Professional Journals and Publishers

This is not intended to be an exhaustive list; however it will be helpful in discerning where to search for assistance during the inquiry and/or when publishing outcomes. To access web information, simply copy/paste the title into your preferred search engine.

HEALTHCARE ADMINISTRATION

Administration and Policy in Mental Health and Mental Health Service Research

Journal of Healthcare Management

Hospitals and Health Networks

Journal of Long-Term Care Administration

Journal of Rehabilitation Administration

Modern Healthcare

AGING

Activities, Adaptation and Aging

American Journal of Geriatric Psychiatry

Clinical Gerontologist

International Journal of Aging and Human Development

International Journal of Geriatric Psychiatry

Journal of Aging and Physical Activity

Journal of Aging and Social Policy

Journal of Aging Studies

Journal of Applied Gerontology

Journal of Geriatric Psychiatry and Neurology

Journals of Gerontology

Journal of Women and Aging

Physical and Occupational Therapy in Geriatrics

The Gerontologist

HEALTHCARE RELATED COMPUTER TECHNOLOGY

Computers in Human Behavior

Computers in the Schools

Health Management Technology

Journal of Technology in Human Services

HEALTH CARE

Home Health Care Services Quarterly

Home Health Care Management and Practice

Journal of Allied Health

The Journal of Women's Health Care

Occupational Therapy in Health Care

HOSPICE

American Journal of Hospice and Palliative Care

Home Health Care Services Quarterly

Journal of Palliative Care

OCCUPATIONAL HEALTH

International Journal of Sports Medicine

Journal of Health and Social Behavior

Journal of Occupational Rehabilitation

Occupational Health and Safety

Occupational Health Nursing
Occupation, Participation and Health

PEDIATRICS AND EARLY INTERVENTION
Child Development
Infants and Young Children
Journal of Early Intervention
Journal of Pediatric Psychology
Pediatric Physical Therapy
Physical and Occupational Therapy in Pediatrics
Physical Disabilities: Education and Related Services
Topics in Early Childhood Special Education

PHYSICAL MEDICINE AND REHABILITATION
American Journal of Physical Medicine and Rehabilitation
Journal of Occupational Rehabilitation
Journal of Orthopaedics & Sports Physical Therapy
Journal of Rehabilitation Research and Development
Physical Medicine and Rehabilitation Clinics of North America
Physiotherapy Theory and Practice
Rehabilitation Counseling Bulletin
Rehabilitation Research, Policy, and Education
Sexuality and Disability
Work: A Journal of Prevention, Assessment and Rehabilitation

PROFESSIONAL ASSOCIATION JOURNALS
Art Therapy: Journal of the American Art Association
American Journal of Occupational Therapy
American Journal of Medical Technology
British Journal of Occupational Therapy
Clinical Laboratory Science
International Journal of Yoga Therapy
Journal of Allied Health
Journal of the American Academy of Physician Assistants
Journal of Athletic Training

Journal of Hand Therapy
Journal of Rehabilitation Research and Development
Journal of Sport Rehabilitation
Lab Medicine
Massage Therapy Journal
Occupational Therapy International
Physical Therapy
Physiotherapy Journal
Physiotherapy Canada
Public Health Journal
Radiologic Technology Journal
Rehabilitation Counseling Bulletin
Respiratory Care Journal

MENTAL HEALTH & WELL-BEING
American Journal of Health Promotion
Canadian Journal of Community Mental Health
Community Mental Health Journal
International Journal of Qualitative Studies on Health & Well-being
Journal of Family Psychotherapy
Journal of Health and Social Behavior
Journal of Organizational Behavior Management
Occupational Therapy in Mental Health
Residential Treatment for Children and Youth
The Clinical Supervisor

RESEARCH
American Journal of Medicine
Health Services Research Journal
Journal of International Medical Research
Journal of Multidisciplinary Healthcare
Qualitative Health Research
The New England Journal of Medicine
The Qualitative Report

Appendix J

Indexes and Abstracts

This is not intended to be an exhaustive list; however, it will be helpful in discerning where to search for assistance during the inquiry or when publishing outcomes. To access Web information, simply copy and paste the title into your preferred search engine.

Social Work Abstracts. Quarterly. Abstracts from journals of social work under social policy and action, service methods, fields of service, the social work profession, history of social work, and related fields in the social sciences.

Abstracts of Hospital Management Studies. Quarterly. International abstracts of studies on management, planning, and public policy related to healthcare delivery.

Ageline. Produced by American Association for Retired Persons. More than 16,500 documents on all aspects of gerontology. Bimonthly updates.

Bibliography of Bioethics. Since 1975, covers English-language literature on ethical issues related to health care. Includes journals, court decisions, government documents, audiovisuals, newspapers, and books. Published annually.

Biological Abstracts. Semimonthly. International abstracts of periodicals including behavioral sciences, bioinstrumentation, environmental biology, genetics, nutrition, and public health.

Child Development Abstracts. Three times per year. Abstracts of articles and books in a wide variety of fields as they relate to infancy and child development.

Combined Health Information Database. Produced by National Institutes of Health. More than 24,000 documents combining four health-related databases: arthritis, diabetes, health education, and digestive diseases. Quarterly updates.

Compendex. Produced by Engineering Information Inc. More than 1,102,100 documents on all aspects of engineering and technology including rehabilitation engineering. Monthly updates.

Cumulative Index to Nursing and Allied Health Literature (CINAHL). Print version from 1956 to present; online version from 1982 to present. Indexes all major nursing journals and over 125 allied health journals, plus book reviews, pamphlets, films, and recordings. Bimonthly updates.

Current Index to Journals in Education (CIJE). Paper abstracts of education-related journals by subject, author, and journal content. Usually used in conjunction with RIE and ECER; these three form the online version, ERIC.

Dissertation Abstracts International. Comprehensive paper abstracts of dissertations by title, author, and subject. Volumes divided into sciences or engineering and humanities or social sciences.

DSH Abstracts. Quarterly from Deafness, Speech and Hearing Publications, Inc., Gallaudet College, Washington, DC. Abstracts articles related to hearing, hearing disorders, speech, and speech disorders. Includes foreign journals. Education Index. From 1932 to the present. Indexes articles from educational periodicals, conference proceedings, and yearbooks.

ERIC (Educational Resources Information Center). Produced by Council for Exceptional Children. More than 589,000 documents on special education materials. Monthly updates. Compilation of paper indexes: RIE, CUE, and ECER.

Exceptional Child Educational Resources (ECER). Abstracts education materials related to children with special needs, by subject and author. Usually used in conjunction with RIE and CUE; these three form the online version, ERIC.

Excerpta Medica. A subsidiary of Elsevier Science Publishing in the Netherlands, first published in 1946. Covers both research and clinical biomedical literature on a worldwide basis. Fifty-two sections including Rehabilitation and Physical Medicine, Gerontology and Geriatrics, Psychiatry, Occupational Health, and Industrial Medicine.

Hospital Literature Index. From 1945 to the present. Indexes studies on administration, planning, and financing of hospitals and related healthcare institutions. All types of healthcare facilities are included. Published quarterly and cumulated annually.

Index Medicus. Full and abridged versions available. Documents from approximately 4,680 medically related journals. Updated monthly and cumulated annually. Online version is **MEDLINE.**

International Nursing Index. From 1966 to present. Indexes 270 international nursing journals and nursing articles from 2,600 nonnursing materials listed in Index Medicus. Published quarterly and cumulated annually.

Linguistics and Language Behaviors Abstracts. Produced by Sociological Abstracts, Inc. More than 72,000 documents on language problems, speech and hearing problems, learning disabilities, and special education. Quarterly updates.

MEDLINE. Online version of Index Medicus. More than 1,600,000 entries on medicine, including biomedicine, and humanities as they relate to medicine. Includes occupational and physical therapy, nursing, social work, biology and physiology, and so forth. Updated monthly and cumulated annually.

OT Search. Online information system with literature in database. Organized by author, subject, and title.

ProQuest. Designed to support the needs of academic researchers; they offer the greatest expanse of high-quality research and curricula-aligned content in a wide-range of subjects.

PsycINFO. Online version of Psychological Abstracts. Entries listed by title, author, and subject; divides psychology into 16 major categories.

PsychLit. Online database of psychology books, journals, and other materials. Comprehensive. Organized by author and subject.

PubMed. Sponsored by the National Library of Medicine of the National Institutes of Health (NIH). PubMed comprises millions of citations of biomedical literature from MEDLINE, life science journals, and online books.

REHABDATA. Produced by National Rehabilitation Information Center (NARIC). More than 16,000 documents on rehabilitation including commercial publications, government reports, journals, and unpublished documents. Monthly updates.

Research Education Complete. Database encompassing scholarly research in all areas of education.

Research Quarterly, American Alliance for Health, Physical Education, and Recreation. Covers literature pertaining to physical health, physical education, and recreation. Cumulative in 10-year indexes from 1930 to present.

Science Citation Index. Indexes literature from the scientific disciplines including medicine, behavioral sciences, substance abuse, and some nursing journals. Published bimonthly with an annual cumulation from 1955.

Social Services Abstracts. Social Services Abstracts provides bibliographic coverage of current research focused on social work, human services, and related areas, including social welfare and social policy. The database abstracts and indexes over 1,300 serial publications, and includes journal articles, dissertations and book reviews. Searches link to Community of Scholars: Social Sciences

Social Science Citation Index. Social Sciences Citation Index®, accessed via Web of Science™ Core Collection, provides researchers, administrators, faculty, and students with quick, powerful access to the bibliographic and citation information they need to find research data, analyze trends, journals and researchers, and share their findings. Overcome information overload and focus on essential data from 3,000 of the world's leading social sciences journals across 50 disciplines.

Sociological Abstracts. 1952 - present. Updated monthly, with approximately 30,000 records added per year. Abstracts and indexes the international literature in sociology and related disciplines in the social and behavioral sciences. Provides abstracts of journal articles and citations to book reviews drawn from over 1,800+ serials publications, and also provides abstracts of books, book chapters, dissertations, and conference papers.

U.S. Superintendent of Documents, Monthly Catalog of United States Government Publications. 1895 to present. Lists publications issued by all branches of the U.S. government, both the Congressional and the department and bureau publications. Current issues indexed by author, title, subject, and series or report.

Appendix K

Evidence-Based Practice Resources by Healthcare Discipline

The following list of resources, separated by healthcare discipline, provides a starting point for anyone beginning the evidence-based practice process. An Internet search of any resource titles will guide you in obtaining these recommended resources.

GENERAL HEALTH CARE

Hall, H. R., & Roussel, L. A. (2012). *Evidence-based practice: An integrative guide to research, administration, and practice.* Burlington, MA: Jones & Bartlett Learning.

Houser, J., & Oman, K. S. (2010). *Evidence-based practice: An implementation guide for healthcare organizations.* Sudbury, MA: Jones & Bartlett.

Rubin, A., & Bellamy, J. (2012). *Practitioner's guide to using research for evidence-based practice.* Hoboken, NJ: John Wiley & Sons, Inc.

HEALTH AND FITNESS OR SPORTS MEDICINE

Dugdill, L., Crone, D., & Murphy, R. (2009). *Physical activity and health promotion: Evidence-based approaches to practice.* United Kingdom: Blackwell Publishing Ltd.

Higdon, J., & Drake, V. J. (2011). *An evidence-based approach to vitamins and minerals: Health benefits and intake recommendations.* New York, NY: Thieme Medical Publishers.

MacAuley, D., & Best, T. (2007). *Evidence-based sports medicine* (2nd ed.). Malden, MA: Blackwell Publishing.

Martin, L., Haskard-Zolnierek, K., & Dimatteo, M. R. (2010). *Health behavior change and treatment adherence: Evidence-based guidelines for improving healthcare.* New York, NY: Oxford University Press, Inc.

LABORATORY SCIENCE

Laboratory Medicine Best Practices. Retrieved from www.futurelabmedicine.org

Marchevsky, A. M., & Wick, M. (2011). *Evidence based pathology and laboratory medicine.* New York: Springer Science + Business Media, LLC.

Price, C. P., Glenn, J. L., & Christenson, R. H. (2009). *Applying evidence-based laboratory medicine: A step-by-step guide.* Washington, DC: American Association for Clinical Chemistry.

MASSAGE THERAPY

Andrade, C., & Clifford, P. (2008). *Outcome-based massage: From evidence to practice* (2nd ed.). Baltimore, MD: Lippincott Williams & Wilkins.

Dryden, T., & Moyer, C. (2012). *Massage therapy: Integrating research and practice.* Champaign, IL: Human Kinetics.

Holey, E. A., & Cook, E. M. (2011). *Evidence-based therapeutic massage: A practical guide for therapists* (3rd ed.). Philadelphia, PA: Churchill Livingstone Elsevier.

NURSING

Brown, S. J. (2010). *Evidence-based nursing: The research-practice connection.* Sudbury, MA: Jones & Bartlett.

Melnyk, B. M., & Fineout-Overholt, E. (2010). *Evidence-based practice in nursing & healthcare: A guide to best practice* (2nd ed.). Philadelphia, PA: Lippincott Williams & Wilkins.

Schmidt, N. A., & Brown, J. M. (2011). *Evidence-based practice for nurses: Appraisal and application research.* Sudbury, MA: Jones & Bartlett.

OCCUPATIONAL THERAPY

Kielhofner, G. (Ed.). (2006). *Research in occupational therapy: Methods of inquiry for enhancing practice* (Section 9, pp. 656–706). Philadelphia, PA: F.A. Davis.

Law, M., & MacDermid, J. (Eds.). (2014). *Evidence-based rehabilitation: A guide to practice* (3rd ed.). Thorofare, NJ: SLACK Incorporated.

Taylor, M. C. (2008). *Evidence-based practice for occupational therapists* (2nd ed.). Malden, MA: Blackwell Publishing.

PHYSICAL THERAPY

Cameron, M. H., & Monroe, L. (2007). *Physical rehabilitation: Evidence-based examination, evaluation, and intervention.* St. Louis, MO: Saunders Elsevier.

Fetters, L., & Tilson, J. (2012). *Evidence based physical therapy.* Philadelphia, PA: F.A. Davis.

Jewell, D. V. (2010). *Guide to evidence-based physical therapist practice* (2nd ed.). Sudbury, MA: Jones & Bartlett.

PHYSICIAN ASSISTANT

Pines, J. M., Carpenter, C. R., Raja, A. S., & Schuur, J. D. (2013). *Evidence-based emergency care: Diagnostic testing and clinical decision rules.* Hoboken, NJ: John Wiley & Sons, Ltd.

Straus, S. E., Glasziou, P., Richardson, W. S., & Haynes, R. B. (2011). *Evidence-based medicine: How to practice and teach it* (4th ed.). Maryland Heights, MO: Elsevier Churchill Livingstone.

RADIOLOGIC SCIENCE

Medina, L. S., Blackmore, C. C., & Applegate, K. (2011). *Evidence-based imaging: Improving the quality of imaging in patient care* (revised ed.). New York: Springer Science + Business Media, LLC.

Medina, L. S., Sanelli, P. C., & Jarvik, J. C. (2013). *Evidence-based neuroimaging diagnosis and treatment: Improving quality of neuroimaging in patient care.* New York: Springer Science + Business Media, LLC.

SOCIAL WORK

Grinnell, Jr., R. M., & Unrau, Y. A. (2010). *Social work research and evaluation: Foundations of evidence-based practice.* New York, NY: Oxford University Press, Inc.

Petr, C. G. (2008). *Multidimensional evidence-based practice: Synthesizing knowledge, research, and values.* New York, NY: Routledge.

Thyer, B. A., Dulmus, C. N., & Sowers, K. M. (Eds.). (2013). *Developing evidence-based generalist practice skills.* Hoboken, NJ: John Wiley & Sons, Ltd.

Author Guidelines for Health Professional Journals and Publications

Below are direct links to peer-reviewed journals and practice-related publications.
The purpose of the list is to give the reader a starting point to review author guidelines—it is by no means an exhaustive list of opportunities to publish one's work.

Athletic Training

International Journal of Athletic Therapy & Training
http://journals.humankinetics.com/authorship-guidelines-for-ijatt/authorship-guidelines-for-ijatt/apaq-authorship-guidelines

Journal of Athletic Training
http://www.nata.org/journal-of-athletic-training

Journal of Sports and Exercise Psychology
http://journals.humankinetics.com/for-jsep-authors

Clinical Laboratory Sciences

Clinical Chemistry
www.aacc.org/publications/clin_chem/

Journal of Clinical Laboratory Analysis
http://onlinelibrary.wiley.com/journal/10.1002/(ISSN)1098-2825

Journal of Clinical Laboratory Sciences
http://www.ascls.org/professional-development/publications/instructions-for-authors-reviewers

Laboratory Medicine
http://labmed.ascpjournals.org/

Society for Laboratory Automation and Screening
http://www.slas.org/publications/journals.cfm

Massage Therapy

American Massage Therapy Association
http://www.amtamassage.org/articles/3/mtj/index.html

International Journal of Therapeutic Massage and Bodywork: Research, Education & Practice
http://www.massagetherapyfoundation.org/massage-research/ijtmb/

Nursing

American Journal of Nursing

http://journals.lww.com/ajnonline/_layouts/1033/
oaks.journals/informationforauthors.aspx

Journal of Professional Nursing

http://www.professionalnursing.org/authorinfo

Occupational Therapy

American Journal of Occupational Therapy

http://ajot.submit2aota.org/journals/ajot/forms/
Ajot_guidelines.pdf

Australian Journal of Occupational Therapy

http://onlinelibrary.wiley.com/journal/10.1111/(ISSN)
1440-1630/homepage/ForAuthors.html

British Journal of Occupational Therapy

http://www.cot.co.uk/contribute-and-submit-
bjot/publish-bjot

Canadian Journal of Occupational Therapy

http://www.caot.ca/default.asp?pageid=162

Occupational Therapy Practice

http://www.aota.org/Publications-News/otp/
Author.aspx

Physician Assistant

Journal of the American Academy of Physician Assistants

http://journals.lww.com/jaapa/Pages/author-
guidelines.aspx

Physical Therapy

Journal of American Physical Therapy Association
http://ptjournal.apta.org/

Journal of Orthopaedic and Sports Physical Therapy
http://www.jospt.org/aboutus/for_authors.asp

Pediatric Physical Therapy

http://journals.lww.com/pedpt/Pages/
InformationforAuthors.aspx

Physical Therapy in Sport

http://www.elsevier.com/journals/physical-
therapy-in-sport/1466-853X/guide-for-authors

Radiologic Technology

American Society of Radiologic Technologists

http://www.asrt.org/main/news-research/
asrt-journals-magazines

Social Work

National Association of Social Work Press

http://www.naswpress.org/authors/index.html

Yoga and Bodywork

International Journal of Yoga

http://www.ijoy.org.in/

Journal of Bodywork and Movement Therapies

http://www.journals.elsevier.com/journal-
of-bodywork-and-movement-therapies/

Yoga Journal

http://www.yogajournal.com/

Appendix M

Guidelines for Contributors to *American Journal of Occupational Therapy*

Note. The *Guidelines for Contributors* is also available at the *American Journal of Occupational Therapy* manuscript processing system website; go to **http://ajot.submit2aota.org** and click on "Instructions for Authors."

The *American Journal of Occupational Therapy (AJOT)* is the official peer-reviewed journal of the American Occupational Therapy Association (AOTA). We welcome the submission of manuscripts that are relevant to the study of occupation and the practice of occupational therapy. Categories of peer-reviewed articles include feature-length articles, case reports, brief reports, and issue papers.

Publication goals include the following:

- Effectiveness studies (outcome studies), systematic reviews, and meta-analyses
- Efficiency studies (studies assessing interventions for such things as patient satisfaction or cost and time efficiency)
- Studies establishing the reliability and validity of occupational therapy instruments
- Studies linking occupational engagement to participation and health
- Studies exploring a currently debated topical or professional issue (The *Issue Is* articles).

AJOT uses the sixth edition of the *Publication Manual of the American Psychological Association* (APA, 2010) as the style guide. Consult this manual for style questions unless specified otherwise in these guidelines.

To submit manuscripts, go to **http://ajot.submit2aota.org/** and follow the online instructions.

Manuscripts must be submitted with the authors' explicit written assurance that the manuscript is not simultaneously under consideration by any other publication. The journal cannot assume responsibility for the loss of manuscripts.

Authors' Responsibilities

Signatures. Before publication of any accepted manuscript, **all authors** must provide original signatures for the statement of authorship responsibility, the statement of financial disclosure, and the statement of copyright release. The Copyright Transfer/ Author Certification/Financial Disclosure Form may be downloaded from the *AJOT* submission website. Signed forms must be submitted upon acceptance of a manuscript for publication.

The statement of authorship responsibility is certification that each author has made substantial contributions to (1) the study conception and design, acquisition of data, or analysis and interpretation of data; (2) the drafting and revision of the article; and (3) the approval of the final version. Moreover, each author takes public responsibility for the work.

Author order. The order of authors in the byline follows APA guidelines. The principal contributor appears first, and subsequent names are in order of decreasing contribution. Authors are encouraged to limit the number of coauthors to six or fewer.

Types of Articles

Feature-Length Article

Feature-length articles include (1) original research reports that focus on philosophical, theoretical, educational, or practice topics and (2) critical reviews (including meta-analyses) that offer systematic review and critical analysis of a body of literature as related to occupation and occupational therapy. Feature-length articles should include a section summarizing the implications of the research for occupational therapy practice; this section should include a bulleted list of the key points. (25 pages maximum or 5,000 words, including title page, abstract, acknowledgments, references, tables, figures, and illustrations)

Brief Report

A Brief Report is a short report of original research that is of a pilot or exploratory nature or that addresses a discrete research question and lacks broad implications. (15 pages maximum or 3,000 words, including title page, abstract, acknowledgments, references, tables, figures, and illustrations)

Case Report

A Case Report is a short report of original work that focuses on a case example of a clinical situation using baseline and outcome measures. The focus can be on a patient or client, a family, an institution, or any other defined unit. The case should represent elements of practice that are not already represented in the literature. (20 pages maximum or 4,000 words, including title page, abstract, acknowledgments, references tables, figures, and illustrations)

The Issue Is

The Issue Is articles address timely issues, policies, or professional trends or express opinions that are supported by cogent argument from the literature. (18 pages maximum or 3,500 words, including title page, abstract, acknowledgments references, tables, figures, and illustrations)

Letters to the Editor (published online)

Letters discussing a recent *AJOT* article or other broad issue relative to the journal are welcome. Letters should not exceed two double-spaced typed pages and can be submitted by going to *AJOT* online at **http://ajot.aotapress.net/**, navigating to the article, and clicking on "submit a response." Letters may be edited for length and to conform with *AJOT* editorial style.

Manuscripts for all categories above, except Letters to the Editor, are peer reviewed.

Note: Consistent with the *Guidelines for Supervision, Roles, and Responsibilities During the Delivery of Occupational Therapy Services* (AOTA, 2009), the roles of the occupational therapist and occupational therapy assistant shall be considered, and when appropriate, role distinctions shall be clarified.

Manuscript Preparation

For format and reference style, consult the APA style manual and recent issues of *AJOT*. Careful attention to style details will expedite the peer review process.

Authors are responsible for ensuring that a blind review process can take place by submitting a masked version of the manuscript, which contains no identifying information, including names and affiliations of all authors and acknowledgments. Unmasked articles will be returned for masking before they are reviewed. Authors of manuscripts that are accepted will be asked to provide an unmasked version.

Double-space the entire manuscript, including abstract, text, quotations, acknowledgments, tables, figure captions, and references. Leave 1-inch margins on all sides, and keep the right side unjustified. Number all pages, starting with the title page, and use line numbering in the text. Use only Times New Roman 12-point font. Manuscripts are compiled and converted to pdf format during the online submission process. Specific instructions are provided at **http://ajot.submit2aota.org/**.

Title Page

The title should be short (no more than 10 words) and reflect the primary focus of the article. On the unmasked copy (which will be requested if the manuscript is accepted for publication), list full names, degrees, titles, and affiliations of all authors. Designate the corresponding author by providing his or her full address, telephone and fax numbers, and e-mail address.

Abstract and Key Words

An abstract of no more than 150 words and at least 3 MeSH key words are required for all articles. Abstracts may be structured (organized with the subheadings Objective, Method, Results, and Conclusion) or unstructured (narrative description of the focus and key content of the article). Note that MeSH key words are reviewed by an indexer and may be edited.

Implications for Occupational Therapy Practice Section

Feature-length articles, including evidence reviews, should include a separate section summarizing the implications of the research for occupational therapy practice. This section should consist of a short paragraph followed by a bulleted list of the practice implications.

Acknowledgments Page

The acknowledgments page is in- cluded in the un-masked copy only. This page follows the last page of the text and precedes the reference list. Brief acknowl- edgments may include names of persons who contributed to the research or article but who are not authors (e.g., a statistician) followed by acknowledgments of grant support. Prior presentation of the paper at a meeting should be briefly described last.

References

Follow the sixth edition of the *Publication Manual of the American Psychological Association* (APA, 2010) for referencing. List references in alphabetical order starting on the page after the last page of text (in the masked version) or after the acknowledgments (in the unmasked version). In-text citations should use author-date format. Personal communications or other nonretrievable citations are described in the text only; provide a name and date for a person and a name, date, and address for an organization. Authors are solely responsible for the accuracy and completeness of their references and for correct text citation.

Below are examples of commonly used reference listings:

- *Journal Article (hard copy or not available online)*:
Dunton, W. R., Jr. (1926). An historical note. *Occupational Therapy and Rehabilitation, 5*(6), 427–439.

- *Journal Article (online version, with digital object identifier*
Arbesman, M., & Lieberman, D. (2011). Methodology for the systematic reviews on occupational therapy for adults with Alzheimer's disease and related dementias. *American Journal of Occupational Therapy, 65*, 490-496. http://dx.doi.org/10.5014/ajot.2011.00257

- *Journal Article (online version, no DOI)*:
Gram, M., & Smed, K. (2011). We can drink our coffee more slowly: Discursive uses of age in relation to holiday consumption—Examples among Danish and German mature travellers. *E-Journal of Applied Psychology, 7*(1), 2-7. Retrieved from http://ojs.lib.swin.edu.au/index.php/ejap/article/view/229/241

- *Book With Corporate Author and Author as Publisher*:
American Psychiatric Association. (2000). *Diagnostic and statistical manual of mental disorders* (4th ed., text rev.). Washington, DC: Author.

- *Book With Author(s)*:
Frank, G. (2000). *Venus on wheels: Two decades of dialogue on disability, biography, and being female in America*. Los Angeles: University of California Press.

- *Edited Book*:
Law, M. (Ed.). (1998). *Client-centered occupational therapy*. Thorofare, NJ: Slack.

- *Chapter in Edited Book*:
Case-Smith, J. (2010). Evidence-based practice in occupational therapy for children with an autism spectrum disorder. In H. M. Kuhaneck & R. Watling (Eds.), *Autism: A comprehensive occupational therapy approach* (3rd ed., pp. 701–742). Bethesda, MD: AOTA Press.

Tables

Provide full titles and begin each table on a new page following the references. Number the tables consecutively as they appear in the text. Data appearing in tables should supplement, not duplicate, the text. Double-check column totals. Be sure that any numbers repeated in the text match the numbers that appear in the table. Define all abbreviations and explain any empty cells in a footnote to each table.

Figures and Illustrations

Number figures in order of mention in the text. Figures (including charts, diagrams, and photographs) must be submitted as high-resolution digitized electronic files (minimum 600 dpi). Figures must be submitted in black and white. Each figure should be uploaded to the BenchPress system as a separate file that is named in accordance with the figure number (e.g., "Figure 1. tif").

Provide a caption for each figure. List all captions on one page, double-spaced. Place the figure caption page after the references. Provide source information for photographs and line art, and ensure that permission has been obtained to reprint figures that have been previously published or have not been created by the article authors (see "Permissions" below).

Note: Limit on Number of Tables and Figures

No more than four art elements—that is, any combination of tables and figures—may be submitted with each article. Authors who submit more than four items total will be asked to edit their submission accordingly. Authors who believe readers will benefit from additional tables or figures may submit those items as supplemental materials. Supplemental materials are not typeset and are posted, at the editor-in-chief's discretion, with the online version of the article exactly as they are submitted.

Statistics

Authors must provide references for statistical tests used or described in the article. When reporting F and x^2 statistics, provide degrees of freedom (df).

Tests and Assessment Tools

Authors must provide references for all tests and assessment tools mentioned in the article or used in the research being described, including tools mentioned in tables or lists of assessments. Tests and assessment tools listed in supplemental evidence tables, however, do not need to be referenced.

Abbreviations

Do not use abbreviations in the title or abstract of the article; the use of abbreviations in the text should be kept to a minimum.

Permissions

Authors who wish to reprint tables, figures, or long quotations from other sources are responsible for obtaining permission from the copyright holder. Letters of permission with original signatures from the copyright holder or an authorized representative must be submitted to the editor at the time of the initial submission. AOTA does not reimburse authors for any expense incurred when obtaining permission to reprint. The need for permission applies to adapted tables and figures as well as to exact copies.

Signed statements of permission to publish must accompany all photographs of identifiable persons at the time of submission.

Authors must provide signed statements of permission from people cited for personal communications at the time of submission.

Derivative Work

Authors who are submitting derivative work using a data set from which other papers were published must provide the publication information for those other papers in the cover letter.

Manuscript Review

Manuscripts and reviews are confidential materials. The existence of a manuscript under review is not revealed to anyone beyond the editorial staff. All submitted manuscripts are initially reviewed by the editor for suitability for the journal. Suitable manuscripts are then sent to editorial board members or guest reviewers for peer review. The identities of the reviewers and of the authors are kept confidential. Initial and subsequent review takes approximately 3 months. All accepted manuscripts are subject to copyediting. Authors will receive a copy of the edited manuscript for review and final approval, as well as reprint order forms, before publication. The authors assume final responsibility for the content of articles, including changes made in copyediting.

Copyright and Patent

On acceptance of the manuscript, authors are required to convey copyright ownership to AOTA.

Manuscripts published in the journal are copyrighted by AOTA and may not be published elsewhere without permission. To obtain permission to reprint journal material, go to the Copyright Clearance Center website at **www.copyright.com**.

Any device, equipment, splint, or other item described with explicit directions for construction in an article submitted to *AJOT* for publication is not protected by AOTA copyright and can be produced for commercial purposes and patented by others, unless the item was already patented or its patent is pending at the time the article is submitted.

Checklist for Authors

- Register at **http://ajot.submit2aota.org/** and follow on-line submission instructions.
- Submitted manuscript contains no identifying information about specific people and places.
- All references are in APA (sixth ed.) style and have been checked for accuracy and completeness and for exact match between list and text.
- Pages are numbered, starting with abstract and key words on page 2.
- Lines are numbered in the main text.
- A section including a bulleted list summarizing the implications of the research for occupational therapy practice is included.
- Written permissions have been obtained as needed for photographs, personal communications, and copyrighted material.
- Digital files and captions are provided for all figures.
- All material is double-spaced (including abstract, references, quotations, figure captions).
- The Copyright Transfer/Author Certification/Financial Disclosure Form as been signed by each author.

REFERENCES

American Occupational Therapy Association. (2009). Guidelines for supervision, roles, and responsibilities during the delivery of occupational therapy services. *American Journal of Occupational Therapy, 63,* 797-803. http://dx.doi.org/10.5014/ajot.63.6.797

American Psychological Association. (2010). *Publication manual of the American Psychological Association* (6th ed.). Washington, DC: Author.

Appendix N

Author Guidelines for *International Journal of Yoga Therapy*

Instructions to Contributors

International Journal of Yoga Therapy publishes scholarly articles about yoga therapy, yoga practice, and yoga philosophy. We encourage submissions from researchers, scholars, yoga therapists, yoga teachers, and healthcare professionals. The journal aims to represent views, practices, and research from all major traditions in yoga and from modern health care, integrative medicine, and psychology.

Research

The journal publishes high-quality reports of original empirical research. Manuscripts must adhere to conventional reporting guidelines and include a title, abstract, introduction, methods section, results, and discussion. We welcome scientific articles regarding pilot studies and encourage authors to publish findings that may benefit other researchers and practitioners. Case studies are empirical reports using a very small sample. They should be reported in the context of a thorough review of the relevant literature, include quantitative or qualitative results, and a broad discussion of the cases' implications for future research or practice. Names and other identifying information must be changed to protect individuals' privacy. All research involving human participants **must** have received prior approval by an Institutional Review Board for the protection of human subjects. Study protocols and previously published materials cannot be considered.

Issues in Yoga Therapy

The journal welcomes scholarly articles that address issues, challenges, and controversies in the research and practice of yoga therapy. Articles in this category include, but are not limited to, considerations of policy issues related to the integration of yoga and health care, explorations of common challenges that yoga therapists and teachers face in their work, and discussions of yoga philosophy as it relates to contemporary yoga therapy practice. Articles in this category must include references to relevant yogic texts and supporting materials, all of which are to be cited using APA format, and should not be based largely on the experience or opinions of the author(s).

Yoga Therapy in Practice/The Yoga Tradition

Yoga Therapy in Practice/The Yoga Tradition articles should review a topic of importance and relevance to practicing yoga teachers, yoga therapists, and healthcare providers. Articles in this category include, but are not limited to, discussions of specific populations or medical conditions and recommended best practices, reviews of research on a topic of relevance to yoga therapy, or reviews of the history of some aspect of yoga therapy or yoga philosophy. Articles must be supported by published research, research in progress, established interventions at yoga therapy clinics, classical yoga texts, or original interviews, all of which are to be cited using APA format. They should not be based largely on the experience or opinions of the author(s). Review articles must contribute something new to the literature.

Perspectives

The journal invites submissions of Perspectives regarding any topic relevant to the research and practice of yoga therapy. Perspectives are not peer reviewed and are limited to 500–1,500 words. Perspectives should be written in a scholarly style. First person narratives and personal accounts are discouraged. Perspectives are typically solicited by the editor. Please contact the editor for guidance before submitting a Perspective, at editor@iayt.org

Review and Selection of Manuscripts

All articles are initially evaluated by the editor for suitability of topic and format. Articles that meet the basic requirements are assigned to a minimum of two peer reviewers chosen on the basis of their expertise and experience. Peer review is blind, meaning that the author's identity is not revealed to reviewers. Reviewers and the editor evaluate the article's contribution to the field of yoga therapy and make specific suggestions for revisions. When making a recommendation to publish or reject an article, reviewers take into account the quality of scholarship, the use of writing that is appropriate for a scholarly journal, and the relevance of the topic to yoga therapists, researchers, and practitioners. Potential authors wishing to view the current peer review guidelines for the type of article they plan to submit should e-mail the editor (editor@iayt.org) and indicate which article category the intended submission falls into. The editor makes the final decision to accept or reject a manuscript. Most manuscripts go through multiple rounds of revisions before they are accepted. Following acceptance, articles are edited for clarity and adherence to journal style guidelines.

Preparation and Submission of Manuscripts

All articles are to be submitted via e-mail to editor@iayt.org. Include a brief introductory note and article abstract in the body of the e-mail and attach the manuscript as a Word document. **All manuscripts must be written and formatted according to the *APA Publication Manual*, sixth edition (www.apastyle.org)**. Research articles must include a note acknowledging any funding sources or potential conflicts of interest, a statement of adherence to ethical guidelines for the use of human participants, and informed consent to use photographs of or publish case information about students or clients. We encourage authors to provide a limited number of high-resolution photos and well-drawn figures, particularly for descriptions of yoga practices or discussions of anatomy. Please do **not** e-mail photos, figures, reference sections, or appendixes as separate files. **Articles are limited to 4,000 to 6,000 words unless authors have received prior approval from the editor**.

Reprinted with permission from Dr. Grace Bullock, PhD, RYT, Editor in Chief. Weblink: http://www.iayt.org/?page=IJYTSubGuidelines.

Appendix O

Outline of a Grant Proposal

Grant Proposal Format

Proposals should adhere **closely** to the following directions and include all of the components listed.

A. ABSTRACT

Include a brief abstract that provides a summary of the proposal (a brief rationale for the project, the methods to be used, and the expected results and outcomes). *Abstracts should be understandable by someone who is not necessarily in the field of expertise of the proposer.*

The abstract should answer the following questions:

a. Why should the project be funded?
b. What problem is the project trying to solve or what are the issues being addressed?
c. How will the proposal go about solving the problem or addressing the issue?
d. What are the expected findings?
e. What are the implications of the findings?
f. How will these be disseminated?

B. NARRATIVE

Include the following components (maximum five pages):

a. Central question being explored or objective being pursued.
b. Rationale and significance of project: how this project will contribute to the applicant's discipline, overall research agenda, or university initiatives.
c. Description of project methodology.

d. If applicable, names of other faculty or students who will participate in this project; location of research site.
e. Plans for disseminating the project's results, such as conferences, workshops, exhibitions and publications, or other appropriate venues.
f. Potential sources of external monies to which you anticipate applying for further funding.
g. An explanation of the candidate's prior work in the field and how the current project fits within the larger scholarly or professional agenda.
h. A description of the contribution that the successfully completed project will make to the candidate's scholarly or professional field.

C. ATTACHMENTS

a. Project budget (use form provided below)
b. Brief resume

Grant Proposal Budget	
BUDGET ITEM	**AMOUNT**
Personnel	
Equipment ■ *List items with prices.* ■ Include a rationale for items.	
Travel	
TOTAL BUDGET REQUESTED	

Index